Children's Intonation

A Framework for Practice and Research

The *'Children's Speech and Literacy Difficulties'* series

Other books in the series:

Children's Speech and Literacy Difficulties: A Psycholinguistic Framework, Book 1
ISBN: 978-1-86156-030-8

Children's Speech and Literacy Difficulties: Identification and Intervention, Book 2
ISBN: 978-1-86156-131-2

Persisting Speech Difficulties in Children: Children's Speech and Literacy Difficulties, Book 3
ISBN: 978-0-470-02744-8

Compendium of Auditory and Speech Tasks: Children's Speech and Literacy Difficulties, Book 4
ISBN: 978-0-470-51659-1

For more information on any of these titles, visit www.wiley.com

Children's Intonation

A Framework for Practice and Research

Bill Wells and Joy Stackhouse

Department of Human Communication Sciences
University of Sheffield, Sheffield, UK

WILEY Blackwell

This edition first published 2016 © 2016 by John Wiley & Sons, Ltd

Registered Office
John Wiley & Sons, Ltd, The Atrium, Southern Gate, Chichester, West Sussex, PO19 8SQ, UK

Editorial Offices
9600 Garsington Road, Oxford, OX4 2DQ, UK
The Atrium, Southern Gate, Chichester, West Sussex, PO19 8SQ, UK
111 River Street, Hoboken, NJ 07030-5774, USA

For details of our global editorial offices, for customer services and for information about how to apply for permission to reuse the copyright material in this book please see our website at www.wiley.com/wiley-blackwell

The right of the authors to be identified as the authors of this work has been asserted in accordance with the UK Copyright, Designs and Patents Act 1988.

Library of Congress Cataloging-in-Publication Data

Wells, Bill (Clinical linguistics)
  Children's intonation : a framework for practice and research / Bill Wells, Professor, Department of Human Communication Sciences University of Sheffield, Joy Stackhouse, Professor, Department of Human Communication Sciences, University of Sheffield.
    pages   cm
  Includes bibliographical references and index.
  ISBN 978-1-118-94762-3 (paperback)
1. Language disorders in children.   2. Linguistics.   3. Children–Language.   4. Prosodic analysis (Linguistics)
I. Stackhouse, Joy.   II. Title.
  RJ496.L35W45 2016
  618.92'855–dc23
                                    2015024893

A catalogue record for this book is available from the British Library.

Wiley also publishes its books in a variety of electronic formats. Some content that appears in print may not be available in electronic books.

Cover image: GettyImages-536053013/skynesher

Set in 9/11pt Meridien by SPi Global, Pondicherry, India
Printed and bound in Malaysia by Vivar Printing Sdn Bhd

1   2016

Contents

Foreword

Intonation is one of the crucial linguistic resources that children need to be able to communicate effectively. The natural home of intonation is spontaneous everyday interaction. Intonation and prosodic features generally play a key role in shaping the meaning of what is said, how it is said and how conversational interaction works. They shape the flow of turns at talk and help configure both the actions those turns perform and the topics being talked about.

Children's Intonation: A Framework for Practice and Research, by Bill Wells and Joy Stackhouse, presents an exciting, interactionally-driven approach to understanding how children develop intonation and exploit it in their speech. Through a series of detailed case studies and practical analytic exercises, the authors show how it is possible to profile children's intonational behaviour based on a careful consideration of talk in interaction. There are two key elements to this approach:

1 the need to examine the location of particular intonation patterns in their sequential context, in order to understand how the pattern that a speaker uses is influenced by the previous speaker's pattern;

2 the need to demonstrate the meaning of intonational and prosodic features with reference to the observable behaviour of other participants in the interaction itself rather than relying on the researcher's or the clinician's own intuitions.

This methodology, developed from the discipline of Conversation Analysis, has a number of advantages over other approaches. It enables practitioners and researchers to study the intonational behaviour of *any* child in *any* interactional setting, irrespective of whether they are deemed to be typical or atypical in their linguistic development. Because the focus of analysis is on turns and sequences of talk, all aspects of a given turn, including its lexical and syntactic characteristics, can be examined, integrated and taken into account. Moreover, because the interactional analysis makes no assumptions as to whether 'unusual' prosody reflects an underlying problem or processing deficit, it also enables the identification of individual children's practices and any compensatory mechanisms they may deploy.

Everyday conversational interaction is the basic, fundamental environment for children's development, use and learning of ordinary language. The sophisticated interactional approach to prosodic features advocated by Wells and Stackhouse in this book provides an important tool for therapists and researchers. It will enable them to develop a more nuanced appreciation of intonational form and function in both typically and atypically developing children, including children with speech, language or hearing impairments and those on the autistic spectrum. It will also significantly enhance the ability of therapists and researchers to give a robust account of both the functional aspects of intonation and the cognitive processes involved in its production and understanding. The models of intonational profiling and psycholinguistic processing that are proposed should moreover permit the development of effective and sensitive strategies for intervention.

This excellent book should be in the hands of anyone who is interested in how children learn to communicate through conversational interaction.

John Local
Emeritus Professor of Phonetics and Linguistics
Department of Language and Linguistic Science
University of York, UK

Preface

Every time we speak, we have to do something with the pitch, loudness and length of our utterances – the prosodic features of speech which combine in patterns of rhythm and intonation. This is as true of the infant taking his or her first vocal turns with a caregiver, as it is of a caregiver interacting with an infant, or of an adult talking to other adults. Nevertheless, compared with other aspects of speech and language development, intonation has received less attention and is rarely seen as a priority for developmental research or for speech and language therapy assessment and intervention. There are several possible reasons for this.

- *Intonation is easy for children*. Relatively few children seem to have problems learning to use intonation patterns. If this is so, the case for studying its development is less obvious compared with other areas of spoken language, such as consonant production or inflectional morphology, which are known to be affected by developmental problems.
- *Intonation is hard to learn about*. Even though as native speakers most of us have no problems in using intonation patterns effectively in our everyday lives, students of child language development, including speech and language pathology students, come to their studies with little explicit awareness of intonation. Students frequently report difficulties in identifying and labelling these patterns in an academic context.
- *Intonation is hard to read about*. Writing systems generally focus on words and their organization into sentences. Western orthographies focus on consonants and vowels, largely ignoring prosodic features. In order to understand a book about intonation, the reader therefore needs to invest some effort in learning a new notation and terminology.

We think that there are nevertheless good reasons to study children's intonation. Our broad aim is to highlight the importance of intonation for everyday conversational interaction and the implications of this for teaching and therapy contexts. We do this by addressing questions such as the following:

- If the intonation of the mother tongue really is relatively easy to learn for the vast majority of children, what is it that makes it easier than other aspects of language?
- How and when do children learn to use intonation for the purposes of interaction?
- As children get older, does intonation become more important or less important for communication?
- Some children with developmental difficulties present with unusual intonation. What form can this take? Why might it occur?
- Other children, whose intonation does not sound atypical, have difficulties in understanding the meanings that others are trying to convey through intonation. How can we identify such problems?
- If intonation is a relative strength for most children with developmental speech and language difficulties, how might intonation be used to support or compensate for other aspects of language?

- Given the importance of intonation in spoken communication, what are the implications for practitioners, parents and caregivers when interacting with young children, particularly children who have speech, language and communication needs?

In order to answer these questions, we have adopted a similar approach to previous books in our series on Children's Speech and Literacy Difficulties. This book shares the same basic orientation towards clinical application and includes:

- a tool for profiling children's intonation skills;
- a developmental phase model to explain typical and atypical intonation development;
- a psycholinguistic model of intonation processing;
- an interactional perspective on intonation use;
- consideration of intonation in relation to both written and spoken language;
- case studies to illustrate key points and clinical application;
- activities for the reader to complete with keys to check answers.

How this book is organized

Following an introduction to the study of English intonation in Chapter 1, Chapters 2–4 present a way to approach the assessment of a child's intonation from a functional perspective, in order to find out whether the child is able to communicate and understand the meanings that intonation conveys in conversation. The material that informs this approach is naturally occurring talk, including talk that occurs in typical play activities. The essential points of these chapters are synthesized in Chapter 5 in the *Intonation in Interaction Profile (IIP)*, a tool for assessing children's intonation through analysis of recorded conversation. These first five chapters are intended to be accessible to anyone interested in intonation from an interactional perspective, and not only those with developmental interests. The emphasis is on the role of intonation systems in handling transitions in conversational interaction, notably transitions between speakers through turn-taking, transitions between topics and transitions between social actions.

In Chapters 6–8 this framework provides the theoretical basis for evaluating and synthesizing research into the development of intonation from birth through to the school years. In Chapter 9, developmental and processing models of intonation are described that incorporate interactional and psycholinguistic perspectives. In the final three chapters (Chapters 10–12), research into the intonation of children with developmental difficulties is described and our assessment approach is illustrated through case studies. In Chapter 10, the focus is on children with speech, language and literacy difficulties. In Chapter 11, we consider children with autism spectrum disorders, Williams syndrome and Down syndrome. Finally, in Chapter 12, we turn to children with hearing impairments, including children who use cochlear implants. These three chapters, which do not need to be read sequentially, offer some pointers in relation to therapy intervention and suggest possible directions for further research.

The book contains numerous transcribed extracts from real conversations involving children. Many of these are illustrated by recordings that can be accessed from the accompanying website, available at: www.stackhousewells.uk. These are either the original recordings or else have been recorded by actors. In all cases, the transcriptions were made from the original recordings.

As in the previous four books in the series, each chapter contains activities and keys to these activities. For some activities it is useful, though rarely essential, to be able to access the accompanying recording. The activities give the reader the opportunity to work with concepts and techniques introduced in the chapter. Undertaking the activity as a joint venture with a colleague is recommended. It is hoped that teachers of child language and speech and language therapy may also find them useful.

Notational conventions are explained in the text and listed in Appendix 1. Key terms are defined in the text. Page references for these definitions are highlighted in bold in the Index.

Pointers for the future

As in the previous books in the series, though some reference will be made to studies of children learning intonation in other languages, the focus is almost exclusively on children learning English as their first language. This reflects the authors' own experience and the state of research more widely: there have been fewer published studies of typical and atypical intonation development in other languages. We nevertheless hope that the framework presented may be of some value for researchers and practitioners who work with other languages.

From a clinical perspective, this book focusses on issues of the nature, causes and assessment of intonation problems. We have included little explicitly about intonation as a part of speech and language therapy interventions. The main reason for this omission is that little has been published on intonation interventions for children. An important aim of this book is therefore to lay a foundation for principled intervention to take place by developing an understanding of children's intonation development, how to assess it, and how to use this knowledge when interacting with children and their carers both informally and in teaching and therapy contexts.

Bill Wells
Joy Stackhouse

Acknowledgements

Some of the research described here was supported by the Economic and Social Sciences Research Council (grant numbers R000271063, R000236696, R000222809). We thank Guy J. Brown (Department of Computer Science, University of Sheffield) for preparing the figures in Chapter 1 and the simulations in Chapter 6. Many speech and language therapists, fellow researchers, former students and colleagues have contributed indirectly and directly to the genesis and production of the book, in some cases by allowing us to make use of their recordings. While it is not possible to list them all, the following merit specific mention: Julie Anstey, Jana Dankovičová, Anna Filipi, Emina Kurtić, Merle Mahon, Tom Muskett, and Jenny Thomson.

The ideas in the book have been shaped through discussion with two long-term collaborators in particular: Juliette Corrin and Sue Peppé. A special debt of gratitude is due to John Local, not only for writing the Foreword but also for developing the theory and methods that underpin our interactional approach to children's intonation. Finally, we would like to thank the children and families whose talk is the subject matter of this book.

About the companion website

The book is accompanied by a companion website:

www.wiley.com/go/childintonation

The website contains a link to the authors' website where you can find:
- Charts from the book for downloading
- Tables from the book for downloading

CHAPTER 1

Intonation

Pitch, loudness and length are among the most salient of the properties of speech perceived by the listener. Linguists sometimes refer to these features as suprasegmental, suggesting that they are somehow 'above' the string of consonants and vowels. This connotation is misleading: rather, in speech, the string of consonants and vowels is overlaid onto a base of phonation. Phonation, or voicing, is generated by an airstream from the lungs passing through the larynx, which results in the perception of fluctuations in pitch and loudness distributed over chunks of varying durations. The term *prosody*, and the related adjective *prosodic*, commonly refer in a broad sense to features of pitch, loudness and duration in speech, encompassing their use in individual words and their component syllables, as well as the use of these features over longer stretches of speech, i.e. phrases, complete utterances, conversational turns. These longer stretches are the main focus of this book. Over such longer stretches, the meaningful patterning of pitch, along with related patterning of loudness and length features, is commonly referred to as *intonation* – hence the title of the book. While some authors restrict the use of this term to the patterning of pitch alone, we use it as a shorthand to refer to communicatively relevant systems, operating over stretches of speech consisting minimally of a single word but usually longer, which are realized primarily through features of pitch, also often of loudness and length, and sometimes of voice quality and articulation.

From the very beginning, long before words made up of consonants and vowels can be identified, infants produce the prosodic features that are used for intonation. Moreover, adult carers respond to them as signalling various kinds of meaning. Infants, in their turn, appear to react to the prosodic components of adults' speech addressed to them; indeed, adults systematically exaggerate some of these prosodic features when addressing infants and young children (see Chapter 6). These observations appear to be true of all cultures that have been studied so far, although the degree of modification varies across cultures. It appears then, that from birth, prosodic features form a set of resources that the child can exploit for communicative purposes, even though in different mature adult languages, prosodic features turn out to be organized in a wide variety of ways. Some of the differences will be described later.

Some children's intonation develops in ways that are unusual for their linguistic environment. The basis for postulating an impairment in intonation is likely to be the listener's auditory impression that the child's use of prosodic features is in some way different from that of the speech community and cannot be attributed to other causes, e.g. being a

Children's Intonation: A Framework for Practice and Research, First Edition. Bill Wells and Joy Stackhouse.
© 2016 John Wiley & Sons, Ltd. Published 2016 by John Wiley & Sons, Ltd.
Companion website: www.wiley.com/go/childintonation

non-native speaker whose intonation in the second language is affected by the mother tongue. Beyond that, the identification, description and explanation of the impairment are influenced by the approach to analysis taken by the investigator, who may be a speech and language pathology practitioner or a researcher, for example. The basic tools of description are phonetic and linguistic. These complementary approaches will now be explained.

The phonetic approach

Typical and atypical prosodic development can be explored by using a range of methodologies that are based on auditory-perceptual and instrumental techniques. Instrumental techniques enable features of the speech signal to be recorded and measured reliably. Some of these techniques measure speech production directly. For example, using electrodes attached to the neck close to the larynx, the laryngograph (or electroglottograph) monitors the vibration of the vocal folds directly as they produce voicing (Abberton & Fourcin, 1997). While this can produce an accurate signal, and is not subject to interference from other noises (unlike a microphone recording), the need to wear a neckband attached by a wire to a computer militates against the recording of natural conversational speech, not least with young children.

For such reasons, the most common type of instrumental analysis used in intonation research is acoustic. An audio recording of the speakers is made via microphones. This can be done using digital audio or video tape recorders, a solid state digital audio recorder, or direct onto a PC or laptop. Conventional audio or video cassette recorders produce an analogue recording, which can subsequently be digitized using special software. The resulting digital audio files can then be analysed using one of the many computer speech analysis packages available. A much-used and freely downloadable program for acoustic analysis is Praat (Boersma & Weenink, 2014), which can be used to display and measure prosodic parameters.

However, acoustic analysis has its limitations too. The first, already mentioned, is that as soon as recording moves outside the artificial environment of the speech laboratory into children's everyday talking environments, for example, home and school, then there will be sources of noise that may be difficult to control – traffic, clattering of play bricks, and so on. It can be difficult and time-consuming to remove such noises from the recorded signal. One particularly important and tricky source of noise is voices of speakers involved in background conversations or even in the same conversation: in a review of the occurrence of overlapping talk, Kurtić, Brown, and Wells (2013) report that, even in relatively formal meetings, for up to 10% of the time, two or more speakers will be talking at the same time and that, in spontaneous adult conversation, up to 45% of all changes of turn contain overlap between the speakers. Overlap is thus a natural part of human spoken interaction; it can only be suppressed by using an artificial speech elicitation task such as a monologue or reading aloud. Although speech research is making progress in developing techniques for separating out the voices of different talkers in overlap, at present, the only satisfactory procedure is to record talkers on separate channels, with each talker using a close-fitting microphone attached to a headset. While this has been done successfully when recording adults in meetings, it is too invasive for research with young children. A commonly adopted response to this issue in child language research has been to omit instances of overlapping talk from analysis. However, this is not a satisfactory solution when analysing intonation because, as will be seen later, the occurrence of overlap is an important source of evidence in revealing how intonation works.

ACTIVITY 1.1

Aim: To explore the extent to which you can track different voices speaking in overlap.

This activity involves listening to a fragment from a recording of spontaneous conversation between English students. Listen to Media File 1.1. If possible, use headphones. You will hear two female adults, Daisy and Beth (these are not their real names), speaking at the same time. Daisy speaks first. Using normal orthography, write down what each speaker says.
    To check how you did, refer to the Key to Activity 1.1 at the end of the chapter, where you will find a transcript of the recording, presented as Extract (1.1).

For these reasons, the auditory perceptual analysis and transcription of intonation remain important research and clinical tools. Although not as reliable as instrumental analysis for identifying the individual phonetic parameters of speech which has been recorded under ideal conditions, the human ear is able to track with some accuracy different voices speaking in noise, including in overlap. In the following activity you can decide how far you agree with that statement.

If you managed to transcribe some of the speech accurately from the mixed file, you may (after congratulating yourself!) like to consider why the task you have just done is extremely difficult for a computer-based speech recognition system. Thus, one of the skills that you possess is the ability to at least sort out the contributing voices when two or more speakers are talking simultaneously, even if it remains hard to work out the words being spoken. Most children appear to develop this skill, and it is likely that one of the aspects of speech that we learn to attend to in order to manage this is intonation. You can listen to the same extract again but this time, listen to each speaker separately. Daisy's contribution is presented as Extract (1.2), Beth's as Extract (1.3):

(1.2) used to hang out in Stevenage when I was younger summer yeah
(1.3) that'd be good we should do that over like summer

Unlike acoustic analysis software, the human listener does not habitually attend to separate phonetic parameters but to speech as an integrated whole. A skilled listener is able to take into consideration a range of different parameters that may be relevant to the realization of an intonation pattern on a particular occasion, for example, variations in loudness, duration, voice quality (such as creak or whisper), and even the way in which word-final consonants are released. Such features will only be evident in the results of acoustic analysis if the analyst is on the lookout for them and so has chosen the relevant instrumental settings for the analysis process. For these reasons, as when analysing other aspects of speech, a combination of instrumental and perceptual methods is ideal (Howard & Heselwood, 2011).

The perception of pitch is mainly determined by fundamental frequency (F0), which is a property of the acoustic signal. In the case of speech, F0 relates to the number of periods of vocal fold vibration per second. It is most commonly measured in Herz (cycles per second) and forms an important part of the investigation of intonation. Figure 1.1 depicts an acoustic analysis of Beth's contribution to the conversational fragment from Activity 1.1. The dark line depicts changes in F0 in the course of the utterance, the F0 scale in Herz being given on the left-hand vertical axis of the graph. The most noticeable features are the big jump-up in F0, of about 80 Hz, from "should" to "do" and the subsequent fall of approximately 100 Hz from "do" through "that".

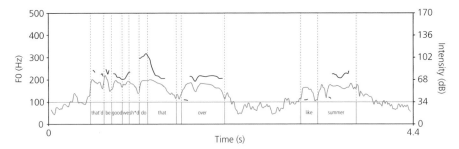

Figure 1.1 Acoustic analysis of Beth's turn from Activity 1.1 (Extract 1.3).

There is a disadvantage to using the linear Herz scale, particularly when dealing with children's intonation: the problem is that the relationship between F0 and the perception of pitch is not linear. This means that a greater Herz interval is needed when high in the pitch range, in order to produce a perceived pitch step, compared to the same pitch step produced low in the pitch range. Thus, a semitone interval produced by an adult male in the lower end of his usual pitch range may be around 5 Hz, while a semitone interval produced by a young child in the upper part of his usual pitch range may be around 20 Hz. In order to facilitate comparison between child and adult intonation throughout this book, F0 measurements are therefore usually expressed in semitones, which is a nonlinear scale, rather than in Herz. In Figure 1.1, the fall on "do that" is approximately seven semitones.

Just as the perception of pitch is determined to a large extent by the fundamental frequency of the signal, so the perception of loudness is largely determined by the intensity of the signal. This can be quantified in a number of ways for collections of utterances, such as mean, median or range of intensity, measured in decibels. When studying the intonation of an individual utterance, it is the loudness of a syllable relative to the rest of that utterance that is most relevant, since key elements of intonation are linked to rhythmically prominent syllables and loudness is one factor in perceived rhythmic prominence.

Intensity measurements outside the laboratory are not very reliable, since reliability depends on a constant distance between mouth and microphone. While this can be achieved by using a close-talking microphone mounted on a headset, as was the case when recording the conversation between Beth and Daisy used in Activity 1.1, this is rarely feasible when recording children in a naturalistic setting. Nevertheless, over the course of a short utterance, the speaker's distance from the microphone is unlikely to vary greatly, so the intensity trace, in combination with careful listening, can be used to help identify the words or syllables that are relatively loud. In Figure 1.1, variation in intensity within the utterance is depicted by the pale grey line beneath the dark F0 line. For example, the intensity on the stressed syllable of the word "over" is about 5 dB lower that on the accented syllables ("that", "good", "do") of the preceding stretch; it drops approximately 3 dB more to the final two words "like summer".

The third main aspect of prosody relates to the temporal domain of speech, and includes the duration of whole utterances, of words, syllables, consonants and vowels; the duration and location of pauses; articulation rate (often measured by number of syllables per second, excluding pauses), including the speeding up and slowing down of rate. Where a clear signal can be obtained for acoustic analysis, it is relatively straightforward to measure most of these temporal parameters using a speech analysis package like Praat. In Figure 1.1, for example, there is a silent interval of around 0.8 seconds between "over" and "like summer". There are also variations in the articulation rate (Dankovičcová, 1997). The phrase "that'd be good we should do that" is produced in just one second, i.e. a rate of 8 syllables per second. By contrast, even if we ignore the pause between "over" and "like", the five-syllable phrase "over like summer" has a rate of approximately 4 syllables per second, which is half the rate of the first phrase. At the bottom of Figure 1.1, spacing reflects the relative length of each word.

The prosodic transcription

Measurement of aspects of the speech signal using acoustic analysis is a valuable aid to the accurate description of prosodic features. It is essential where the aim is to make statistical generalizations from large amounts of data, for example, about the habitual fundamental frequency range or the average articulation rate of an individual speaker or of a group. However, auditory perceptual judgement is also an invaluable tool. Most of the examples discussed in this book are taken from more or less naturalistic interactions involving children and adults, where overlapping talk is frequent and where the recordings were made under less-than-ideal conditions. Prosodic features were first transcribed impressionistically, as were segmental aspects of the talk in some cases, particularly where the child has immature or atypical speech. Key portions of the recordings were later subjected to acoustic analysis, using Praat. However, because of the quality of the original recordings and characteristics of the children's vocal productions, it was not always possible to obtain a reliable acoustic record. The transcripts represent the convergence of results from both these procedures, with the aim of keeping them readable. The International Phonetic Alphabet (IPA), and the conventions used in Conversation Analysis, provide ways of notating these prosodic features in a transcription. Pitch height and pitch movements are presented iconically between staves, the staves representing the upper and lower limits of the speaker's habitual pitch range. Loudness, pause, duration and tempo features are notated using symbols and diacritics of the IPA, including extensions. Examples of this approach to transcription will be found later in the chapter. A full list of transcription conventions can be found in Appendix 1.

The linguistic approach

While the phonetic approach is concerned with the accurate description of prosodic parameters in speech, using auditory perceptual and instrumental techniques, the linguistic approach to intonation shows how these features communicate meaning. Prosodic features serve to realize linguistic systems such as tone (in tone languages), stress and intonation. From this perspective a prosodic impairment impacts on the linguistic system in question, with the result that the speaker's meaning, in its broadest sense, may be obscured. Identification of a linguistic impairment of intonation is therefore dependent on the analyst having a description of the intonation system of the language. The intonation of English has probably received more scholarly attention than that of any other language, though systematic descriptions are now available for a large number of different languages (Hirst & Di Cristo, 1998; Jun, 2005).

Various approaches to the systematic description of intonation have been adopted. The ToBI notation, derived from autosegmental-metrical theory, has been widely adopted in phonetic and speech technology research (Jun, 2005; Ladd, 2008). However, it has so far been little applied to clinical analysis or to studies of children's intonation development, where versions of more traditional analyses have tended to be used, following the lead of David Crystal (Crystal, 1987; Snow & Balog, 2002). As a necessary foundation for the rest of the book, the next part of this chapter provides a descriptive framework for English intonation, based on this more traditional approach.

English intonation: a brief introduction

The term *intonation* is generally used to refer to the linguistic patterning of pitch height and movement, together with loudness and duration, to realize meanings that are additional to the meanings conveyed by words and grammar. When pitch is used in lexical and/or morphological systems, for example, to distinguish word meanings, we talk of a *tone language*. Well-known examples include Thai and Mandarin Chinese, which will be discussed in Chapter 6 in the context of young children's need to work out whether or not the language they are having to learn is a tone language. The linguistic use of pitch in almost all varieties of English is intonational only. This description applies to Southern Standard British English. While many accents of English, including General American, have systems that are very similar, others are very different, for example, in Northern Ireland or among many speakers of Afro-Caribbean ethnicity. Dialect variation is discussed at various points in the course of the book, in relation to children's development.

Traditional approaches to English intonation generally identify basic intonation patterns from which the speaker can select. These patterns will be referred to as (nuclear) Tones. In some current research on intonation, it is usual to talk about pitch accents rather than Tones. Ladd (2008) discusses equivalences between the two descriptions. However, in this account we will follow the tradition of using descriptive labels and iconic diacritics, as in Table 1.1.

As illustrated in Table 1.1, the diacritic representing the Tone is placed in front of the Tonic syllable (described below). The number of meaningfully different Tones in English intonation continues to be the subject of debate (Cruttenden, 1997; Gussenhoven, 2004; Ladd, 2008). Our own approach to this issue is presented in Chapter 4. When the word 'Tone' is used with an initial upper case letter, as here, it signifies that the word is being used with a specific meaning as defined in this book. The convention also applies to other technical terms that are defined in this chapter.

The unit of intonation at which the Tone system operates is now usually referred to as the Intonation Phrase (IP), although tone unit or tone group used to be common alternatives. Its boundaries are marked by double vertical lines ‖, the IPA symbol for a major intonation boundary.

To illustrate the transcription of English intonation, we return to Daisy's turn from the fragment of conversation used in Activity 1.1. An acoustic trace is presented in Figure 1.2.

Table 1.1 Diacritic notation for Tones in English intonation, as used in reading transcriptions in this book.

Fall	Rise	Fall-rise	Rise-fall
ˋYES	ˊYES	ˇYES	ˆYES

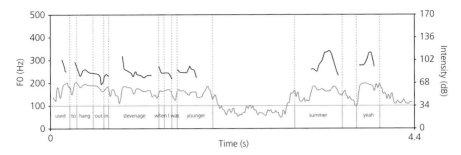

Figure 1.2 Acoustic analysis of Daisy's turn from Activity 1.1 (Extract 1.2).

The Intonation Phrase (IP) is the fundamental structural unit of intonation, and indeed may be viewed as the basic unit of speech production. In Extract (1.2.1) there are three Intonation Phrases:

(1.2.1) ‖used to hang out in Stevenage when I was younger ‖ summer ‖ yeah ‖

IP boundaries are realized by the following features, in varying combinations (cf. Cruttenden, 1997):

1 occurrence of the Tonic, which carries the Tone (see below). The Tonic is not always located at the end of the IP, but it must have occurred for the IP to be heard as complete.

2 lengthening of final syllable(s) of the IP;

3 pause following the IP;

4 jump in pitch from the end of one IP to the start of the next IP.

Feature (3), a silence of around one second, is evident following "younger", suggesting a boundary there. Feature (1), the Tonic, is the one criterion for an IP that is obligatory. The Tonic is recognized primarily by the Tone, a noticeable pitch movement on the stressed syllable of a word which makes that syllable stand out from what precedes and follows it. In addition, the Tonic is often relatively long and loud compared to surrounding words. In the first IP, the word "Stevenage" is a good candidate for a Tonic, as it has a fall of five semitones on the first (stressed) syllable; no other syllable has a comparably large pitch movement until we get to "summer" (rise-fall over five semitones) and "yeah" (rise-fall spanning three semitones). "Stevenage" is relatively loud compared to the preceding and following words and also its first syllable, measuring 150 milliseconds, is 50% longer than any other syllable in the IP until "younger", which itself illustrates feature (2). On this basis, we have added Tone diacritics in (1.2.2), which indicate not only the pitch direction but also the fact that the following word is the Tonic:

(1.2.2) ‖ used to hang out in `Stevenage when I was younger ‖ˆsummer ‖ˆyeah ‖

In the transcription system used here, a distinction is made between an ordinary Tonic and a Supertonic, notated by ⇑ placed before the Tone diacritic. The Supertonic has extra prominence, often from a combination of a particularly big pitch movement, noticeable loudness and extra lengthening, compared to an ordinary Tonic; while the surrounding words may be correspondingly quiet and fast, with very little pitch movement. In many publications, the presence of a Supertonic is indicated by under-lining, italics or capitals, inviting the reader to use the features just listed if reading aloud. Here is an example from the novel *Atonement* by Ian McEwan. Bryony, aged 13, is coaching her young cousin to read the lines of a play she has written:

(1.4) "It's a question", Bryony cut in. "Don't you see? It goes up at the end."
"What do you mean?"
"There. You just did it. You start low and end high. It's a *question*."

(McEwan, 2001: 33–34)

The italics on the final word of the final sentence contrast with the earlier presenta-tion of the same words at the beginning of the extract. They can be transcribed as in (1.4.1):

(1.4.1) ‖ 'its a `question ‖ **versus** ‖ 'its a ⇑`question ‖

The functions of the Supertonic will be explained in Chapter 3, while Bryony's misapprehension about the intonation of questions will be discussed in Chapter 4.

The IP can be subdivided into constituent parts. Minimally, it must have a Tonic. Any syllables that follow the Tonic are known as the Tail. The pitch of the Tail generally continues the direction of the pitch of the Tone, thus if the Tone is a rise, then the syllables of the Tail will continue to step up. Conversely, if the Tone is a fall, the syllables of the Tail will continue to fall until reaching the base of the speaker's normal pitch range. In the first IP of Extract (1.2), the Tail consists of "when I was younger".

The first prominent syllable of the IP is called the Onset. It is useful to make a distinction between a (neutral) Onset and a High Onset because this contrast has a specific role to play in the organization of talk, as will be explained in Chapter 2. In our transcription system, a High Onset is marked ↑, whereas a neutral onset is simply marked with the IPA stress symbol ' (see next section: Stress and Rhythm, for further explanation). Any words from the Onset, up to but not including the Tonic, form the Head. Any syllables preceding the Onset are known as the Pre-head. This gives the following structure:

‖ (Pre-head) ' (Onset + rest of Head) ` Tonic (Tail) ‖

Elements in brackets are optional. This means that a short utterance of a single mono-syllabic word can be intonationally complete, that is, it can constitute a complete IP, if it carries a Tone, since it thereby becomes a Tonic, which is the minimal element for an IP. The final two IPs in (1.2.3) are examples of single-word IPs. The top row of (1.2.3) presents a systematic reading transcription of Daisy's turn; beneath it is an indication of how it maps onto the constituent parts of the IPs:

(1.2.3)

‖'used	to hang out in	'Stevenage	when I was 'younger‖	‖ ^summer‖	‖ ^yeah ‖
Onset	rest of Head......	Tonic	Tail.....................	Tonic	Tonic

IP boundaries frequently indicate a potential place for a change of speaker, referred to as a turn transition relevance place (TRP). For this reason, intonation is important for the regulation of turn-exchange. This is explained in detail in Chapter 2. Now complete Activity 1.2 before reading further.

ACTIVITY 1.2

Aim: To discover how some of the concepts introduced in this section can be used when analysing talk involving a young child.

Study Extract (1.5), a short interchange between Robin (CA 1;9), and his mother. Then answer the questions that follow. Robin and his mother are engaged in play with a jigsaw puzzle board, into which pieces are to be fitted. At this point, his mother is quizzing him about one particular piece, depicting a train. Mother's turns are transcribed using the system for adult English intonation described under 'The linguistic approach'. Robin's turns are transcribed in the way described under 'The phonetic approach', since at this point in his development we cannot assume that he is operating with the mature adult intonation system.

(1.5)

```
1   M:   ‖↑ 'whats ⇑`this bit 'called though ‖
```

```
2   R:   çi:j akəlᵛ
             {f}
3   M:   ‖ it `isnt ‖ its 'called a ⇑`funnel ‖
```

```
4   R:   f ɑ f a
             {f}
5   M:   ‖ thats 'right ‖ n ↑'what comes 'out of the `funnel ‖
```

```
6   R:   ʔə mɛ ʊ kʰ
```

1 Where is the Tonic located in line 1? Why do you think that Robin's mother has placed it there?
2 In line 3, there are two IPs. Why do you think the boundary between them occurs where it does?
3 In line 3, the two IPs have different Tones. Why do you think Robin's mother has chosen these Tones?
4 It is sometimes said that questions in English have rising intonation. In Extract (1.4), is there evidence to support this claim?
5 Turn exchange proceeds smoothly through the extract: Robin's mother does not start talking before Robin has finished. Why do you think there are no overlaps?
Compare your answer to the key to Activity 1.2 at the end of this chapter.

Stress and rhythm

Smaller units may be identified within an IP. This can be appreciated by reading aloud the phrases in Extracts (1.6) and (1.7):

(1.6) CHOCOLATE-CAKE AND HONEY
(1.7) CHOCOLATE, CAKE AND HONEY

Syntactically, (1.6) consists of a compound noun (cake made with chocolate) followed by another noun (honey). You are likely to have read it with an intonation structure such as in (1.6.1):

(1.6.1) ‖ 'chocolate cake and `honey ‖

Syntactically, in (1.7) there are three separate nouns, referring to three separate items of food. You may have read it with an intonation structure as in (1.7.1):

(1.7.1) ‖ 'chocolate 'cake and `honey ‖

There is a separate peak of prominence on "cake" that was not present in the compound noun in (1.6.1). The difference can be described in terms of number of units within the Head. In (1.6.1), the Head consists of a single unit, "chocolate-cake and". In (1.7.1), the Head consists of two units: "chocolate", then "cake and". In order to provide a helpful characterization of these smaller units, it is necessary to consider the role of stress and rhythm, and their relationship to intonation.

Word stress

In English and many other languages, part of the stored phonological representation of a word of two syllables or more is its (word) stress pattern. This pattern is an abstract property of the word, deriving from the opposition between stressed and unstressed syllables. Most words have one stressed syllable, the remaining being unstressed. The IPA symbol for (primary) stress is the superscript vertical stroke ' positioned in front of the stressed syllable; unstressed syllables are not marked. In English, stress is fixed for each word, but the position of stress varies on different words. Because English has words of different numbers of syllables, ranging from one to five or more, when these are combined with different stress locations, the number of possible, and indeed actual, patterns is considerable. Some examples are presented in Table 1.2.

The stress pattern of a word is very salient: along with number of syllables, it is one of the features most likely to be retained, for example, when we make a slip of the

Table 1.2 Examples of English lexical stress patterns.

	Stress on 1st	Stress on 2nd	Stress on 3rd
1 syllable	'CHEESE	–	–
2 syllables	'POSTMAN	GUI 'TAR	–
3 syllables	'TELEPHONE	BA 'NANA	KANGA 'ROO
4 syllables	'CATERPILLAR	KA 'LEIDOSCOPE	PANO 'RAMA
5 syllables	–	EX 'TERMINATOR	UNBE 'LIEVABLE

ACTIVITY 1.3

Aim: To investigate informally the effects on pronunciation of increasing speech rate.

For this activity, ideally you will have access to an audio recording device, so that you can record and listen to your performance. If that is not available, just observe your performance in real time.
　　Repeat the following phrase five times, starting slow and careful, getting faster on each repetition, ending at your maximum speed:

(1.8) THE TELEPHONE IS LIKE A BANANA.

What happens to your pronunciation as you speed up?
　　Check your observations with the Key to Activity 1.3 at the end of the chapter.

tongue. To some extent, the position of the stress is predictable from the segmental content of the word (Roach, 2009) but overall the position of word stress is far less predictable in English than in many other languages, for example, Polish, where the stress is almost always on the penultimate syllable, or Czech, where it is generally on the first syllable (Laver, 1994).

This abstract pattern of word stress is realized phonetically when a speaker produces the word in an utterance. More strongly stressed syllables tend to be relatively loud. There is also a natural tendency for a syllable with strong stress to be longer in duration and higher in pitch, though these tendencies can be overridden in particular languages or dialects, for example, for speakers of the West Midlands accent of English, around Birmingham, the stressed syllable is characteristically lower in pitch than adjacent unstressed syllables. Thus loudness, pitch prominence and relative length are the main auditory correlates of stress. As we have seen, these are also the main auditory correlates of the Tonic.

Lexically unstressed syllables are realized phonetically as less prominent than stressed syllables. They are likely to be quieter, shorter in duration and less obtrusive in pitch: they are unlikely to carry much dynamic pitch change and are usually not far away, in the speaker's pitch range, from the preceding and/or following syllables. In addition, in English, the vowel in an unstressed syllable frequently has a more central quality, and is often schwa [ə]. While stressed syllables generally remain salient, unstressed syllables or their vowel nuclei may not always be realized phonetically in actual speech, particularly when the tempo of speech is increased or a more casual style is used.

Rhythm

In speech, phonetically prominent and non-prominent syllables are organized into patterns, which constitute the rhythm of the utterance. The phonetic features that convey rhythmic prominence include pitch, loudness, duration and vowel quality. These features were mentioned in the context of word stress in the previous section. It is important to make a distinction between, on the one hand, word stress as an abstract property of a word, that is, part of our phonological representation for that word, that we draw on for comprehension as well as production, and, on the other hand, the phonetic realization of stress within a particular utterance, as a peak of prosodic prominence that contributes to the rhythm of the whole utterance. It is the latter that provides the basis for the intonation structure of the IP. Rhythmic patterns are thus a property of actual utterances rather than of individual words. The inherent stress pattern of a word may relate in various ways to the rhythm of an utterance in which that word occurs.

Rhythmic patterns vary widely across different languages and are often one of the most striking features of a foreign accent. There is also an increasing recognition of the importance of rhythm in young children's perception and acquisition of their first language (see Chapter 6).

The Foot

The unit of rhythm is the Foot. A Foot consists of one strong syllable, which may be followed by weak syllables. Foot boundaries can be marked by the IPA symbol for stress, a vertical stroke ', which precedes the strong syllable beginning the Foot. Since the Tonic syllable, marked with a Tone diacritic, is always rhythmically strong, there is no need to mark it separately with a stress diacritic: it is implied in the Tone diacritic.

An IP can consist of a single Foot, e.g. a single word, of one or more syllables, as in (1.9) and (1.10):

(1.9) ‖ `this ‖
(1.10) ‖ `funnel ‖

The Foot that contains the Tonic can be preceded by one or more Feet, forming the Head. In (1.9.1), there is one Foot, "whats", preceding the Tonic, while in (1.10.1) there are two Feet before the Tonic: "what comes" and "out of the":

(1.9.1) ‖ 'whats `this ‖
(1.10.1) ‖ 'what comes 'out of the `funnel‖

The Foot beginning with the Tonic may be followed by one or more Feet, which form the Tail. In (1.9.2), "called though" is a Foot that forms the Tail of the IP:

(1.9.2) ‖ 'whats `this bit 'called though ‖

It is possible to have a silent beat, where there is no audible strong syllable at the beginning of the Foot but nevertheless both speaker and listener perceive a beat. The speaker may signal it by a gesture or nod. In this transcription system, the silent beat is symbolized by an underlined space, preceded by the Foot boundary mark. Such a Foot would constitute a Pre-head, as in (1.11):

(1.11) ‖ '_its 'called a `funnel ‖

Rhythm and grammar

In general, the rhythmically strong syllables in an utterance are more likely to belong to lexical items (noun, lexical verb, adjective or adverb) rather than function words (pronoun, preposition, auxiliary verb, article, etc.). In (1.11), CALLED is a verb and FUNNEL is a noun. In (1.12), TEDDY and NECK are both nouns:

(1.12) ‖ whats 'teddy got round his `neck ‖

FUNNEL and TEDDY are both disyllabic, the first syllable having the lexical stress. This then becomes the strong syllable of the Foot. Where the lexical item has more than one syllable, the strong syllable is (almost always) the syllable that is marked for word stress in the word's phonological representation. CALLED and NECK are monosyllabic and so their phonological representations are not specified for word stress. However, in these utterances, they are realized as the strong syllable of their Foot.

Although it is most often the lexical words in an utterance that appear in rhythmically strong positions, there are plenty of occasions when function words occur in a strong position too. In such cases, the function word often has a contrastive implication, in which case it is likely to be realized with a Supertonic. An example, already discussed, is "this" in (1.9.3), reproduced from Extract (1.9.2) in Activity 1.2.

(1.9.3) ‖↑ ˈwhats ⇑ˋthis bit ˈcalled though ‖

In Activity 1.3, we considered different realizations of the sentence THE TELEPHONE IS LIKE A BANANA. The uncontracted form of IS, namely [ɪz], is most likely to be found when IS forms the Tonic, as shown in (1.8.5), for instance, when the speaker is correcting the previous speaker who had denied the resemblance between telephone and banana:

(1.8.5) ‖ the ˈtelephone ⇑ˋis like a baˈnana ‖

Intonation and meaning

The aim of these sections has been to present a simple and usable notation system for English intonation, as spoken by mature speakers. The exposition has covered intonation structure, through its relation to the rhythmic structure of utterances, which includes links with the abstract patterns of word stress. From this presentation, it may be apparent that the main role of the prosodic features of speech (notably pitch, loudness and length) is to integrate two types of meaning.

First, an utterance is made up of words, each of which has a stress pattern that is a major cue to its accurate recognition by listeners. This abstract pattern therefore has to be realized in the utterance in such a way as to make it identifiable. Clearly, one aspect of phonological learning for young children is to learn the correct stress pattern and how to realize it. The importance and salience of this aspect of a word's phonology are implicit in Extract (1.5), the exchange between Robin and his mother studied in Activity 1.2 and reproduced here:

Robin: circle

(1.5)
1   M: ‖↑ ˈwhats ⇑ˋthis bit ˈcalled though ‖

        ⋀
        —
        _____

2   R: çiːj akəlˠ
                { f }

3   M: ‖ it ˇisnt ‖ its ꞌcalled a ⇑ˋfunnel ‖

      ⌃＼

4   R: f ɑ f a
          {f}

5   M: ‖ thats ꞌright ‖ n ↑ꞌwhat comes ꞌout of the ˋfunnel ‖

      ⌃＼

6   R: ʔə mɛ ʊ kʰ

In line 3, Robin's mother explicitly corrects his attempt at labelling the item in line 2. In line 4, Robin duly has another attempt. This is accepted by his mother in line 5, even though it is clearly still quite a long way from her own pronunciation of FUNNEL. It is interesting to note the features that his and her pronunciations share: they both have two syllables, the same word-initial consonant, and in both, it is the first syllable that is prominent in terms of pitch and loudness. By contrast, if we compare Robin's word in line 2 with his mother's pronunciation of FUNNEL, we can note that Robin's word has three syllables, a different initial consonant, and prominence on the second syllable. On the other hand, the final syllable is very similar to the final syllable of FUNNEL as produced by his mother – a similarity that is lost when he produces his revised attempt in line 4. This example suggests that not all phonological features are equal, when speakers are concerned to ensure the recognizability of a word, and that conveying the word's stress pattern may be particularly important.

The second type of meaning conveyed by prosodic features is meaning that is associated with intonation. Some aspects of intonational meaning, such as the ability to mark the end of the turn and to highlight important parts of the utterance, have been briefly touched on in this chapter. The most important task for the young child with regard to intonation is to learn to understand and convey its meanings. The next three chapters therefore address the three main types of meaning that English intonation serves: to organize the orderly exchange of speaking turns (Chapter 2); to highlight what is important or new in a turn that the listener should attend to (Chapter 3); and to initiate a new action in the talk, or to display alignment with an action that is underway (Chapter 4). These three areas of meaning are particularly relevant to carer–child interaction where, as we have seen, the meanings that young children try to convey through words are often obscured as a result of limited linguistic knowledge and ability. For this reason, we will continue to draw on the interactions between Robin and his mother when explicating these three areas of meaning and the role of intonation in communicating them.

Key to Activity 1.1

A transcript of this extract of overlapping talk is presented as Extract (1.1). Start and end of overlap are marked with [ ]. Silences are indicated in tenths of a second, that is, (0.8) signifies 800 milliseconds:

```
(1.1)
Daisy used to ha[ng out in Stevenage when I was younger]
Beth            [that'd be good we should  do   that   o]ver
      (0.8)
Beth  [like summer]
Daisy [  summer   ](.)yeah
```

Key to Activity 1.2

1 There is a Supertonic on "this", which suggests that they have just been talking about a different bit of the train piece, and the mother is now highlighting a new bit. This function of Supertonic placement is discussed further in Chapter 3.

2 The IP boundary occurs after the end of one clause, "it isn't", and before the start of the next clause. IP boundaries most often occur at the end of a major grammatical unit such as a clause. Research has shown that while there is no deterministic relation between IP boundary and the boundaries of grammatical units, IPs tend not to be greater than a sentence and most often coincide with a clause (Crystal, 1969).

3 The Tone in the first IP is a fall-rise, a Tone that often projects that the speaker is going to continue talking, as here. The Tone in the second IP is a fall, which often projects a TRP, that is, the end of the current speaker's turn, as here. The relationship between IP boundaries and turn construction is considered in Chapter 2.

4 There are two syntactic questions, in line 1 and line 5. The Tone is a fall on each occasion. This does not support the notion that in English, questions are routinely spoken with a rising Tone.

5 Robin seems to display ability to mark the end of his turn, by a (rise-)fall pitch movement (lines 2, 4). For this reason he can be credited with the ability to produce an IP. As noted under (3) above, falling Tones (including rise-falls) in Southern British English often mark a TRP. Robin's mother displays an orientation to Robin's IP boundary and falling Tones as marking a TRP, i.e. the end of his turn, by starting her own turn (lines 3, 5).

Key to Activity 1.3

1 It is likely that one of your first changes was to use the contracted form of is, i.e. [z] rather than [ɪz]. In most positions other than the very beginning or end of the IP, contraction of this copula/auxiliary verb form is usual, even at a relatively slow speech rate. Here this would create a coda cluster [nz]; though in connected speech it is very likely that the alveolar nasal itself will no longer be articulated, being marked just by nasality on the preceding vowel: [fəõz]

2 Many grammatical items (often known as function words) consist of a single weak syllable. This includes determiners, auxiliary verbs and pronouns. In this sentence, at a fast speech rate the definite article. THE is likely to lose its vowel, leaving perhaps just a weakly articulated and voiceless dental fricative before the voiceless plosive at the beginning of TELEPHONE: [θtʰ]. The indefinite article A is quite likely to be devoiced too, and even to disappear almost entirely, perhaps just audible as a brief aspiration, sandwiched between the voiceless plosive at the end of LIKE and the plosive at the start of BANANA.

3 The first vowel of BANANA is likely to disappear at a fast speech rate, a common fate for an initial unstressed syllable that immediately precedes the stressed syllable in the word. It is well known that syllables in this position are particularly vulnerable in the speech of young children: ˈNANA is a very common child pronunciation of the word.

4 Similarly, the middle, unstressed vowel of TELEPHONE, sandwiched between the stressed syllable and a relatively prominent final syllable, is likely to be lost at a faster rate.

One possible outcome of the increase in rate is therefore something like:

(1.8.1)
TH ˈTEL PHONES LIKE B ˈNANA
[θˈtʰɛlʲfəõzlaɪkə̥ˈpnɑnə]

You can listen to a pronunciation of this sentence at slow and fast rates.

(1.8.2)
‖ [ðəˈtʰɛlʲɪfəõnzlaɪkəbə ˋnɑnə] ‖

(1.8.3)
‖ [θˈtʰɛlʲfəõzlaɪkə̥ ˋpnɑnə] ‖

In the slower pronunciation, there are two stressed syllables, the second forming the Tonic, and seven unstressed syllables. In the faster pronunciation, there are again two stressed syllables, the second forming again the Tonic, but just five unstressed syllables. Because the stressed syllables are the same in both versions, both retain the same basic intonation structure:

(1.8.4)
‖ THE ˈTELEPHONE IS LIKE A BA ˋNANA ‖

CHAPTER 2

Turns

In Chapter 1, it was suggested that one of the key functions of intonation is to help regulate the exchange of speaking turns. We saw that Robin at the age of 1;9, was apparently able to signal unambiguously to his mother that his turn was complete and that she could take a turn herself. Furthermore, he seemed to be able to identify without difficulty the point at which she had completed her turn. In this chapter we delve more deeply into turn-taking, exploring what it is that the young child has to learn about intonation in order to participate in orderly conversation.

The basic organizing principle of social interaction is that the participants take turns. This is evident when people play a board game, get off a plane, negotiate a crossroads and, above all, when they have a conversation. Research in Conversation Analysis since the 1960s has taken the turn to be the building block of talk-in-interaction (Sacks, Schegloff, & Jefferson, 1974). In this chapter, we will show how intonation is used in the design of speaking turns; and how, conversely, the business of taking turns provides the young child with rich opportunities to discover the structure of intonation.

The purpose of turn-taking varies according to the activity in question, for example, in a board game, it increases the likelihood of an enjoyable time being had by the players; at a crossroads, it decreases the likelihood of traffic accidents. Each of these activities has a set of conventions to regulate the taking of turns, which may be more or less explicit. The turn-taking rules of a board game like Monopoly are set out in print, in the rules of the game. Similarly, the turn-taking conventions of traffic at a roundabout or a crossroads, including, for example, the rules of how traffic light signals must be interpreted, are set out in the highway code for the country in question. The turn-taking procedures that regulate passengers getting off a plane are not usually written down. For talk-in-interaction, the conventions are generally more like those for getting off the plane, in that they are not codified. This is particularly true of conversation; other types of talk-in-interaction, such as in school lessons, have more institutionalized turn-taking procedures.

The first job that the turn-taking conventions need to do is regulate how turns are allocated to participants in the activity. In the case of Monopoly, the rules state that each player throws the dice in sequence, the order being determined by position round the table. In the case of a crossroads, turn allocation may be regulated by traffic lights or by signs and markings on the road that indicate who has right of way. For

Children's Intonation: A Framework for Practice and Research, First Edition. Bill Wells and Joy Stackhouse.
© 2016 John Wiley & Sons, Ltd. Published 2016 by John Wiley & Sons, Ltd.
Companion website: www.wiley.com/go/childintonation

disembarkation from a plane, in some cultures at least, there is a convention whereby the passengers in the row nearest the exit are (implicitly) allocated a turn to make their way to the exit before passengers seated one row further from the exit, and so on. However, this is not compulsory. In conversation, the allocation of turns depends on the number of participants. If there are only two, there is a simple alternation: if one speaker indicates the end of his turn, then the next turn is allocated by default to the other speaker. Where there are more than two speakers, the current speaker can select the next speaker. This can be done by linguistic means, for example, by naming a participant. In Extract (2.1), a speech and language therapist (T) is conducting a session with two 9-year-old boys, Len (L) and Patrick (P), who have language difficulties. Len is talking about at trip he made to a theme park:

(2.1)
```
58   L: er and when lady was about to read one (.) one bit
59      it was too fast because it went like this (makes noise)
60   T: did it
61   L: yeah mm and she said it was too fast
62   T: mm
63   P: what
64   L: but (.) wu- uh one of the boards
65   T: Len can you see Patrick's looking at you and he's listen-
        ing to you
66      but you're [not looking at him at all]
67   L:            [o h  y e s   I    forgot] I forgot I nearly
```

In line 65, the therapist nominates Len, rather than Patrick, to take the next turn. She does this by specifically naming him at the beginning of her turn, which takes the form of a question. Len duly takes the next turn in line 68. Nomination of the next speaker can also be done by current speaker directing their gaze to a particular person. It can be seen from this extract that turn-allocation by nomination can be a powerful means for controlling the direction of the talk. Here, the therapist moves the talk away from the exchange between the two boys about Len's visit to the theme park. She obliges Len to engage in some meta-reflection about his own interaction, apparently alluding to a therapy agenda that has been established earlier in this session or in an earlier session, as evidenced by line 67 where Len says "I forgot."

The current speaker does not have to nominate a next speaker. In such cases, another speaker can self-select to take the next turn. As a result, sometimes more than one new speaker starts talking at the same time. On the other hand, it may transpire that no new speaker takes up the opportunity provided by the current speaker. In this situation, the conventions of turn allocation allow the current speaker to continue.

While intonation does not have a large role in turn allocation, it is central to the second component of turn-organization: how turns are constructed. In the case of Monopoly, each turn starts with a single throw of the dice which determines how many squares the player's piece can move. Depending on where the piece lands, various other activities come into play that can extend the turn. Once these actions are completed, then the turn ends. In the case of the crossroads, turn construction is regulated by the convention that the driver's turn will consist of moving across the crossroads and proceeding along one of the other roads. Turns could in theory be constructed in other ways, such as moving forward to the middle of a crossroads then parking and getting out of the car; or not moving forward at all when one's turn has been allocated (e.g. by a green traffic light). However, such unconventional turns are sanctionable by other road users or even by the law. Turns at talk are built principally out of turn constructional units (TCUs) and, like the turns in a board game or at a crossroads, have recognizable beginnings, middles and ends. A turn at talk may be constructed from visible behaviours such as gaze and gestures, as well as audible linguistic resources of grammar, vocabulary and intonation. The construction of turns in talk is considered in more detail below, in relation to intonation in particular.

A newcomer to a shared activity needs to learn the turn-taking conventions. Sometimes the newcomer can read about them, as for Monopoly or when preparing for a driving test, although this is often secondary to being inducted into the conventions by more experienced practitioners. In the case of disembarking from the plane, where nothing is written down, induction may occur if travelling with a more experienced passenger; otherwise the newcomer is dependent on observation of others' behaviour. In the case of talk-in-interaction, the infant usually has access to a carer willing to induct him into turn-taking practices, as well as ample opportunity for observation. However, the infant wishing to learn the conventions of conversational turn-taking differs from newcomers to these other activities in that as yet he has no language through which he can be inducted into those conventions. Because the turn-taking conventions of talk-in-interaction are implemented largely by means of language, and the structure of the language is to a significant extent shaped by the requirements of these conventions, the infant has to draw on his or her growing knowledge of each to support his or her learning of the other.

In this chapter, it will be shown how intonation is centrally involved in the construction of turns at talk. The different parts of turns will be related to the different elements of the intonation phrase (IP) that were described in Chapter 1. Observations of a young child, Robin, talking and playing with his mother between the ages of 19–21 months, illustrate that the collaborative activity of taking turns is managed mainly because the participants share an understanding of how intonation works. Talk involving young children is particularly useful in uncovering the relationship between intonation and turn construction, because at this stage the child's stock of words is limited, pronunciation is often very divergent from the adult form and the child has only the most rudimentary resources for combining words. The reliance on other means, particularly intonation, to manage turn-taking is therefore more apparent than in adult talk, where more evidence for the completion of a turn may be available from its grammar and semantics. Further details about the recordings of Robin and his mother can be found in Appendix 2.

Turn constructional units

According to Sacks et al. (1974), turns are built out of turn constructional units, henceforth referred to as TCUs. Each turn must comprise at least one TCU. Quite often, a TCU will coincide with a grammatical sentence, as in (2.2), where Robin's mother produces a turn consisting of a single sentence, made up of a single clause:

(2.2) M: is that the funnel

Here, her turn is not grammatically complete until the final word, "funnel"; the string of words "is that the" is not a TCU, because it is not grammatically complete. Because a TCU is, by definition, complete, it can project the end of the turn, where another speaker has the opportunity to start talking. The place where this can happen is at the end of the TCU, in this case, following the word "funnel". This place is called the Transition Relevance Place (TRP), so called because at this place it becomes relevant for another speaker to take the floor, that is, for turn transition to occur. It is analogous to a system of traffic lights: from the point of view of the listener, the lights are on red until the speaker produces the word that renders the TCU complete. That word could be considered as the yellow light: once it is over, the listener can take a turn. Anything that follows, e.g. a silence, is then interpretable as a green light, indicating the Transition Relevance Place. In (2.2.1) and throughout this book, the red light is symbolized by dark grey shading and the yellow (or amber) light by a lighter grey shading, while the green light is not marked. These conventions are listed in Appendix 1.

(2.2.1)   is that the funnel (.)

However, the mapping between grammar and TCU is not always straightforward. Another turn produced by Robin's mother is shown in (2.3):

(2.3) whats teddy got round his neck (.)

Again, this is a complete sentence consisting of a single clause, so there is a TRP after "neck". In terms of traffic lights, this can be shown as (2.3.1):

(2.3.1)   whats teddy got round his neck (.)

However, there is (at least) one earlier point of possible grammatical completion. This is after "got", implying an earlier yellow light, as in (2.3.2):

(2.3.2)   whats teddy got round his neck (.)

A listener who is solely monitoring for grammatical completion could legitimately start talking after "got". This would mean that the two speakers would be talking at the same time - a situation that for the most part participants in talk-in-interaction avoid.

ACTIVITY 2.1

Aim: This activity provides an opportunity to further investigate the concept of the turn-constructional unit (TCU). The following turn, produced by Robin's mother, is taken from an extract studied in Chapter 1:

(2.4)   whats this bit called though (.)

Like (2.2) and (2.3), this is a complete sentence consisting of a single clause, and so there is a TRP after "though". However, in this case, there are more points of possible grammatical completion earlier on.
1 Write out three other possibly complete sentences contained in this turn.
2 Colour the words in each of the four possible sentences, using the traffic light code (see Appendix 1). Check your answers with the Key to Activity 2.1 at the end of this chapter.

Because there are many occasions where the end of a clause is not a clear guide to the onset of the TRP, it is not possible to find direct correspondences between TCUs and particular units of grammar: a purely grammatical definition of the TCU is not tenable. Sacks et al. (1974) concluded that other features, including intonation, are also involved in marking a TCU.

In the next section, it will be shown that intonation plays an important role, in conjunction with grammar, in indicating where the TRP may start. It is for this reason that young children need to be able to deploy and react to intonation appropriately, if they are to take part in orderly turn-taking.

The Intonation Phrase: a system of traffic lights for turn-taking

In Chapter 1, it was suggested that that the Intonation Phrase (IP) is not only the basis of intonation structure but also can be thought of as the fundamental unit of speech production in talk-in-interaction. In relation to turns, there is a great deal of evidence that for a turn to be treated as complete, it must consist of a complete IP. In this sense, intonation provides a powerful means for participants to overcome the potential limitations of grammar as a way of marking TCU boundaries. We saw in Chapter 1 that the IP can vary considerably in length and structural complexity. It has one obligatory element, the Tonic, and a number of optional elements, as shown in (2.5):

(2.5) ‖ (Pre-head) ' (onset + rest of Head) ` Tonic (Tail) ‖

This structure provides for IPs, and therefore turns, of varying length and complexity. Each will be potentially complete, because it contains a Tonic.

IP boundaries frequently indicate a potential place for change of speaker, i.e. a turn transition relevance place (TRP). For this reason, intonation is important for the regulation of turn-exchange, as has been shown in studies of different varieties of English, including General American English (Ford & Thompson, 1996) and Standard Southern British English (Walker, 2004) as well as other British English varieties including Tyneside (Local, Kelly, & Wells, 1986), Ulster (Wells & Peppé, 1996), West Midlands (Wells & Macfarlane, 1998) and Afro-Caribbean (Local, Wells, & Sebba, 1985).

In the previous section, the idea of a system of traffic lights to regulate turn-taking was introduced in relation to grammar but it transpired that grammatical completion was not very reliable as a signal for the onset of the TRP. In English, intonation provides a system of traffic lights that is rather more reliable. The default mapping between IP structure and turn construction is shown in (2.5.1):

(2.5.1)   ‖ (Pre-head) ' (Onset + rest of Head) ` Tonic (Tail) ‖

While the current speaker is still in the Head of the IP, the lights are on red (dark grey shading here), even if the speaker pauses: if someone else starts talking now, they will be heard as competing with her for the floor. Once the current speaker reaches her Tonic, the lights change to amber (light grey shading), at which point other potential speakers may gear up to start talking. If the current speaker now stops talking, this is the green light: it will usually be treated as a TRP, i.e. a legitimate place for a new speaker to start up. The new speaker may also start up in overlap with a Tail produced by the current speaker, though more often the new speaker waits till the current speaker has finished talking. Now complete Activity 2.2 before reading further.

ACTIVITY 2.2

Aim: To gain some experience in analysing talk-in-interaction from the point of view of intonational traffic lights.

For this activity, it is useful to have red, yellow and green highlighter pens.

In carer–child interaction, both child and adult can be seen to orient to intonation as a system of traffic lights. Study the transcript of the recorded interaction in Extract (2.6), which is between Robin (CA 1;9) and his mother (M). You have already worked with this extract in Activity 1.2 in Chapter 1. This time, the aim of the activity is to discover how the system of intonation traffic lights operates.

(2.6)

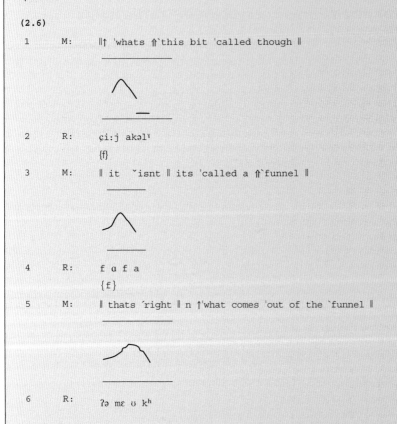

```
1     M:     ‖↑ 'whats ⇑`this bit 'called though ‖
```



```
2     R:     çi:j akəlˠ
              {f}
3     M:     ‖ it  ˇisnt ‖ its 'called a ⇑`funnel ‖
```



```
4     R:     f ɑ f a
              {f}
5     M:     ‖ thats ´right ‖ n ↑'what comes 'out of the `funnel ‖
```



```
6     R:     ʔə mɛ ʊ kʰ
```

1 Assuming the default mapping from intonation structure to turn-taking traffic lights, as described above, mark the traffic light structure of each IP produced by Robin's mother in lines 1, 3 and 5. NB. Lines 3 and 5 each contain two IPs.
2 Robin produces single word turns in lines 2, 4 and 6. Taking his mother's response (in lines 3 and 5) as evidence, what colour of traffic light would you use to mark Robin's turns?
3 What would you expect to happen following line 6?
Check your answers with the Key to Activity 2.2 at the end of this chapter.

Gaining and giving away the floor

Although adults occasionally produce turns consisting of an IP of a single word only, for instance, when repeating a child's attempt at a word, most of the time the turn is more elaborate, as in lines 1, 3 and 5 of (2.6). The mother's turns in lines 3 and 5 each consist of two IPs; in each case, the Tonic of the final IP is on the last word and is a fall. It is at this point that Robin starts his turn, i.e. straight after a yellow light; he does not start in the course of the Head of his mother's second IP, i.e. not during a red light. This suggests that Robin is aware when her turn has ended and that this awareness derives, at least in part, from recognition of the intonation structure of his mother's turns. He is thus able to gain the floor with a straightforward change of speaker turn.

In the same way, we can see that Robin's mother responds to his single word utterances in lines 2 and 4 as complete turns: following his utterance, she immediately starts her own turn (lines 3, 5). In line 2 ‖ çi:j akəlˠ ‖ and in line 4 ‖ f ɑ f a ‖, Robin's single word utterance is delivered with a rising-falling pitch contour that can be heard as equivalent to the rise-fall Tone used by his mother and other speakers of her accent. By starting to talk, his mother gives Robin feedback that a rise-fall ending at the bottom of his pitch range is an effective way of showing others that he has finished his turn. On this evidence, Robin can be credited with the ability to create a TCU consisting of a single word by producing an IP. The TCU serves as a complete turn and also serves to surrender the floor. It can therefore be notated as ‖ çi:j akəlˠ ‖, with a yellow traffic light.

As described so far, the system of intonation for giving away and gaining the floor is simple: the current speaker produces some talk and marks the end of it with a Tonic, which signals to the listeners that they may now take a turn. This is an intonational equivalent to the convention in military radio-transmitted interaction, whereby each speaker says the word "over" at the end of a turn to signal that the turn is finished. A prosodic system of this kind is found in at least one variety of English: in Afro-Caribbean English, it has been reported that the end of the speaker's turn is routinely marked by a fall in pitch on the final syllable of the turn (Local et al., 1985).

However, in most varieties of English, including the variety of Southern British Standard English spoken by Robin's mother, things are more complicated. This is evident in line 1 of Extract (2.6), where the Tonic is located on "this", which is not the final word of the IP. The reasons for such variations in Tonic placement were mentioned in Chapter 1, and will be explored in depth in Chapter 3. For the purposes of the present discussion, it is sufficient to note that this results in a yellow light well before the end of the TCU, followed by a green light that is co-extensive with the Tail of the IP: "bit called though".

From the point of view of signalling the Transition Relevance Place (TRP), the possibility that English offers for varying Tonic placement represents an additional challenge for the young child. This is evident in the talk that follows on from the extract we studied in Activity 2.2, presented here as Extract (2.7), where confusion arises as to whether or not Robin has signalled the end of his turn. In lines 6, 7 and 12 of the transcript, the pitch pattern is represented directly above the words associated with it:

(2.7)

5   M: ‖ thats ʹright ‖ n ↑ʹwhat comes ʹout of the ˋfunnel ‖

6   R: ʔə mɛ ʊ kʰ   [f ɑ f ə]
          {f   f}(0.5){f}

7   M: [smoke-]
                          ((M nods))
                     (0.5)

8   M: ‖ˇsmoke comes out of the ʹfunnel‖ ˋdoesnt it‖
          ((Mother nods))
                     (1.5)

9   M: ‖ˆhm‖
                     (1.6)

10 M: ‖s that ʹright‖
                     (2.1)

11 R: (unintelligible whisper)
                     (1.0)

12 R: m̥mɵk ə   fɐ fɐː

13 M:‖   ‖ˈthats ˆrightˈ‖ ˆsmoke out of the funnel‖ ˆsgood‖

In line 6, Robin produces a turn that is more elaborate than lines 2 and 4 of (2.6), in that it consists of two words. The first, SMOKE, has the same rise-fall pitch as in lines 2 and 4, and could be reasonably interpreted by his mother as a Tonic. As the transcript indicates, he seems to have shown her a yellow light (see Key to Activity 2.2, Question 3). His mother starts to speak (line 7). However, Robin continues his turn with [ɑfə] (FUNNEL), again with a rise-fall. As a result, Robin and his mother are speaking in overlap. We can see that this interactional problem was caused by Robin breaking a traffic light rule: having signalled to his mother that he had stopped, with SMOKE, he continued to talk, with FUNNEL. To return to the crossroads analogy: Robin stops his car at the crossroads, allowing the other driver (his mother) to set off; but then Robin sets off again before his mother has completed her turn and reached the other side of the crossroads. The result is a collision; Robin and his mother end up talking at the same time, as if in competition with one another. The remainder of the extract, which will be discussed in the next section, can be seen as an attempt to recover the situation, following this crash.

Holding the floor

This occurrence of overlap, which we have compared to a collision, can be attributed to Robin's attempt to extend his occupancy of the floor, by extending his turn beyond a single word. As mature speakers, most of the time we use turns that are longer than a single word. We therefore need ways of securing the floor so that we are not interrupted before we have finished our turn. Since the Tonic announces a transition relevance place, then every time we produce a Tonic, our occupation of the floor is at risk: someone else may take over. This is what happened to Robin in lines 6–7 of (2.7).

However, speakers have access to a variety of resources that help them hold on to the floor. For instance, I can announce that I am going to tell a joke. This would normally secure me the floor until I get to the punch line, no matter how many Tonics I produce. Young children can also enjoy an extended turn of this kind, when playing. For example, Corrin (2002) presents sequences where children of Robin's age produce several TCUs, separated by pauses, which accompany the child's manipulation of play toys, without any intervention by the mother. One such sequence will be discussed in Chapter 7.

In conversational interaction, the current speaker can enhance his chances of keeping the floor by deploying a range of resources, singly or in combination. One resource is to avoid making eye contact with the listeners, since re-establishing eye contact generally projects a TRP (Filipi, 2009). The spoken language itself also provides various lexical resources for extending the turn. Here, we focus on three resources provided by intonation: the Tail, the Head, and Multiple Intonation Phrases.

The Tail
One way to extend the IP beyond a single word is to add material after the Tonic. Robin's mother does this in line 1 of Extract (2.6.1), reproduced here as (2.6.2):

(2.6.2)   ‖↑ 'whats ⇑`this bit 'called though ‖

The post-Tonic words "bit called though" form the Tail; as such, it displays a green light as a default. This is because in English, Tails are vulnerable to terminal overlap by another speaker (Wells & Macfarlane, 1998): listeners are liable to treat the material in the Tail as semantically predictable, and so it is not always necessary to hear it out.

This predictability is evident in (2.6.2): if the words "bit called though" had been omitted or overlapped, "what's this" on its own may well have sufficed to elicit a fitted response from Robin. Because of their semantic predictability, though Tails do extend the IP and therefore the TCU, they do not reliably serve to keep the floor.

Nevertheless, speakers do produce Tails, and as in (2.6.2), they are often produced without being overlapped. Indeed, Extract (2.6.1) concluded with Robin producing a turn in line 12 that has a Tonic + Tail IP structure, which is then confirmed by his mother, who uses the same Tonic + Tail IP structure in line 13 while expanding Robin's grammatical structure. These turns are reproduced as Extract (2.6.3):

(2.6.3)

| 12 | R: | m̥mɵk ɔ   fɐ fɐː |
| 13 | M: | ‖'thats ^right‖ ^smoke out of the funnel‖ ^sgood‖ |

The Head

It might be assumed that, leaving intonation aside, grammar on its own is a robust resource for holding onto the floor. It is true that if a point of grammatical completion has not been reached, listeners generally do not treat the turn as complete. This being so, the speaker can hold onto the floor by avoiding syntactic closure. However, as was seen earlier, grammar is not infallible as a guide, since points of possible grammatical completion often occur before the end of the TCU (Schegloff, 1996; Local & Walker, 2012). The example was (2.3):

(2.3) whats teddy got round his neck (.)

Here, there is a possible completion point after "got". Intonation can help the speaker overcome the risk of losing the floor at a premature juncture, for example, after "got", by incorporating the possible completion point into the Head, as Robin's mother did on this occasion, shown in (2.3.1):

(2.3.1) ‖ whats	'teddy	got round his	`neck
Pre-Head	Onset	rest of Head	Tonic

The default mapping of a red light onto the Head then alters the TCU structure projected by the syntax, to reduce the risk of an early incoming. By allowing for words prior to the Tonic, the Head of the IP provides one effective way to extend the TCU.

Speakers can combine these two resources of intonation to extend their turn, producing both a Head and a Tail. Extract (2.8), again from Robin's mother, illustrates this:

(2.8) ‖ so	'where	does the	`teddy	go‖
Pre-Head	Onset	rest of Head	Tonic	Tail

Turning to Robin, it is noteworthy that even at this early stage of linguistic development, as Extract (2.9) shows, there is evidence of the child using a Head + Tonic structure and that this enables him to produce a turn longer than a single word, without being interrupted.

(2.9)

1   M: ‖now 'whats (.) 'whats `this‖
          ((handing a TOP piece to R))

2   M: ‖can you re'member what `this is‖

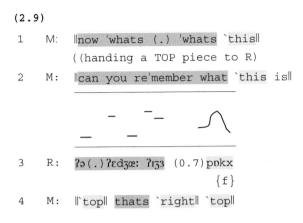

3   R: ʔə(.)ʔɛdʒœː ʔɪ˥˧˧ (0.7)pɒkx
                              {f}

4   M: ‖`top‖ thats `right‖ `top‖

In line 3, Robin produces six syllables. The first five have level pitch, around the middle of his speaking range. The sixth has a large rising falling pitch movement and is louder – it is clearly the most prominent syllable. His mother does not start talking until after the sixth syllable, even though there is a substantial pause between the fifth and the sixth. This strongly suggests that she is responding to Robin's use of mid-level pitch as a turn-holding device: she waits until after his 'Tonic' before she starts her own turn. Similar instances from Robin and other children at this developmental stage are presented by Corrin, Tarplee, & Wells, (2001), offering evidence for the claim that mid-level pitch functions as a turn-continuation device for the child.

Multiple intonation phrases

Speakers often produce turns that consist of more than one Intonation Phrase. Because the occurrence of the Tonic announces a turn transition relevance place (TRP), such turns are in theory vulnerable to an interruption from a potential next speaker following the first IP. In many cases, this may not be a problem, because multi-IP turns are not necessarily planned to be multi-unit turns from the outset. On the contrary, they may arise only because a new speaker does not come in after the first IP. The turn-taking mechanisms described by Sacks et al. (1974) allow for this: if no other speaker comes in at a TRP, then the current speaker may continue. There is a striking case in Extract (2.7) where, having begun at line 8, Robin's mother's turn extends until line 10, as there is no response from Robin. It could be transcribed as a single extended turn of four IPs, as in (2.10):

(2.10) M: ‖ `smoke comes out of the 'funnel ‖ `doesnt it ‖ (1.5) ‖ ʰm ‖ (1.6)
          ‖s that ´right ‖ (2.1)

It is evident from the intervening silences that the last two TCUs, "hm" and "is that right", realized as separate IPs, are produced as a follow-up to the lack of response from Robin. Their wording too makes it clear that she is pursuing a response. Robin's mother almost certainly did not plan this multiple IP turn at the outset to be a single extended turn; rather, it was constructed incrementally in the light of the unfolding interaction with Robin. In such cases, there is no reason to expect IPs that are not turn-final to be different in their intonation design from turn-final IPs, since each IP is potentially turn-final anyway, at the moment of its production.

Alternatively, the speaker may design the first turn-constructional unit in such a way as to project another immediately following, i.e. to secure a turn that extends beyond the end of the first unit. Phonetic resources, including intonation, have been shown to be particularly important here (Schegloff, 1996; Local & Walker, 2004; Walker, 2010). As was noted in Activity 2.2, Robin's mother's turns in lines 3 and 5 of Extract (2.6) each have two IPs. Each IP coincides with a grammatically complete turn constructional unit. In line 3, reproduced here as (2.11), there is a distinct rising pitch movement on "isn't", interpretable as a Tonic:

(2.11)

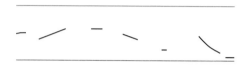

3 M: it isnt   its called a   funnel

However, there is no break at all between "isn't" and "it's", pronounced [ˈɪznˈɪʔs]: there is no final [t] on "isn't", and no slowing down over syllables of "isn't". These are features that Walker (2010) identifies as characterizing a rush-through, where the speaker holds onto the turn by hastening into the next IP. In the present notation, a rush-through is represented by ‖⇒ : a double arrow pointing rightwards from the IP boundary into the next IP, as in (2.11.1):

(2.11.1)   3 M: ‖ it ´isnt‖⇒ ʹit's ʹcalled a `funnel‖

Very similar features are evident in line 5 of (2.6), reproduced here as (2.12): the first IP has a rising tone on "right", which constitutes the Tonic; however, there is no [t] at the end of "right", and no slowing down. The syllabic nasal representing "and" at the beginning of the next IP belongs to the Foot that starts with "right", so the Foot ʹright n   crosses the IP boundary, joining the two IPs rhythmically.

(2.12)

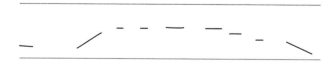

‖ thats ´right‖⇒ n ʹwhat comes ʹout of the `funnel‖

Similarly in (2.13), which is line 13 of Extract (2.7), there is no pause between IPs, though this time there is a Foot boundary. In terms of pitch, "right" and "smoke" both have rise-falls, each starting higher than the last. The pitch contour of the first IP finishes in the middle of the speaker's range, whereas the second IP ends at the base of her range.

(2.13)

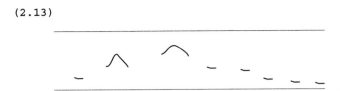

8 M: ‖ˈthats ˆright‖⇒ˆsmoke out of the funnel‖

Listening to each of these turns, it is evident that there are some recurrent prosodic characteristics. There is no pause between the two adjacent IP's: the first flows directly into the second. This may be enhanced by rhythmic integration, where a Foot straddles the IP boundary. The Tonic of the first IP frequently ends around the middle of the speaker's pitch range, rather than reaching the base or top of the range. These three turns (2.11, 2.12, 2.13) share a similar structure, in that the first TCU, which is shorter than the second, provides a direct confirmation or disconfirmation of Robin's preceding turn: or "it isn't", before moving onto a longer second TCU. Where there are two adjacent IPs in this type of turn, it is often the case that the first will be located, or at least end up, in the middle of the speaker's pitch range. In combination with the rhythmic integration that was mentioned, this has the effect of gluing the two IPs in such a way that it would be difficult for another speaker to gain the floor following the first IP.

Extract (2.14), which is line 8 from (2.7), has a rather different structure. Here, the first IP is the longer of the two, followed by a short tag question "doesn't it".

(2.14)

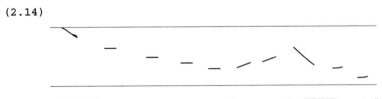

8 M: ‖ ˋsmoke comes out of the ˈfunnel ‖⇒ˋdoesnt it‖

The Tonic of the first IP is on "smoke", which potentially projects an upcoming TRP; the following stretch "comes out of the funnel" continues the descending pitch movement of "smoke", reaching its lowest point on "the", although this is not at the base of the speakers' range. On the final word of the IP, "funnel", the pitch climbs again steeply (around ten semitones), connecting forward to the onset of "doesn't it". This second IP starts high in the speakers' range. As in the previous examples, there is no pause between the IPs. The pitch then descends rapidly, clearly marking a TRP.

Thus, in each of these four turns, Robin's mother uses features of pitch and rhythm to ensure that she gets into a second turn constructional unit without interruption. In terms of the traffic lights, these features override the occurrence of the Tonic that marks the first IP, which would otherwise signal a yellow light – as has been shown in the transcript to this point. Instead, they warrant a red light for the entire first IP, as shown in (2.11.1), repeated, to (2.14.1):

(2.11.1) ‖ it ˊisnt ‖⇒ its ˈcalled a ˋfunnel ‖

(2.12.1) ‖ thats ˊright ‖⇒ n ˈwhat comes ˈout of the ˋfunnel ‖

(2.13.1)   ‖ `thats ^right ‖⇒^smoke out of the funnel ‖

(2.14.1)   ‖ `smoke comes out of the 'funnel ‖⇒`doesnt it ‖

This consideration of multi-IP turns brings to light the key point that the intonational phrase (IP) and the turn-constructional unit (TCU) are not always co-extensive: the occurrence of a Tonic does not inevitably announce a transition relevance place. A second important point is that non-final IPs often have a Tonic that ends around the middle of the pitch range. Thus, speakers and listeners seem to orient to mid-pitch as projecting that the turn is not yet complete.

The extended extract that we have been considering, first presented in this chapter as (2.6) and (2.7), illustrates a basic problem that confronts every child as he produces his first multiword utterances: "How can I say more than one word without being interrupted?" If the child produces his first word with a pitch movement that is heard as a Tonic by the adult, then the adult will most likely start talking, as in lines 3, 5 and 7 of (2.6) and (2.7). We have seen that to prevent this happening, mature speakers have two sets of intonation resources. One is to use a Head + Tonic structure, which was described earlier, and which apparently Robin could deploy, as in (2.9.1):

(2.9.1)   ʔə(.)ʔɛdʒœː ʔɪ̣ʒʒ (0.7)pɒkx

This involves avoiding the use of a prominent pitch contour on the first word. The second strategy is the one we have just seen in examples from his mother, namely, to produce the initial IP with a Tonic that is basically in the middle of the pitch range. Research indicates that at this stage, Robin and other children are also able do this. This is discussed in Chapter 7, in the context of typical intonation development.

Overlap and turn-taking

So far, we have considered how speakers, adult or child, can deploy intonation resources to gain, hold and give away their turn in such a way as to minimize the collision that manifests as overlap, when more than one speaker talks at the same time. However, as was noted at the beginning of the chapter, overlap occurs frequently in adult talk. How to deal with the interactional issues presented by the occurrence of overlapping talk, in the ways that are conventional for the language and culture into which they are born, is therefore something that children have to learn. Prosodic features, including intonation, provide a resource for this. The remainder of the present chapter will describe some ways in which intonation is used to manage overlap. In Chapter 7, we will revisit overlap in order to explore the opportunities it provides for the young child to discover how the intonation system works. Conversation Analysis research on overlapping talk provides an analytical apparatus, as well as a wealth of observations about how overlap operates in adult talk. Additionally, there has been work on the prosodic features of various types of overlap.

Accidental overlap

Overlaps of various kinds will happen by accident, due to latitude in the turn-taking system (Jefferson, 1984, 1987). There are overlap resolution practices available to participants to deal with this contingency, such as continuing to talk or immediately dropping out. A frequent occurrence is where, following a TRP, two or more participants start talking simultaneously. An instance of this was discussed earlier in the chapter. It occurred in lines 6 and 7 of Extract (2.7), which is re-presented as (2.15).

(2.15)

```
5    M:    ‖thats ´right ‖ n ↑'what comes 'out of the `funnel‖


6    R:    ʔə mɛ ʊ kʰ      [f ɑ f ə]
           {f      f}(0.5){f}
                         [_____]

                         [  ↘   ]

                         [_____]

7    M:                  [smoke-]
                         ((M nods))

                  (0.5)

8    M:    ‖ˇsmoke comes out of the 'funnel‖ `doesnt it‖
           (( Mother nods))
```

Once speakers find themselves in overlap, as here, they are confronted with the urgent issue of how to get out of it. (Schegloff, 2000) describes the procedures that are available to participants in order to resolve such overlaps. The most common practice is that used by Robin's mother in line 8: one speaker curtails their turn, dropping out after one syllable or beat of overlap. In terms of intonation structure, his mother's turn in line 7 can be described as an incomplete IP, because it does not have a Tonic: as the transcription shows, there is a slight fall, but it does not get lower than a high-mid point in her pitch range. As discussed in the previous section of this chapter, mid-pitch routinely projects that there is more talk to come in the IP, so the TCU is not complete. Unlike his mother, Robin does not break off his turn in line 6: [fafə] forms a complete IP, its pitch reaching the base of his range.

After she has dropped out, Robin's mother uses another practice commonly found in adult-adult talk: the recycled turn beginning (Schegloff, 2000). She recycles SMOKE, which becomes the first element of a new turn (line 8). The accuracy of this recycling is striking: she uses not only the same word and pitch pattern, including pitch height onset; but also repeats her head nod. Now complete Activity 2.3 before reading further.

ACTIVITY 2.3

Aim: To examine the relationship between intonation and overlapping talk.

In Extract (2.16), Robin is talking as he fits pieces into his jigsaw puzzle board. For ease of reading, his presumed target words are presented in standard orthography. Two instances of overlap occur. For each overlap, answer the following questions:
1 Why do the two speakers start talking in overlap at this point?
2 Describe the mother's talk in the overlap, in terms of (i) grammar, and (ii) intonation.
3 Describe Robin's talk in the overlap, in terms of its intonation.
4 What happens after the overlap?
5 Produce a traffic light transcription for each IP in the extract.

(2.16)

```
                    ╲       ─           ╲       [ ─     ]
  ╲                           ─                 [    ─ ]  ╲
1    R:    now push(.) [it]goes  there(.) [it there] (.)push
                         [__]_____[_____]
                         [  ]               [    ─  ]
                         [╰─]_____[ ─_____]
2    M:                  [mm]               [what  go ]

           ─   ─   ─

                         ╲
3    M:    what goes  in  there
```

Check your answer with the Key to Activity 2.3 at the end of this chapter.

Collaboration and competition in overlapping talk

So far we have considered overlap that arises at or soon after the start of the turn. At the opposite end of the spectrum is the type of overlap that is closest to non-overlapping turn exchange. Broadly speaking, this is where the incoming happens following the Tonic of the overlapped turn (Jefferson, 1987; Wells & Macfarlane, 1998). In adult talk, this type of overlap passes off without overt interactional consequence (Schegloff, 2000). Likewise, Robin and his mother do not treat this type of overlap as a problem (Wells & Corrin, 2004). In Extract (2.17) they are attempting to fit a soldier piece into the puzzle:

(2.17)

1   M: and the soldier isnt doing quite right is he yet

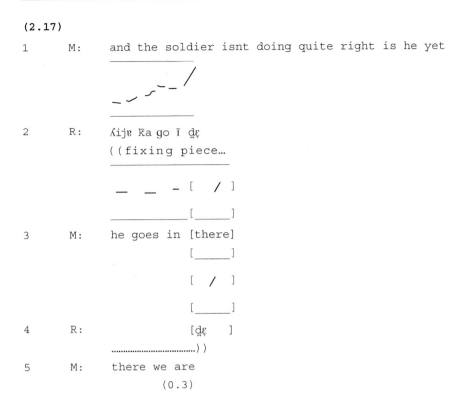

2   R: ʎijʊ ʄa go ĩ d̥ɛ̥
           ((fixing piece...

            ‒   ‒   - [∕]
           _____[_____]
3   M: he goes in [there]
                       [_____]

                      [∕]

                      [_____]
4   R: [d̥ɛ̥   ]
           ....))
5   M: there we are
                 (0.3)

The overlap can be described as collaborative rather than competitive, since Robin and his mother are on the same track with the puzzle. His mother's use of "we" in line 5 provides further evidence of the collaborative nature of this sequence. Intonationally the relevant lines can be transcribed as in (2.17.1):

(2.17.1)

3   M: ‖ he 'goes in ['there] ‖
4   R: ‖['d̥ɛ̥] ‖

Robin's incoming in line 4 overlaps and is identical (lexically, if not in its segmental phonetic detail) with the final word of his mother's turn. Robin's "there" in line 4 has a similar rise to his mother's "there" in line 3, with which it is simultaneous. This suggests that Robin has predicted the pitch pattern that is appropriate to terminate his mother's turn. He is thus providing a Tonic, and a yellow light, to complete his mother's IP and TCU. This enables his mother to take the next turn (line 5) without any problems arising. The coordination of Tone choice (both are rises) may be attributable to the fact that both Robin's rise in line 4 and his mother's rise in line 3 are themselves echoes of Robin's own rise on "there" at the end of line 2. So here is some evidence of Robin's prosodic accomplishment: in line 4 he is able to place his word in the right prosodic and grammatical slot, and also to use a pitch pattern that is appropriate to it (as evidenced by the fact that his mother also uses it).

Competition

In the examples considered so far, the speakers end up talking in overlap, but this has arisen by accident and Robin's mother moves swiftly to resolve the situation. However, it also happens that a participant will deliberately start up in the course of a current speaker's turn. Sometimes this is because the new speaker wants to take over the floor. Competing for the turn is a necessary social skill so it is important for the child to learn how to deploy this intonation in order to compete successfully for the floor, as well as to handle competitive incomings from others. This use of intonation will not be illustrated from the talk of Robin and his mother because no such instances were found of this type of competition, either by Robin or by his mother. It may be that turn competition is not typical of one-to-one carer–child interaction. It also seems likely that children of Robin's age do not compete for the floor in this way, although competitive overlap is evident in recordings of children a few months older and throughout the preschool years, as will be discussed in Chapter 7.

Competitive incomings can sometimes be problematic for participants in interaction, if the incoming is heard as an interruption, i.e. where the current speaker believes they have the right to retain the floor. Thus, the reduction of interruptions that are considered to be inappropriate may be a target for speech and language therapy intervention. An example of this type of interruption was seen at the start of the chapter. In Extract (2.1), a speech and language therapist (T) is conducting a session with two 9-year-old boys, Len (L) and Patrick (P), who have language difficulties. Here we present, as (2.18), the end of that extract, and what immediately follows:

(2.18)

```
65   T:   ‖Len ‖ can you 'see 'Patricks ˇlooking at 'you:‖
          and hes `listening to you ‖⇒ but 'youre

66   T:   [not 'looking at him at ^all]‖

67   L:   [↑o h          ^y e s      ]‖ 'I for`got‖ 'I for`got ‖⇒
          {ff                      ff }

68   L:   I ˇnearly ‖ hh I ˇnearly ‖

69   T:   ‖`mm(.)‖I 'think its `better when you 'look at each other

70        when youre ['tal]king ‖⇒ 'dont `you‖

71   L:             [⇑why]
                    {ff  }

72   P:   ‖↑ 'what 'what 'what

73   T:   ‖↑'then you can `see the 'person‖

74   P:   ‖↑'what would you

75   P:   ‖↑'what 'what did it 'look like in the er: `ghost 'train‖ (0.5)

76   L:   ‖↑'look like in the ˇghost 'train‖

77   P:   ‖ˇyeah ‖
```

In line 67, Len starts talking at a point where it is clear that the therapist has not yet completed her turn in line 66. Although she continues to the end of her turn, Len also continues to talk, ending up as sole occupant of the floor in line 67. His turn trails off ("I nearly") without grammatical completion in line 68, at which point the therapist resumes. Before the therapist has reached a TRP in line 70, Len starts in overlap once again (line 71). On both occasions when Len starts talking in overlap, his pitch is noticeably higher and louder than elsewhere, dropping back to a more usual level once the therapist has stopped.

French and Local (1983) and subsequently Wells and Macfarlane (1998) and Schegloff (2000) have identified several characteristics of turn-competitive incomings that appear to hold for a number of varieties of English:

1 Turn-competitive incomings happen before a TRP. This means that intonationally, they happen prior to the Tonic, i.e. normally during the Head of the IP. In lines 67 and 71, Len starts talking before the therapist has produced a Tonic in that IP.

2 The incoming speaker uses high pitch and extra volume up to the point of the turn-occupant's termination. In the notation presented in Chapter 1, this is represented as a high onset ↑.

3 A high and loud incoming causes the turn-occupant to alter the talk prosodically, in one of three ways:

   i Increase loudness and decrease pace, in which case the turn reaches a TRP. This indicates return of competition, and the incomer may drop out.

   ii Decrease loudness, and fade out. The turn does not reach a TRP. This is represented as moving directly from a red light (turn in progress) to a green light (the floor is surrendered), skipping the yellow light of the Tonic that normally announces an upcoming TRP.

   iii Continue to the end of the turn without noticeably modifying pitch, loudness or tempo. This is exemplified here by speaker T in lines 66 and 70.

Some of these features can be seen in (2.18.1), in which part of (2.18) is transcribed with the traffic light notation.

2.18.1

```
65   T:   ‖Len‖can you 'see 'Patricks ⇑ˇlooking at 'you:
          ‖and hes ⇑ˇlistening to you‖⇒but 'youre

66   T:   [not 'looking at him at ^all] ‖

67   L:   [↑o h          ⇑ˆy  e    s] ‖ 'I for`got‖ 'I for`got‖⇒
          {ff                      ff }

68   L:   Iˇnearly ‖ hh Iˇnearly ‖

69   T:   ‖ˋmm(.)‖I 'think its ⇑ˋbetter when you 'look at each other

70        when youre ['tal]king ‖⇒'dont `you‖ =

71   L:           [⇑why]
```

The overlaps in this extract underline the importance of prosodic features in the management of talk. In line 67, the words of Len's turn suggest that he accepts the point that the therapist has just made, namely that he has neglected to follow the therapy advice that had been given previously, that he should try to maintain eye contact with his interlocutor. One might therefore expect Len to have used a prosodic design that was suitably collaborative, as described in the previous section. However, he designs his turn using noticeably competitive prosodic features: there is a step up in pitch combined with very loud volume: a high (and loud) Onset. Perhaps on account of this mismatch, the therapist does not seem to accept Len's acquiescence at face value, and pursues a further confirmation from him that he has taken her therapy instruction on board. Her doubts turn out to be well-founded, since Len now explicitly challenges the basis for her therapy advice, using a competitively designed overlap with a high and loud Supertonic on the word "why" in line 71.

From line 72 onwards in (2.18), Patrick makes a concerted effort to shift the topic away from the therapy discussion between Len and the therapist. His behaviour suggests that he regards occurrence of two competitive overlaps in quick succession as disruptive to the orderly progress of the interaction. The way in which Len has violated the traffic light conventions is evident from the transcript of the overlapping turns using the traffic light notation, presented in (2.18.1): Len's incomings are placed where the therapist (T) is displaying a red light. At this point Patrick attempts to take the floor (line 72), though in line 73 the therapist provides a response to Len's challenge. Patrick persists in his attempt to take the floor, in lines 74 and 75, and it transpires that he wants to shift the topic back to Len's 'ghost train' narrative that preceded the therapy intervention in line 69. This is successful, as Len picks up on the 'ghost train' topic again in line 76.

In this section on overlapping talk, we have seen that the interactional contingencies that give rise to overlap are complex and varied. Furthermore, they provide opportunities for the child to be inducted into some of the social practices of their community, notably the management of turn-taking. Speakers can start talking at any place relative to the talk of a prior speaker or a current speaker, including in overlap. What the child has to learn about is not so much "where am I allowed to come in?" but, rather, they have to learn which designs of incoming are legitimate at the different possible places, i.e. following or during the current speaker's turn. A key aspect of the incoming turn's design is its intonation. The child also has to learn what the interactional implications are of variously designed incomings at different places. Such implications are: is this incoming meant to compete for the floor, or is it collaborative? In Extract (2.18) it was clear that intonation was central to the competitive overlaps produced by Len. By contrast, Extract (2.17) illustrated an overlap that was collaborative rather than competitive. The collaborative character of this overlap was evident not only in the positioning of Robin's incoming but also in the fact that his rising tone matched his mother's. This observation prefigures the theme of Chapter 4: the interactional factors that lead participants to choose to use one tone rather than another.

Summary

In Chapter 2, an analytical framework has been presented which allows us to address the following questions about turn-taking, in relation to spoken interactions involving a child (C):

Gaining the floor

1 Does C refrain from taking a turn until the current speaker has projected the end of their own turn? (C observes red light.)
2 Does C routinely start a turn with minimal pause, following the prior speaker's turn? (C observes yellow and green lights.)
3 Does C produce an appropriately designed non-competitive turn in overlap, while the current speaker is still talking?
4 Does C produce an appropriately designed competitive turn in overlap, in a bid to capture the floor while the current speaker is still talking?

Holding the floor

1 Does C produce a turn of more than one word by creating an IP with a Head? (C uses red light.)
2 Does C produce a turn of more than a single IP by creating a non-final IP before the final IP? (C keeps red light on.)
3 Does C produce a turn of more than a single IP by rushing through a projected TRP at end of the first IP? (C keeps red light on.)
4 Does C resist a turn-competitive incoming by using intonation features? (C keeps red light on.)

Giving up the floor

1 Does C project the end of the turn by using the Tonic? (C uses yellow light.)
2 Does C break off to give way to a turn-competitive incoming? (C uses green light.)
3 Does C invite collaborative turn completion by producing an incomplete IP as a prompt? (C uses red + green light.)

Key to Activity 2.1

(1)

```
  (i) what's this
 (ii) what's this bit
(iii) what's this bit called
```

(2)

Each of the answers to (1) is a clause, in fact a grammatically complete sentence, and therefore, potentially a TCU, so each would end with a yellow light. Following this grammatical definition of a TCU, the actual turn produced by Robin's mother could be analysed by the listener in any of the ways shown in (2.4.1) to (2.4.4), providing a range of different starting up points for the next turn, involving different amounts of possible overlap:

```
(2.4.1) what's this bit called though (.)
(2.4.2) what's this bit called though (.)
(2.4.3) what's this bit called though (.)
(2.4.4) what's this bit called though (.)
```

Key to Activity 2.2

A suggested traffic light notation for this extract is presented below as (2.6.1).

1 Line 1: Because the Tonic is on "this", the rest of the IP forms the Tail. Such Tails are vulnerable to an overlapping incoming from another speaker, though children of Robin's age are less likely to do so (Wells & Corrin, 2004).

2 Lines 3, 5: In each line, there are two IPs. Both IPs have the default structure, with Tonic, and therefore yellow light, on the final word, "funnel". Turns consisting of more than one IP are discussed later in this chapter.

3 Robin's turns in lines 2 and 4 are highlighted as yellow, because his mother comes in straight afterwards. This suggests that she responds to them as completed turns.

4 Line 6 looks very similar to lines 2 and 4, in that it is a single word with a rise-fall intonation contour. On this basis, one might expect that his mother will again treat this as signalling a TRP, and therefore that the next thing to happen will be that his mother starts talking.

(2.6.1)

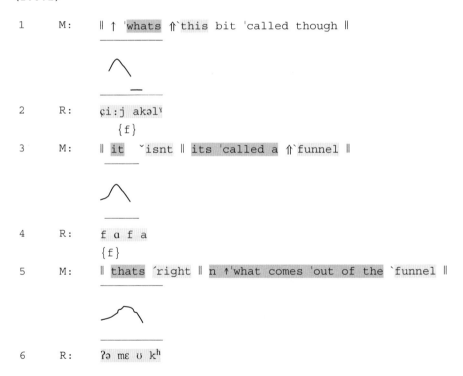

1	M:	‖ ↑ 'whats ⇑`this bit 'called though ‖
2	R:	çi:j akəlˇ {f}
3	M:	‖ it ˇisnt ‖ its 'called a ⇑`funnel ‖
4	R:	f ɑ f a {f}
5	M:	‖ thats ´right ‖ n ↑'what comes 'out of the `funnel ‖
6	R:	ʔə mɛ ʊ kʰ

Key to Activity 2.3

1 Robin's turn is made up of three or four apparently separate IPs: the pitch on the first, second and fourth descends to the base of his pitch range, after each of which his mother starts to talk. The silence between the end of Robin's turn and her talk is very short. We can therefore infer that she treats Robin's pitch falls as yellow traffic

lights, projecting TRPs. By the standard conventions of turn allocation, she therefore has the right to take a turn at his point. However, Robin then produces more talk so they twice end up in overlap.

2 In the first overlap, mother produces a minimal response token "mm" with a low rising pitch. In the second overlap, she starts a TCU beginning with "what goe(s)", breaking off as she finds herself in overlap. As in the "smoke" example in Extract (2.15), the curtailed TCU "what goe(s)" is an incomplete IP. Grammatically, it is an incomplete clause.

3 Robin completes each overlapped IP, by producing a Tonic (falling pitch to the base of his range) on the final syllable.

4 In line 3, Robin's mother recycles the broken-off turn, using the same wording. This time she produces a complete IP and a grammatically complete sentence.

5 A traffic light transcription is presented as (2.16.1):

(2.16.1)

```
1  R: now push (.) [it] goes there (.) [it there    ]    push

2  M:                [mm]                [what go-   ]

3  M: what goes in there
```

CHAPTER 3

Focus

Children live in an environment that is rich in topics to talk about. Children therefore need to identify what the particular topic is that an interactional partner is talking about at a given moment. Equally, they need to indicate to an interactional partner the topic of their own turns at talk. An important non-verbal resource for this is manual pointing, which is used by young children before they gain access to more sophisticated linguistic resources (Filipi, 2009). An important linguistic resource, which mature speakers of English have access to, is provided by the system of Tonic placement (sometimes referred to as Tonicity), which is the vocal equivalent of pointing. Just as physical pointing can be used to indicate the object that the pointer wants to be a Focus for shared attention, so Tonic placement can be used by the speaker to highlight the word in his utterance that the speaker wants the listener to focus on. Like physical pointing, this vocal pointing can sometimes be quite precise, in order to pick out a single word. On other occasions it can be more like a point in the general direction of an object or objects, leaving the listener to work out exactly what is being indicated.

Since Intonation Phrases (IPs) routinely map onto Turn Constructional Units (TCUs), as described in Chapter 2, the Tonic can serve to indicate the Focus of that TCU. This can be seen in Extract (3.1), from a conversation between two female friends at university, talking about a plan to meet up in the vacation.

```
(3.1)
Daisy    we need to do something fun when we're all out in London
         well I I could come up to like Wycombe or wherever  Harrow
         and I could meet [ your          friend]
Beth                      [theyre  pretty  close]  Wycombe  and
                          Harrow
```

Daisy produces a turn consisting of four TCUs. From Daisy's turn, Beth explicitly picks up the two place names Wycombe and Harrow as the topic, on which she comments: "they're pretty close". The falling Tone diacritics in the intonation transcript given in (3.1.1) show that in Daisy's turn, each of these two place names, Wycombe and Harrow, carries a Tonic. However, when Beth repeats the place names, they are in the

---

Children's Intonation: A Framework for Practice and Research, First Edition. Bill Wells and Joy Stackhouse.
© 2016 John Wiley & Sons, Ltd. Published 2016 by John Wiley & Sons, Ltd.
Companion website: www.wiley.com/go/childintonation

Tail of her IP; the Tonic is now on "close", the last word in her new comment that "they're pretty close":

(3.1.1)

```
Daisy  ‖we 'need to do 'something `fun when we're 'all 'out in 'London‖
       ‖well I 'I could come 'up to like `Wycombe or whe'rever ‖
       `Harrow‖
       ‖and 'I could 'meet your          ´friend‖
Beth                       ‖theyre 'pretty `close 'Wycombe and 'Harrow‖
```

By placing the Tonic on a specific word, the speaker can highlight that word, marking it out as the topic, as Daisy does. The listener may then pick up, as Beth does. When Beth, as the new speaker, explicitly repeats the topicalized items, she locates them elsewhere than in the Tonic position. In this instance, she places them in the Tail. This displays that the topicalized item, i.e. Wycombe and Harrow, are not the Focus of Beth's turn: Beth's Focus is on their proximity: "they're pretty close". This system of highlighting the new or focused part of the turn while backgrounding the part that has been previously topicalized, thus enables the progression of topics from one conversational turn to the next.

Focus and Tonic placement

Focus depends on the speaker's use of phonetic prominence, in the form of the Tonic, to highlight the part that is most important in the TCU. The prominence of the Tonic is realized by various combinations of pitch prominence and movement, extra loudness, lengthening and greater articulatory precision. The accomplishment of Focus also entails the converse: the speaker may background the parts of the TCU that are less important, e.g. by narrowing the pitch range, reducing loudness, speeding up the tempo and eliding consonants or vowels. In this section, we will concentrate mainly on the placement of the Tonic, rather than the detail of how it is realized phonetically. Now complete Activity 3.1 before reading further.

In TCUs with maximally broad Focus, like (3.6), the Tonic does not have a function in relation to Focus; its only function is to function as a yellow traffic light for turn-taking, as described in Chapter 2. In adult English talk, this resource is not always necessary or used, since the TRP may be evident from the semantic, pragmatic and grammatical design of the turn (Ford & Thompson, 1996). For this reason, you may have felt less certain about the location of the Tonic in (3.6). In English, the most common, or default, location for the Tonic in IPs with maximally broad Focus is the last content word in the IP, often the final noun. This is the case in (3.6), with "window".

Bob's narrow Focus IP in (3.4) has the same Tonic location as the maximally broad Focus IP in (3.6).Thus, the difference in Focus structure between (3.4) and (3.6) is not reflected in the placement of the Tonic, which in both (3.4.1) and in (3.6.1), is on "window":

(3.4.1) ‖ 'someones broken the `window ‖
(3.6.1) ‖ 'someones 'broken the `window ‖

ACTIVITY 3.1

Aim: To investigate factors that determine the speaker's choice of Focus placement, and thus the location of the Tonic.

In the following constructed conversational exchanges, presented as (3.2)–(3.6), the second speaker (Bob) uses the same words each time: "someone's broken the window". Read each exchange aloud. Treat each exchange as an entirely separate conversation from the exchange that precedes it. If convenient, find another person to take the role of the first speaker (Angela). If possible, make an audio recording of the exchanges.
  For each exchange, do the following:
1 Indicate where you placed the Tonic when you read Bob's turn. You can do this simply by underlining the Tonic; or you can transcribe Bob's turn using the traffic light notation from Chapter 2.
2 Describe how Angela's turn affects Bob's placement of the Tonic.

(3.2) Angela: someone's opened the window, have they?
       Bob: someone's broken the window

(3.3) Angela: just show John the new window in the front room, will you?
       Bob: someone's broken the window

(3.4) Angela: someone's broken the patio door, have they?
       Bob: someone's broken the window

(3.5) Angela: someone's broken the window
       Bob: someone's broken the window?

(3.6) Angela: it's cold in here
       Bob: someone's broken the window

The Key to Activity 3.1 can be found at the end of the chapter.

Nevertheless, there are phonetic differences between broad and narrow Focus. On many occasions the Tone in the narrow Focus case of (3.4) is more perceptually prominent in terms of pitch, e.g. a rise-fall or a fall from higher in the pitch range, as opposed to a narrow fall from the middle of the range in the case of broad Focus. In cases of narrow Focus, the Head is likely to be delivered more rapidly and with less clearly articulated consonants and vowels; and there may be a greater contrast in loudness between Head and Tonic (Wells, 1986). In Chapter 1, we referred to this type of Tonic as *Supertonic*, to reflect its extra prosodic prominence. It is notated as ⇑.

In final position, this distinction is particularly important. Narrow Focus on the final word of the IP, as in (3.4.1), is marked by a Supertonic located on that word, as shown in (3.4.2):

(3.4.2) Angela: someone's broken the patio door, have they?
         Bob: ‖ 'someones 'broken the ⇑`window ‖

By contrast, maximally broad Focus, i.e. Focus over the whole IP, is often realized by an ordinary Tonic located by default on the final word, as originally shown above in (3.6.1):

(3.6.1) Angela: it's cold in here
         Bob: ‖'someones 'broken the `window ‖

The same general principle of default Tonic placement for broad Focus is evident in example (3.3), where the Tonic is in a non-final position:

(3.3) Angela: just show John the new window in the front room, will you?
   Bob: ‖ 'someones `broken the 'window ‖

Where the last content word of the turn (here "window") is not in Focus because it has just been mentioned, then the speaker will usually place the Tonic on the preceding content word. In (3.3), this is "broken". Here "broken" attracts the Tonic not because it is the Focus, but merely as a default location to avoid having the Tonic on "window". This Tonic placement on "broken" thereby shows that there is broad Focus on "someone's broken", but no Focus on "the window". This contrasts with (3.2.3), where the Focus is specifically and uniquely on the word "broken", and therefore has a Supertonic:

(3.2.3) Angela: someone's opened the window, have they?
      Bob: ‖ 'someones ⇑`broken the 'window ‖

To summarize, in English, there is a mapping from Focus (broad or narrow) to Tonic placement (final or non-final) and Tonic type (ordinary Tonic or Supertonic). The speaker who wants to convey narrow Focus uses a Supertonic, with extra pitch prominence, loudness and tempo or durational prominence. The Supertonic is then interpreted by listeners as signalling narrow Focus on the Tonic word, while any words in the Head and/or the Tail therefore have zero Focus. On the other hand, a normal Tonic is interpreted by listeners as signalling Broad Focus over what precedes the Tonic word, i.e. the words in the Head. Thus, the speaker who wants to convey broad Focus will place a (normal) Tonic on the last stressed syllable of the stretch of words that they want to be in Focus. If there are any words in the Tail, they have zero Focus. The dialogues from Activity 3.1, which cover this range of theoretical possibilities, are re-presented below with notations for both Focus and intonation, to demonstrate the mappings between the two.

(3.2.4)
Angela: someone's opened the window, have they?
Bob: ‖ 'someones `broken the 'window ‖

{ -F } { F }   { -F }

(3.3.3)
Angela: just show John the new window in the front room, will you?
Bob: 'someones `broken the 'window ‖

{   F   }   {   -F   }

(3.4.3)
Angela: someone's broken the patio door, have they?
Bob: ‖ 'someones 'broken the⇑`window ‖

{   -F   } { F }

(3.5.2)
Angela: someone's broken the window
Bob: ‖ 'someones 'broken the ´window ‖

{   -F   }

(3.6.2)
Angela: it's cold in here
Bob: ‖'someones 'broken the `window ‖

    {   F   }

Since these exchanges were constructed for experimental purposes, we need to be cautious when generalizing from such data to the real-life situations in which young children learn how to speak their language. The exchanges were designed in order to highlight specifically the role of Tonic placement with regard to Focus. However, in reality, speakers and listeners handle issues to do with Focus by drawing on a wider range of linguistic and non-linguistic resources. From a linguistic perspective, for example, it is very common to omit altogether any items where Focus is absent. In (3.4), one might expect Bob to respond without repeating the previously mentioned item "broken", i.e. to use ellipsis, as in (3.4.4):

(3.4.4) Angela: someone's broken the patio door, have they?
         Bob: it was the window

Pronouns and other anaphoric devices are very often used to indicate that an item has already been mentioned, as in the use of "it" rather than "the window" in (3.3.4).

(3.3.4) Angela: just show John the new window in the front room, will you?
         Bob: someone's broken it

The use of pronouns or of ellipsis reduces the number of items that potentially compete for Focus, and thus reduces the requirement on the speaker to use the Tonic to mark Focus. For this reason, from the perspective of intonation and its development and use by children, the English Focus-Tonic system is best viewed as a resource that may be drawn on by speakers as circumstances dictate, rather than as an inherent feature of every utterance.

Activity 3.2 provides an opportunity to work with the notion of Focus in relation to Topic, using a transcript of an actual conversation. This will lead to a consideration of Focus and Tonic placement in cases of typical and atypical intonation development. Complete this activity before reading further.

In Activity 3.2, we saw that the topical Focus will shift in the course of an interaction, sometimes abruptly (as in line 4), but often more subtly (as in lines 6 and 10). In this way, the conversation can be seen to progress. In this extract, the interaction is around shared picture book reading. Although this may have some distinctive characteristics compared to other kinds of talk, the progression from one topic to a related next topic is typical of mundane conversation and probably of any type of spoken interaction. Indeed, the idea of *progression* in talk is fundamental. Sometimes it is claimed that the main purpose of talking is to exchange information – a notion that underlaid influential theories about speech in the middle of the last century. However, careful study of what people actually do in conversation shows that for much of the time their main preoccupation is to keep the conversation going, and that the apparent exchange of information is subservient

ACTIVITY 3.2

Aim: To investigate linguistic factors that influence Focus placement, and thus the location of the Tonic.

The following transcript, presented as Extract (3.7), is of an interaction between a 19-year-old female student (E) and a 5-year-old boy (David). They are looking at a picture book.

(3.7)

```
1     E:    what d'you think it is David
2     D:    teddy bear
3     E:    yes it could be a teddy bear
4     E:    who's that there coming up the path
5     D:    postman
6     E:    what's he going to do
7     D:    get out a letter
10    E:    and what's he going to do with the letter
11    D:    put it in the letter box
14    E:    and who's this d'you think
15    D:    girl
```

1 Starting at line 2, identify in each turn/line the new word or words that represent a shift of topic in the context of the preceding talk. Mark this underneath with an {F} for Focus, as in Examples (3.2.4)–(3.6.2) in the preceding section. Mark words that are repeated from the preceding one or two lines with {-F}. A suggested notation for lines 2 and 3 is presented in (3.7.1) as an illustration. Do not add intonation or traffic light notation.
2 Make a note of the reason for your decision about each line.

(3.7.1)

```
1         E:       what d'you think it is David
2         D:       teddy bear
                   {    F    }
3         E:       yes it could be a teddy bear
                   {    F    } {    -F    }
```

The Key to Activity 3.2 can be found at the end of the chapter.

to that more social goal. The progression or shifting of topic is one way of ensuring that the conversation itself progresses. Other things happen in conversation, as we shall see shortly, that may temporarily impede the progression of the talk. However, if participants attend to the issue of focussing on topics and shifts of topic, as E and David do in Extract (3.7), then the interaction is able to progress. Intonation has an important role in facilitating Focus and thus the progression of topics. We will explore this role in Activity 3.3. Complete this activity before reading further.

Activity 3.3 illustrates the point made at the start of this chapter, that Tonic placement is the vocal equivalent of pointing. Like manual pointing, vocal pointing can sometimes be quite precise, picking out just one word. This is narrow Focus. On other occasions it is more like a point in the general direction of an object or objects. This is broad Focus, which requires more work from the listener to work out the scope or extent of what the speaker is focussing on. The power of the system of vocal pointing, as well as some of its limitations, can be gauged if we delete all those parts of the IP other than the Tonic, as in (3.9).

ACTIVITY 3.3

Aim: To investigate how the location of the Tonic relates to Focus and topics in conversation.

The following transcript, presented as Extract (3.8), is of an interaction between a 19-year-old female student (E) and David, a 5-year-old boy (D). They are talking about a picture book that they are looking at. It is the same interaction as in Activity 3.2. However, certain lines that were omitted from (3.7) are included in (3.8).

(3.8)

```
1     E:    what d'you think it is David
2     D:    teddy bear
3     E:    yes it could be a teddy bear
4     E:    who's that there coming up the path
5     D:    Postman
6     E:    what's he going to do
7     D:    get out a letter
8     E:    get out a letter
9     D:    Yes
10    E:    and what's he going to do with the letter
11    D:    put it in the letter box
12    E:    he's going to put it in the letter box
13    D:    Yes
14    E:    and who's this d'you think
15    D:    girl
16    E:    is it a girl
17    D:    I already said that
```

1 Read the transcript aloud, ideally with another person so that one of you reads E, the other D. If possible, make an audio recording.
2 On the transcript, indicate where you placed the Tonic in each turn when acting the parts of E and D. Start at line 1. You can do this simply by underlining the Tonic syllable. As explained in Chapter 1, the Tonic syllable is the syllable within the Intonation Phrase where the main pitch movement starts; it is often louder and longer than other syllables in the IP. Where you think the Tonic is particularly prominent in terms of its pitch, loudness, duration or other features, mark it as a Supertonic with ⇑. You may find it helpful to mark IP boundaries too.
3 Consider the relationship between Tonic placement and Focus, by comparing your transcript for this activity (Activity 3.3), to the transcript you produced for Activity 3.2.

The Key to Activity 3.3 can be found at the end of the chapter.

(3.9)

```
1     E:    what dyou think it is David
2     D:    teddy bear
3     E:    could
4     E:    path
5     D:    postman
6     E:    do
```

7	D:	letter
8	E:	letter
9	D:	yes
10	E:	do
11	D:	letterbox
12	E:	letterbox
13	D:	yes
14	E:	this
15	D:	girl
16	E:	girl
17	D:	said

In (3.9), by tracking the 'Tonic' words alone, it is possible to get some idea of the topical content of the conversation, although the way in which one topic shifts to the next - from PATH to POSTMAN to LETTER, via LETTER BOX to GIRL – remains hazy. In this condition, all the listener has to go on is the information conveyed by a few salient syllables – one word per IP. However, we have seen that in English the Tonic does not always highlight solely the word where it is located, as in narrow Focus. In cases of broad Focus, the scope of potential Focus extends back to words preceding the Tonic. This was illustrated in Activity 3.1, Example (3.6):

(3.6)   Angela: its cold in here
        Bob: someones broken the <u>win</u>dow

In Bob's turn, there is broad Focus, extending over the whole utterance. However, the same Tonic placement may point to narrow Focus, just on the final word, as shown in (3.4):

(3.4)   Angela: someones broken the patio door, have they?
        Bob: someones broken the <u>win</u>dow

Thus the skilled listener of English will be aware that when speakers 'point' by placing the Tonic on a word, they may be pointing just to that word, as in (3.4); or they may be pointing to a bigger phrase that ends with that word, as in (3.5). Thus, in line 4 of (3.8.2), presented here as (3.10), the Tonic on the final word, "path", may signal broad Focus, i.e. Focus on the whole of the Head as well as the Tonic:

(3.10)

4	E:	‖who's that there coming up the <u>path</u>‖
		{ **F** }

The transcript in (3.8.1) showed the Focus structure of each TCU, as identified in Activity 3.2 on the basis of what information in each TCU is new with reference to the immediately preceding context. For some lines with a final Tonic, e.g. lines 4,7 and 11, the context suggests broad Focus over the whole TCU, as was illustrated in Bob's turn in (3.6). Thus, by placing the Tonic on a particular word, the speaker may be pointing not just to that 'Tonic' word, but to part or all of the Head as well. So in terms of IP structure, the only words that are indisputably not in Focus are the words that make up the Tail, i.e. following the Tonic word, as in line 10 of (3.8.2) , shown here as (3.11):

(3.11)

```
10       E:      ‖and what's he going to do with the letter‖
                 {            - F          } { F } { - F    }
```

Here, "the letter" does not receive Focus.

    The relationship between Focus and intonation can be summarized as follows:

1 The word representing the key, often new, item of the turn constructional unit (TCU) normally carries the Tonic.

2 The Focus of the TCU may be restricted to the word carrying the Tonic. This is narrow Focus.

3 However, the Focus of the TCU may also incorporate material that immediately precedes the Tonic, giving broad Focus. This material will form part or the whole of the Head of the IP.

4 Material in the Tail of the IP will not be in Focus.

5 Some TCUs may have no (i.e. zero) Focus. In this case, the Tonic serves simply to delimit the end of the turn or TCU.

In the next part of this chapter, the emergence of the system of Tonic placement and Focus will be investigated by examining naturalistic interactions between Robin and his mother. The aim is to identify what it is that the child needs to learn about Focus and intonation and to explore how the co-participants, like Robin's mother, may facilitate the process.

Turn-final Tonic and Focus

In the extracts presented in Chapter 2 we saw that Robin, at the age of 19–21 months, sometimes produces a turn that seems to consist of more than a single word. In such turns there is the potential to highlight a part of the utterance and background the remainder, for the purposes of Focus. The question we will explore in this section is: does Robin demonstrate competence in using this system?

    In Extract (3.12), originally presented as (2.9) in Chapter 2, Robin and his mother are completing a jigsaw. Robin's turn comprises six phonetically different syllables, obliging the listener to treat the turn as consisting of more than just one word, since it is highly unlikely that a child of Robin's age would have a word of five or six syllables in his vocabulary.

(3.12)

```
1   M:   ‖ now 'whats (.) 'whats `this ‖
         ((handing a spinning top piece to R))
2   M:   ‖ can you re'member what `this is ‖
```

```
3   R:   ʔə(.)ʔɛdʒœː ʔɪ̯ʒʒ  (0.7)pɒkx
                              {f}
```

```
4   M:   ‖ `top ‖ thats `right ‖ `top ‖
              {f}                    {p}
                  (1.2)
5   M:   and where does that `go
6   M:   does that go in ´there
            ((Robin tries to fit TOP piece into puzzle board))
```

Robin's syllable sequence in line 3 does not contain any words that are readily recognizable from their phonetic shape. Nevertheless, in line 4, his mother displays that she has recognized a version of the word TOP. She also topicalizes TOP rather than any of the preceding words: she produces the word TOP twice, yet does not reproduce a version of the other five syllables from Robin's turn. Her turn serves as an affirmatory repeat (Tarplee, 1996), closing the short labelling sequence. Then in lines 5 and 6, she shifts the topic to the place where the piece fits into the puzzle.

How is Robin's mother able to identify the word TOP from his turn in line 3? Clearly she is primed to hear it, having in line 2 asked him, albeit indirectly, to name it. Nevertheless, the syllable that he produced that is closest to TOP phonetically, namely [pɒkx], has onset and coda consonants that diverge widely from the adult targets in place of articulation. Presumably his mother is helped by the fact that Robin apparently marks this syllable as the narrow Focus of his turn, by making it a Supertonic: it carries a wide rise-fall pitch movement, while his preceding syllables stay within narrow pitch range; it is noticeably louder than those preceding syllables and it is preceded by a pause. Thus, it seems that Robin already uses the resources of intonation to convey narrow Focus on the part of his response that is topically most relevant to his mother's prior question. In line 4 his mother then displays her own orientation to the Tonic–Focus system by twice repeating the word that Robin has highlighted. In line 5, she moves the topic on by taking that item out of Focus, using a pronoun THAT to replace TOP and placing the Tonic on the verb GO. The transcript in (3.12.1) shows the Focus and traffic light structure of this exchange.

(3.12.1)

```
2        M:   ‖ can you re´member what this is ‖
3             ʔə(.) ʔɛdʒœː ʔɪʒʒ (0.7) ⇑pɒkx
                                              {F}
4        M:   ‖ top ‖ thats right ‖ top ‖
              {F}
```

A similar sequence is found in Extract (3.13). Again, Robin's mother asks him to label objects that they both can see.

(3.13)

```
1        M:   and what are these
              (2.5)
```

```
2      R:       ə nʌ::    bʊkʰ
3      M:       that's right there's a book
                (1.5)
4                theres a book
                {p            p}
```

Following Robin's turn in line 2, his mother displays recognition of the expected label in line 3, by her affirmatory repeat of the word BOOK. This time, however, we cannot tell whether in THERE'S A in line 4 she is also recasting the syllables that Robin produced before the word BOOK in line 2.

It is noteworthy that in (3.12) and (3.13), the word that his mother topicalizes occurred in the final position in Robin's prior turn. It will be recalled from Activity 3.1, that when the Tonic is located on the final word in the TCU, this may indicate that the Focus is narrow, just on that specific word. On the other hand, it may also indicate broad Focus, i.e. that the speaker is not highlighting any item in particular. So does Robin actually know how to place the Tonic on a word to give it Focus? Perhaps it is just a happy accident: he is simply placing the Tonic on the final syllable of his turn in order to mark his turn as complete (cf. Chapter 2) but his mother treats him as having competently identified the topic of his turn. She displays this by reiterating the apparently highlighted item. But is she simply projecting the adult system onto Robin? Some evidence that this may indeed be the case, and that Robin may not yet be competent in the Tonic-Focus system after all, comes from instances where he produces turns which do not meet his mother's expectation.

Learning to (De)Focus

As we saw in Activity 3.1, a key feature of the Tonic-Focus system is, where possible, to avoid placing the Tonic on a word that has been mentioned in the immediately prior context, because a repeated item may not have Focus. So if a speaker's turn consists of two items, one of which has just been mentioned, the Focus, and thus the Tonic, should be on the new item. This is evident in Extract (3.14), where Robin is holding a jigsaw piece depicting a ball. On the floor, there is also an actual ball.

(3.14)

```
        ((R, holding jigsaw ball, walks from jigsaw puzzle to
        near M))
        ─────


        ∧
        ──
4    R:  bɔ ((looking at real ball on floor, drops jigsaw ball))
        {p}
        ─────────────

        ∧
        ──
```

5   εjə dɔkʰ ((R picks up real ball with lh , transfers it to
            rh))

_____

                                          ⌡
              ‿   ‿
            _____

6   M: theres your ball
            _____

            ∧

            _____

7   R: bɔ ((R picks up jigsaw ball with lh))
            {f}
            _____

              ‿

                    ‿
            _____

8   M: two balls
9   R: Heh
            ((R turns round, walks back to jigsaw holding real and
            jigsaw ball))

In his words (lines 4 and 7), and his accompanying actions, Robin makes it clear that
his topic is BALL, but he does not apparently have the linguistic resources to express the
more complex notion that he is engaged with two different balls: in line 7, Robin, holding the 'ball' piece from his jigsaw in one hand and a real ball in the other hand, simply
produces another version of the word BALL, though this time it is louder and has a wider
pitch span than in line 4, thus more like a Supertonic, compared to the ordinary Tonic
in line 4. As a way of marking plural nouns in English for a child who cannot produce
a word-final alveolar fricative, this Supertonic-like device has been observed in a case
study by Camarata and Gandour (1985) of a boy aged 3;8 with expressive speech and
language difficulties, summarized in Chapter 10 of this book.

In line 8, Robin's mother topicalizes BALL from his immediately prior turn by incorporating it into her turn but she places the word in the Tail of her two-word IP, as BALL
has just been mentioned. By default "two", her addition to the topic, therefore turns
up in Tonic position, giving the structure shown in (3.14.1):

(3.14.1) ‖ `two` balls ‖
             {F} {-F}

Her turn can therefore be interpreted as a recast and expansion of Robin's turn in
line 7, with the appropriate Focus and Tonic structure for what Robin had apparently
intended.

Extract (3.14) thus demonstrates that Robin's mother uses the simple manipulation
of Tonic placement to indicate Focus in her interaction with Robin. The question then
arises as to whether Robin can do the same, when producing his first multiword utterances. The following extract shows that this is not necessarily a straightforward or

automatic procedure for Robin. Extract (3.15) was considered in some detail in Chapter 2, with reference to Robin's ability to construct more complex Intonation Phrases.

In line 6, Robin produces a turn that consists of two words. The first, SMOKE, has a rise-fall pitch and could reasonably be interpreted by his mother as a Tonic. He seems to have shown her a yellow light, whereupon his mother starts to speak (line 7). However, as Robin continues his turn with [fɑfə] (FUNNEL), Robin and his mother end up talking in overlap (lines 6 and 7).

(3.15)

5   M: ‖that's ´right ‖ n ↑'what comes 'out of the `funnel‖

6   R: ʔə mɛ ʊ kʰ   [f ɑ f ə]
           {f   f}(0.5){f}

7   M: [smoke-]
                             ((M nods))
                        (0.5)
8   M: ‖ˇsmoke comes out of the 'funnel‖ `doesnt it‖
           ((Mother nods))
                        (1.5)
9   M: ‖ˊhm‖
                        (1.6)
10   M: ‖s that ´right‖
                        (2.1)
11   R: (unintelligible whisper)
                        (1.0)

12   R: m̥mɒk ə fɐ fɐː
13   M:‖ 'that's ^right‖ ^smoke out of the funnel‖ ^sgood‖

In Chapter 2, we saw that this interactional problem is caused by Robin breaking a traffic light rule: having signalled to his mother that he had stopped, with SMOKE, he continued to talk, with FUNNEL. In the context of this chapter, we can add that with his first word SMOKE, he has supplied a topically relevant answer to M's question. If he wants to produce a longer TCU, then the issue of Focus will arise: as SMOKE is the Focus, then any following material has to be shown to be not in Focus, by being in the Tail.

This is what his mother did with "<u>two</u> balls" in (3.14). It is what the context demands in (3.15), since the further material that Robin produces, FUNNEL, has just been mentioned by his mother in the previous turn and so is not a candidate for Focus. However, Robin produces FUNNEL with high, dynamic pitch and loudness prominence. Far from marking a Tail, these features are ones that are associated with the Supertonic. When used in overlap with another speaker, these features can also signal competition for the floor (see Chapter 2, also French & Local, 1983; Kurtić et al., 2013), which is presumably why Robin's mother cuts off her turn in line 7. Yet there is no subsequent evidence in the interaction that Robin really wanted to secure the floor at this point: he does not say anything further until line 12, despite three attempts from his mother to elicit something from him. We can therefore reasonably conclude that the prominence on FUNNEL is evidence of a Focus-Tonic error on the part of Robin, suggesting that he has not yet mastered the system of associating lack of Focus with absence of Tonic features.

For a perspective on how children might learn about intonation, and the Tonic-Focus system specifically, the latter part of Extract (3.15) is of considerable interest. When Robin's mother recycles and completes her interrupted turn in line 8, she produces it as a recast and expansion of Robin's turn in line 6, but with the intonation structure of Tonic + Tail that ensures that only SMOKE is prominent and therefore in Focus. Thus, this is effectively a repair of Robin's intonation. She pursues a response from Robin with "doesn't it", and, on getting no response, with further prompts in lines 9 and 10. When he does eventually speak, in line 12, his turn is very similar in terms of its segmental phonetics to his original version in line 6, apart from the addition of a schwa between the two words. Intonationally, however, line 12 is quite different: the first word is again prominent, but the second, FUNNEL, is produced this time with relatively low pitch. In line 13, his mother accepts this as a correct version with "that's right", even though in terms of grammar and segmental phonology it is clearly a long way from being right. She repeats a truncated version of her own line 8, again with the Tonic + Tail structure, and assesses that, and therefore presumably also Robin's version in line 12, as "good". This analysis is reflected in the transcript given in (3.15.1):

(3.15.1)

```
5    M:    ‖thats ˌright‖ n 'what comes 'out of the  `funnel‖
6    R:    ʔə ⇑meʊ kʰ        [⇑fafə]
               {F}              {F}
7    M:                  [smoke-]
                  (0.5)
8    M:    ‖ˇsmoke comes out of the 'funnel‖ `doesn't it‖
             { F}  {            - F              }
                  (1.5)
9    M:    ‖ˆhm‖
                  (1.6)
10   M:    ‖s that ´right‖
                  (2.1)
```

```
11    R:    (unintelligible whisper)
                (1.0)
12    R:    m̩mək ə fɐ fɐ:
            {F}    {-F}
13    M:‖   'that's ˆright‖ ˆsmoke out of the funnel‖ ˆsgood‖
                    { F}  {              -F             }
```

This extract indicates that working on Focus, in relation to intonation structure, is a relevant linguistic issue for Robin's mother at this stage in Robin's development. It suggests that the child's mastery of intonation is not something that can be taken for granted, even in typical development - a theme that will be returned to in Chapter 7.

Focus and Tonic placement in atypical intonation development

In this section, the clinical relevance of Focus is illustrated from the case of a child for whom the manipulation of Tonic placement in order to accomplish Focus happened much later than for Robin. David, from the West Midlands of England (near Birmingham), was receiving therapy for his expressive speech and language difficulties, although the therapy was not targeted at prosodic features. At CA 5;04 he was recorded with a speech and language therapy student, who is asking him about a story in pictures. Extract (3.16), which is an excerpt from data originally analysed by Wells and Local (1993), illustrates the pattern that David uses on all his utterances. In the picture, a postman is holding a letter. It is the same transcript as the one used in Activity (3.3), with the addition of the intonation transcribed from the original recording. Because his intonation is atypical, we have transcribed it impressionistically. David's words are transcribed using IPA symbols, with a gloss underneath.

(3.16)

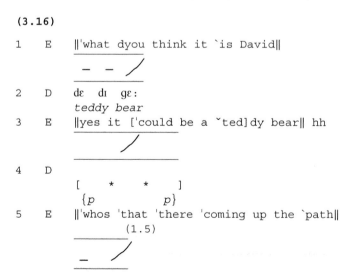

```
1    E    ‖'what dyou think it `is David‖

2    D    dɛ  dɪ  gɛ:
          teddy bear
3    E    ‖yes it ['could be a ˇted]dy bear‖ hh

4    D
          [    *     *    ]
          {p          p}
5    E    ‖'whos 'that 'there 'coming up the `path‖
                (1.5)
```

6 D bəʊsmad̥
      postman

7 E ‖'whats he 'going to ´do ‖

    —   — — — ⟋

8 D gɛd ag ə gɛ ta
      get out a letter
                    (1.0)

9 E ‖get 'out a `letter‖

      ⟋
      —

10 D yes

11 E ‖and 'whats he 'going to ´do with the 'letter‖
                    (1.0)

    — — —   — — —   — —   ⟋

12 D dʌd ɪt ɪn   dʌd ɪt dʊ   gɛ ta   bɒks
      put it in (1.7) *put it the letter   box*
                    (0.8)

13 E ‖hes 'going to 'put it 'in the `letter 'box‖

      ⟋
      —

14 D Yes
                    (1.0)

15 E ‖and 'whos ´this d'you 'think‖
                    (1.0)

      ⟋
      —

16 D gɜ ::
      girl
                    (1.0)

17 E ‖s it a `girl‖

    — — - -   —   ⟋

18 D aɪ ɔ wɛ dɪ gɛd ðatʰ
      I already said that
                    (0.8)

19 E ‖shes 'already ‖
                    (0.5)

    — — - -— ⟍ ⟋

20   D   aɪ ɔ wɛ dɪ dɛd ðatʰ
         I already said that
                  (0.3)

21   D   aɪ ɡɪd
         I did

David invariably locates the main pitch movement on the final syllable of his turn, and it is invariably a rising pitch of at least 9 semitones. Words preceding this final syllable are produced with level pitch around the middle of his pitch range. His IPs can therefore be interpreted as having an invariant Head + Tonic structure.

On the positive side, David's idiosyncratic prosodic pattern serves to mark the end of his turns in a clear, consistent and unambiguous way, which is useful for him and his co-participants, given the unintelligibility of his speech. By clearly signalling the end of his turn, David manages to maintain interactions with others without undue overlap or interruption by others: the Head + Tonic structure provides David with the interactional space to produce turns that consist of several words rather than just a single word. In Extract (3.12), Robin displayed this emergent ability at the age of 21 months.

David's invariable location of the Tonic on the final syllable of the utterance is not typical for the West Midlands variety of English, nor for Standard Southern British English or many other varieties. This has a negative consequence for his marking of word stress: on utterance-final words, the stress is invariably heard to be on the final syllable. This affects the stress pattern of multisyllabic nouns, including compound nouns, e.g. LETTER BOX, which in line 11 he produces with final instead of initial stress.

More importantly for the theme of this chapter, David is not using the Tonic-Focus system. There is no real evidence that David can highlight a non-final word through Tonic prominence in the way that Robin does at the end of Extract (3.15), even when this would be expected from the context. Before discussing the consequences of this atypical pattern for David, we should note how his co-participant E handles Focus and topic issues in this extract. In lines 5, 7, 11 and 15, she progresses the topic of the talk by introducing new elements: she asks David about new aspects of the picture in front of them. However, this is not always so: in lines 9, 13, 17, she simply repeats part or all of David's immediately prior turn, not contributing anything that is topically new. David eventually displays his annoyance with this aspect of E's behaviour, explicitly pointing out in line 18 and again in line 20 that she is just repeating what he has already said!

The consequences of David's atypical intonation pattern for signalling his intended Focus and thus to contribute the development of topics in the conversation can be seen if we compare the expected semantic Focus with the Focus that is implied by his atypical Tonics. One expected distribution of semantic Focus in this passage was presented in Extract (3.7.2). In Extract (3.17), that transcription is shown as the bold **SF** (Semantic Focus) beneath the transcript, indicating the word or words that can be expected to be semantically focused, usually because they represent new information; while information that has already been mentioned is marked with –**SF**. As in (3.7.2), the semantic Focus has been assigned without reference to intonation, but solely on the basis of the semantics of each turn.

In (3.17) in addition to the semantic focus, notated **SF**, we present the Tonic Focus, notated **TF**. Tonic Focus refers to the type and scope of Focus that is implied to the listener by the speaker's placement of the Tonic. Using the traffic light notation from Chapter 2, the Tonic is marked by pale shading, the Head by dark shading. The Supertonic, with its implication of narrow Focus, is signified by ⇑.

(3.17)

```
1   E    what dyou think it is David

2   D    teddy ⇑bear
                 { TF }
         {    SF    }
3   E    yes it [could be a ted]dy bear hh
         {              TF              }
         {      SF       }
4   D            [    *      *      ]

5   E    whos that there  coming up the path
         {               TF                }
         {               SF                }
6   D    post⇑man
                {TF}
         {  SF  }
7   E    whats he going to do
         {        TF        }
         { SF}      {-SF}{   SF   }
8   D    get out a lett⇑er
                     {TF}
         {       SF       }
9   E    get out a letter
         {     TF      }
         {    -SF      }
10  D    ⇑yes
         {TF}
         {  }
11  E    and whats he going to ⇑do with the letter
                               {TF}
         {         -SF         } { SF }{     - SF     }
12  D    put it in put it the letter⇑box
                                    {TF}
                  {         SF         }
13  E    hes going to put it in the letterbox
         {                TF                }
         {               -SF                }
14  D    ⇑yes
15  E    and whos this dyou think
         {    TF    }
         {    SF    }
```

```
16  D    ⇑girl
         { TF }
         { SF }
17  E    s it a girl
         {     TF   }
         {   -SF    }
18  D    I already said    ⇑that
                            {TF}
         {        SF    }
19  E    shes already
         {     -TF    }
         {    -SF     }
20  D    I already   said  ⇑ that
                            {TF}
         {              -SF      }
21  D    I ⇑did
           {TF}
         {  -SF}
```

It was explained earlier in this chapter that usually the Tonic provides a pointer to the listener as to what the speaker is focusing on. If the Tonic is very prominent (notated as ⇑ for 'Supertonic'), e.g. a wide pitch movement that is louder and longer than anything in the rest of the IP, then this indicates that the Focus is solely on that word: this is narrow Focus. This being the case, in Extract (3.17), we have assigned narrow (Tonic) Focus to the final word of each of David's turns.

Turning now to E, earlier in this chapter we saw that in adult English the convention is that where the Tonic is not especially prominent, and when it occurs at the end of the IP, it signals that the whole of the IP is in Focus. This is broad Focus, where no element in the IP is more important than any other one. Sometimes for E, Tonic Focus (TF) and Semantic Focus (SF) are co-extensive. For example, in line 5, the Tonic is on the final word, "path", implying that the whole of the IP is in broad Focus; contextually, the whole of E's turn in line 5 is new, since she has shifted the topic from the teddy bear to the postman. In such cases the Tonic-Focus system is functioning optimally. This is equally true in line 11, a case of narrow Focus: E uses a Supertonic on "do", which is the only new element in her turn.

However, even for typical mature speakers such as E, this is not always the case. One striking discrepancy is found in line 3, where there is apparent disregard for the basic relationship between Tonic Placement and Focus in English. Here the Tonic is on the final word, "teddy bear", implying broad Focus over the whole IP; however, "teddy bear" has just been mentioned by David in line 2 so is no longer new. The semantic Focus is "it could be", so to conform to the Tonic-Focus system, the Tonic should be on "could". This kind of discrepancy shows that the 'rules' are not absolute and that speakers have latitude to deviate from the expected pattern. Other apparent discrepancies are in fact systematic. This is particularly the case where E repeats David's turn, in lines 9, 13 and 17. As was noted earlier, these turns contain no semantic Focus at all and in such cases final Tonic placement is the default pattern, simply marking a yellow traffic light, i.e. the end of the turn.

For David, discrepancies between semantic Focus and Tonic Focus are the norm rather than the exception. In line 8, for example, he places a Supertonic on the final word, which implies narrow (Tonic) Focus on "letter", whereas the semantic Focus is broader: it includes the action "get out", since this has not been mentioned before. The same applies in line 12. In line 18, the discrepancy is even more striking: David places a Supertonic, implying narrow Focus, on "that", a pronoun presenting what is already known from line 16 ("girl"); and simultaneously not signalling any Focus on the new part. "I already said". These examples show that David is not making use of the usual Tonic-Focus system at all.

Summary

In Chapter 3, we have attempted to provide a coherent approach to the relationship between Focus and intonation, specifically Tonic placement and Tonic type. The relationship between intonation, stress and Focus, in English and in other languages, has been the subject of linguistic debate for several decades. A valuable overview of the theoretical issues involved is presented in Chapter 6 of Ladd, (2008). Drawing on some of the key concepts that have been developed in the course of that debate, we have used this approach to describe some features of typical and atypical development in children learning English. The approach allows us to address the following questions about Focus when examining spoken interactions, including interactions involving a child (C).

1 Does C indicate broad Focus over the whole IP by using final Tonic placement?
2 Does C indicate narrow Focus on the final word of the IP by using final Supertonic placement?
3 Does C indicate narrow Focus on a non-final word of the IP by using non-final Supertonic placement?
4 Does C background non-Focus material, by placing it in the Tail after a non-final Tonic?
5 Does C recognize the current speaker's broad and narrow Focus by attending to Tonic and Supertonic placement? Does C design the next turn accordingly?

These questions are incorporated into a profile of intonation in interaction that will be presented in Chapter 5. They inform the analysis of typical development of Focus in Chapters 6–8 and atypical development of Focus in Chapters 10–12.

Key to Activity 3.1

For many speakers, the following description will capture the main differences. It is based on recordings of such exchanges by several pairs of speakers, analysed in Wells, (1988).

(3.2) Angela: someone's opened the window, have they?
      Bob: someone's broken the window

It is very likely that you placed the Tonic on "broken", as shown in (3.2.1). The Tone might be a rise-fall or a fall-rise, or a fall starting relatively high in the pitch range. The Tonic begins on the lexically stressed syllable of the focussed item, i.e. 'brok-'. The Tonic syllable is likely to be relatively loud and long.

(3.2.1) ‖ ¦someones `broken the ¦window ‖

In Bob's turn, one specific word is highlighted: "broken". This is the only new word in the TCU: all the other words are repeated by Bob from Angela's turn, and are therefore 'given', so there is no reason for Bob to put Focus on any of them. By locating the Tonic, and therefore the Focus, on "broken", Bob highlights it as his own topic. Bob progresses the talk by correcting Angela's claim that someone opened the window. It is an example of other-initiated other repair: the source of the trouble to be repaired is in Angela's turn, i.e. "opened", but Angela does not repair it herself. Bob takes it upon himself to initiate the repair and to carry it through, by overtly correcting Angela's claim. This example shows that the system of Tonicity and Focus is a valuable resource for accomplishing repair in conversation. The focussed word can be indicated by a bold capital **F** positioned beneath the word in Focus, as in (3.2.2).

(3.2.2) ‖ ¦someones `broken the ¦window ‖
                    { **F** }

(3.3)   Angela: just show John the new window in the front room,
        will you?
        Bob: someone's broken the window

Again, the Tonic is likely to be located on "broken". The Tonic begins on the lexically stressed syllable of the focussed item, i.e. 'brok-'. The Tone might be a rise-fall or a fall-rise, or a fall, as shown in (3.3.1). However, the Tonic syllable is likely to be less high, loud and long than in (3.2):

(3.3.1) ‖ ¦someones `broken the ¦window ‖

Unlike in (3.2), "broken" is not the only new word in Bob's turn in (3.3). In fact, only "window" has been previously mentioned in Angela's turn. In (3.3), Bob is not explicitly correcting the factual truth of Angela's turn. Rather, Bob is correcting an assumption that underlies Angela's turn, namely that the new window is in a fit state to be shown to John. This distinction between types of correction does not impact on the location of the Tonic: in (3.3), as in (3.2), the Tonic in Bob's turn is on "broken". This shows that the key factor is simply the prior mention of the word "window" by Angela: in English, if a word has just been mentioned, whether by a new speaker or the same speaker, then there is a very strong tendency to avoid marking it with the Tonic. In such circumstances, the speaker has to find another location for the Tonic. This confronts the speaker with the problem of where to put it. In English, the strong tendency is to put the Tonic on another content word in the TCU, such as a noun, verb or adjective, rather than a function word such as a pronoun, preposition, determiner or auxiliary verb. Thus, in this case, the Tonic is more likely to be on "broken" than on "someone", "has" or "the". In such cases as in (3.3), it would be misleading to say that the Focus is on "broken" as it was in (3.2). Rather, the location of the Tonic shows that there is a noticeable absence of Focus on "window", as "window" has just been mentioned. This can be shown as in (3.3.2):

(3.3.2) ‖ 'someones `broken the 'window ‖
                              { -F }

Thus, Bob's turns in (3.2) and (3.3) have the same Tonic placement, but different Focus structures.

(3.4) Angela: someone's broken the patio door, have they?
       Bob: someone's broken the window

It is very likely that you placed the Tonic on "window", as shown in (3.4.1). The Tonic begins on the lexically stressed syllable of the focussed item, i.e. 'win-'. The Tone might be a rise-fall or a fall-rise, or a fall starting relatively high in the pitch range. The Tonic syllable is likely to be relatively loud and long. The Head of the IP, "'someones broken the", may be produced rather quickly, with weak articulation of some consonants and vowels, and little pitch variation or prominence on potentially stressable syllables like the first syllable of 'broken':

(3.4.1) ‖ 'someones broken the `window ‖

Bob's turn in (3.4) is similar to (3.2) in important respects. Again, one specific word is highlighted, although this time it is the final word: "window". This is the only new word in the TCU: all the other words are repeated by Bob from Angela's turn, and are therefore given. There is therefore no reason for Bob to put Focus on any of them. By locating the Tonic, on "window", Bob highlights it as his own topic. Bob progresses the talk by correcting Angela's claim that someone opened the patio door: like (3.2), it is an example of other-initiated other repair.

(3.5) Angela: someone's broken the window
       Bob: someone's broken the window

It is likely that you placed the Tonic on "window" – assuming that Angela had just put her Tonic on "window". If Angela's Tone was a fall, Bob's Tone is quite likely to be a rise, as shown in (3.5.1).

(3.5.1) Angela: ‖ 'someones 'broken the `window ‖
         Bob: ‖ 'someones 'broken the ´window ‖

This choice of a non-matching Tone, which orthographically would be indicated by a question-mark at the end of Bob's sentence, is a way of initiating a new action in the conversation, in this case requesting Angela to give some further explanation. The factors determining a speaker's choice of Tone are discussed fully in Chapter 4.

In terms of semantic content, Bob does not introduce any new items: he repeats Angela's words, word for word. For this reason, turns such as Bob's in (3.5) can be described as having Zero Focus.

(3.6) Angela: it's cold in here
       Bob: someone's broken the window

It is likely that you placed the Tonic on "window". In this case, the Tonic starts on the lexically stressed syllable of the word, i.e. 'win-'. The Tone may be a fall, starting around the mid of the speaker's pitch range. However, you may have felt less sure about where the Tonic is located, compared, for instance, to (3.2), (3.3) and (3.4). The Head may be produced relatively slowly, and with pitch prominence, giving rise to two rhythmic feet prior to the Tonic, as in (3.6.1):

(3.6.1) ‖ ˈsomeones ˈbroken the ˈwindow ‖

Bob does not repeat any of the words used by Angela. He thus has no reason to highlight or avoid any particular word or words: all are equally new. One way of conceptualizing this is that in (3.6) the Focus is maximally *broad*, compared to (3.2) and (3.4) where the Focus is maximally *narrow,* and (3.5) where the Focus is *Zero*.

Key to Activity 3.2

1 Starting at line 2, identify in each turn/line the word or words that represent a shift of topic in the context of the preceding talk. Mark this with an F (for Focus). Mark words that are repeated from the preceding one or two lines with {-F}.
2 Make a note of the reason for your decision about each line.
A suggested transcription of Focus is given in (3.7.2).

(3.7.2)

```
1    E:   what d'you think it is David
2    D:   teddy bear
          {     F     }
3    E:   yes it could be a teddy bear
              {     F     } {    - F    }
4    E:   who's that there coming up the path
          {                      F                    }
5    D:   Postman
          {  F  }
6    E:   what's he going to do
          {           F           }
7    D:   get out a letter
          {     F         }
10   E:   and what's he going to do with the letter
          {              - F          } {   F  } {   - F    }
11   D:   put it in the letter box
          {           F             }
14   E:   and who's this d'you think
               {   F   }
15   D:   girl
          { F }
```

Each line in the transcript will now be considered from the perspective of Focus and Topic.

Line (2): TEDDY BEAR is a single (compound) noun; it represents new information, in response to E's question in line 1, and thus represents a new Topic. It is therefore marked as the Focus.

Line (3): E repeats TEDDY BEAR, which is not now a new topic so is not the Focus. It is therefore marked as {-Focus}. She does, however, introduce an element of uncertainty about the content of the picture, with COULD BE. This has the potential to be picked up as a new topic. For example, in his next turn, David might have reaffirmed his claim with something like "It is! Look at his ears!". We therefore have marked her first words as in Focus.

Line (4): Rather than pursue her uncertainty, E immediately shifts the topic to another part of the picture. She asks David to identify a character, "who's that", specifying verbally (rather than simply by pointing) the particular character she is now focussing on. As the location of the character "there" appears to be essential for David's correct identification of the character, we can infer that E places all the elements of this turn in Focus.

Line (5): David's turn consists of a single new word, which is topically fitted to E's question in the previous turn, and is therefore in Focus.

Line (6): E now shifts the topic slightly away from identifying the character to the character's actions. The new and therefore focussed element is GOING TO DO.

Line (7): David's response is topically fitted, as he specifies the action GET OUT, and the object, A LETTER that is acted upon. Thus, the whole of his turn is in Focus. He does not state the agent, THE POSTMAN / HE, which is already given from the immediately prior context.

Line (10): In this turn E restates the agent HE and the object LETTER, which are therefore not in Focus. Her Focus is on the action DO WITH.

Line (11): David treats line 10 as a request to specify a (further) action by the postman, by supplying a new action PUT (IT) IN THE LETTERBOX, which is thus the Focus of his turn.

Line (14): E changes topic once more, asking David to identify a new character (whom she is presumably pointing to), and which is therefore her Focus.

Line (15): As in line 5, David's turn consists of a single new word, which is topically fitted to E's question in the previous turn, and is therefore the Focus.

Key to Activity 3.3

Possible Tonic placements are presented in transcript (3.8.1).

(3.8.1)

```
1    E:    || what d'you think it is David ||
2    D:    || teddy bear||
3    E:    || yes it ⇑could be a teddy bear ||
4    E:    || who's that there coming up the path ||
5    D:    || postman ||
6    E:    || what's he going to do ||
7    D:    || get out a letter ||
8    E:    || get out a letter ||
9    D:    || yes ||
10   E:    || and what's he going to ⇑do with the letter ||
```

```
11    D:    || put it in the letter box ||
12    E:    || he's going to put it in the letter box ||
13    D:    || yes ||
14    E:    || and who's this d'you think ||
15    D:    || girl ||
16    E:    || is it a girl ||
17    D:    || I already said that ||
```

There are two issues to decide on when transcribing the Tonic. The first is to decide which word the Tonic should be on. This issue will be discussed in conjunction with the next question, as it is closely linked to the assignment of Focus. Once the word has been selected, a further issue is to determine which syllable of that word should bear the Tonic prominence. If the word is monosyllabic, then there is nothing to decide. Examples are PATH in line 4; GIRL in lines 15 and 16. Where the word has two or more syllables, then the Tonic syllable will be the syllable that carries the lexical (word) stress. This was explained in Chapter 1. Thus, in lines 7 and 8, where the Tonic is on the word LETTER, the Tonic syllable is the first syllable, since that is the syllable marked for lexical stress in the phonological representation for letter. This is also the case for three further multisyllabic nouns that carry the Tonic in this extract: TEDDY BEAR (lines 2, 3), POSTMAN (line 5) and LETTER BOX (lines 11, 12). These are compound nouns, in which two separate nouns, e.g. LETTER and BOX, have been fused to form a single lexical item that has a meaning that is related to but distinct from its two parts: a letter box usually refers not to a box for putting letters in but to an aperture in a door designed for the delivery of letters. A compound noun like LETTER BOX is signalled phonologically by lexical stress located on the first of the two compounded nouns: 'LETTER BOX, 'TEDDY BEAR, 'POSTMAN. This can result in related phonological features, such as the schwa vowel in the second syllable of 'POSTMAN. Thus, we can see that accurate positioning of the Tonic depends on the speaker having accurate knowledge of the phonological representation of the word in question, in cases where that word has more than one syllable. This may involve quite specific knowledge of the relationship between phonology and the lexicon, in this case, the particular stress pattern that is associated with compound nouns.

The transcript presented as (3.8.2) combines the Tonic placements of (3.8.1) and the Focus transcript from (3.7.1). We have added the traffic light notation introduced in Chapter 2, to indicate in more detail the structure of each Intonation Phrase. As before, the dark grey shading indicates the Head of the IP; the light grey indicates the Tonic; words with no shading are in the Tail. In this transcript, the choice of Tone (rise, fall, etc.) is not marked on the Tonic syllable, as this is not relevant to issues of Focus. Instead, the underlining is retained to mark the location of the Tonic syllable.

(3.8.2)

```
1    E:    || what d'you think it is David ||
2    D:    || teddy bear ||
           {       F       }
3    E:    || yes it ⇑could be a teddy bear ||
               {         F      } {     - F      }
```

```
4    E:    ‖ who's that there coming up the path ‖
            {                          F                   }
5    D:    ‖ postman ‖
            {   F   }
6    E:    ‖ what's he going to do ‖
            {            F         }
7    D:    ‖ get out a letter ‖
            {       F        }
8    E:    ‖ get out a letter ‖
            {       - F       }
9    D:    ‖ yes ‖

10   E:    ‖ and what's he going to ⇑do with the letter ‖
            {            - F         } {   F   } {    - F    }
11   D:    ‖ put it in the letter box ‖
            {            F            }
12   E:    ‖ he's going to put it in the letter box ‖
            {                      - F               }
13   D:    ‖ yes ‖

14   E:    ‖ and who's this d'you think ‖
                   {   F   }
15   D:    ‖ girl ‖
            {  F  }
16   E:    ‖ is it a girl ‖
            {     - F     }
17   D:    ‖ I already said that ‖
            {         F      } { - F }
```

Each line in the transcript will now be considered from the perspective of the relationship between Tonic placement and Focus.

Line (1): Because we do not have the previous context, i.e. what they have been talking about, the Tonic has been placed on the last item of the IP, IS, indicating broad Focus over the whole IP: no item is signalled out as topically more important than the rest. The Tonic thus functions mainly to signal the end of the turn, as explained in Chapter 2. DAVID, the name of the addressee, used by E to select him as the next speaker (cf. Chapter 2) is presented as the Tail of the IP, as is common in English.

Line (2): David produces a single lexical item, the compound noun TEDDY BEAR, so that is the Focus of the turn (see Key to Activity 3.2); it carries the Tonic, which signals the end of the turn. The Tonic syllable is the first syllable, for the reason explained above.

Line (3): This is a more complex turn, from the perspective of Focus. The relation of the turn to the ongoing topic was explained in the Key to Activity 3.2. With regard to the location of the Tonic, the important consideration for E is to avoid placing the Tonic on the word that has just been mentioned, i.e. TEDDY BEAR, which is now {-Focus}. This is why COULD is a likely candidate as the bearer of the Tonic: it is available as a word that is not {-Focus}. BE is another possible candidate location for the Tonic, for the same reasons.

Line (4): E's turn presents topically entirely new content (see Key to Activity 3.2), so there is no specific Focus. As we saw in Activity 3.1, the Tonic is likely to be located on the last word of the IP, and functions to signal the end of the turn. An alternative for E would be to present the turn as two IPs, e.g: ‖ who's that there ‖ coming up the path ‖.

Line (5): As line 2.

Line (6): E now shifts her Focus to the character's actions. The new, and therefore focussed element is now GOING TO DO, rather than HE, which refers to the postman who was mentioned by David in line 5. When the Focus is on a phrase such as GOING TO DO here, then the Tonic is routinely placed on the final word in the phrase, in this case, DO.

Line (7): David's response, GET OUT A LETTER, is all new content, addressing E's question. It is therefore all in broad Focus. As described for line 4, the Tonic will normally then be on the stressed syllable of the final word.

Line (8): This turn was omitted from Activity 3.2. It is an exact repeat by E of David's prior turn. Thus, it is not serving to progress the topic. Rather, E is checking her understanding of David's turn. This is evidenced by David's next turn, in line 9. While the Tone may be different (as will be discussed in Chapter 4), the repeat is likely to have exactly the same IP structure and Tonic placement as the turn being repeated, unless the repeater is checking one specific part of the prior turn that she thinks she may not have understood or heard right. In the latter case, the repeater may use Tonic placement to identify that item.

Line (9): This is a minimal confirmation, where Focus and Tonic placement are not at issue.

Line (10): This is similar to line 3, in that an important consideration for E is to avoid placing the Tonic on the word that has just been mentioned, i.e. LETTER, which is now {-Focus}. E restates the agent HE as well as the object LETTER, but her Focus on the action DO WITH. For both these reasons, DO or WITH are the most likely locations for the Tonic.

Line (11): David treats line 10 as a request to specify a (further) action by the postman, by supplying a new action PUT (IT) IN THE LETTERBOX, which is thus the broad Focus of his turn. The Tonic is located on the stressed syllable of the last lexical item in the focussed phrase.

Line (12): This turn was omitted from Activity 3.2. It closely resembles line 8, being a slightly expanded repeat by E of David's prior turn. Thus, it is not serving to progress the topic. Rather, E is checking her understanding of David's turn. This is evidenced by David's next turn, in line 13. It is likely to have exactly the same IP structure and Tonic placement as the turn being repeated.

Line (13): Minimal confirming response, cf. line 9.

Line (14): E asks David to identify a new character (presumably she is pointing to this new character). The broad Focus is thus on identifying the new item, represented linguistically by the proposition WHO'S THIS.

Line (15): As in lines 2 and 5, David's turn consists of a single compound noun, which is topically fitted to E's question in the previous turn. It therefore carries both Focus and the Tonic.

Line (16): E produces yet another understanding check by repeating the content of David's previous, this time formulated as an interrogative. There is zero Focus as there are no new sematic items, so the Tonic is located on the final lexical item.

Line (17): In David's turn THAT is a pronominal form standing for GIRL, and as such represents given information, which does not have Focus. There is broad Focus over the preceding words "I already said" so the next available candidate location for the Tonic is SAID.

CHAPTER 4

Actions

In Chapter 1, we saw that intonation is organized in terms of intonation phrases (IP). This provides a flexible resource for the management of turn-exchange in interaction (Chapter 2) and, through the placement of the Tonic, for the identification of the speaker's Focus (Chapter 3). This approach to intonation emphasizes the real-time decisions about intonation that speakers and listeners have to make. For instance, as the speaker, I have to decide whether to continue my turn in progress or to signal that it is complete. As the listener, you have to decide whether or not to take the floor at any particular moment. Your decision will determine whether or not, as a new speaker, your incoming will overlap my turn. Your decision will also influence the intonational design of your incoming. As explained in Chapter 1, the defining feature of an IP is the presence of a Tonic, the place where a major pitch movement occurs. We have already seen that the Tonic may vary in its position, for the purposes of Focus. We have incidentally noted that the Tone, which forms the Tonic, may take different forms, e.g. it may be rising or falling. This is reflected in the notation we have been using, where the Tonic is indicated by the presence of a diacritic immediately before the Tonic syllable. Thus, the speaker has a choice of which Tone to use as the Tonic. This choice is widely viewed as central to the communication of meaning through intonation. The factors that influence a speaker's choice of Tone are the subject matter of this chapter.

Our account of the Tone system is informed by the view that intonation provides a set of flexible resources that can be deployed in real time in response to the demands of talk-in-interaction. According to this view, a speaker's choice of a rising as opposed to a falling Tone is routinely influenced by the obligation to be responsive to the previous speaker's turn. A primary factor determining a speaker's choice of which Tone to use at a particular place in the conversation is whether the speaker is initiating a new action or is continuing with the action already in progress. Conversations, and other forms of talk-in-interaction, consist of action sequences of various kinds (Schegloff, 2007). A participant may initiate an action which entails a potentially very short sequence. An example would be a greeting like "Hi", to which a response with "Hi" would be sufficient to close the greeting sequence. Conversely, the action that the participant initiates might potentially project a much longer sequence, such as inviting the recipient to embark on some kind of narrative, e.g. to talk about what they did at the weekend. Once an action sequence is underway, the participants may go along

Children's Intonation: A Framework for Practice and Research, First Edition. Bill Wells and Joy Stackhouse.
© 2016 John Wiley & Sons, Ltd. Published 2016 by John Wiley & Sons, Ltd.
Companion website: www.wiley.com/go/childintonation

with the action in progress or else at any point may choose to initiate a new action. Where a participant wants to initiate a new action, that participant has to display that this is happening, in a way that is recognizable to the other participants.

This can be illustrated from part of a conversation first presented in Chapter 2, involving Len (L), Patrick and their speech and language therapist (T), presented here as Extract (4.1). At an early point in this interaction, the therapist produces a turn (line 9) that is an invitation to Len to talk about things he likes to do in town. Len aligns with the invitation by immediately producing a list of four things he likes doing (lines 10–13).

(4.1)
```
9   T:   ‖ 'Len 'what dyou like `doing when you 'go into 'town ‖
10  L:   ‖ er 'seeing the ´[bu]ses ‖ 'seeing the ´trains ‖
11  T:                      [mm]
12  L:   and 'seeing the `tills ‖(.)
13  L:   and I (.) 'always `buy 'things ´there ‖
14       (1.5)
15  T:   [mm  ]
16  L:   ‖ [there]‖ so- 'some 'things are ´mine ‖⇒ 'some 'things `arent ‖
17  T:   ‖ `sorry ‖ 'some 'things 'are
18  L:   ‖ 'some 'things (.)'some 'things I 'bought are ´mine ‖⇒
19       'some 'things I 'bought arent ‖
20  T:   ‖ 'some things (.) you 'brought are ˇyours ‖
21  L:   ‖ ˇyeah ‖
22  T:   ‖ and some things`arent for ´you ‖
23  L:   ‖ ´no ‖
24  T:   ‖ ↑ who are the`other things 'for 'then ‖
```

As Len has been given an apparently open-ended opportunity by the therapist to talk about what he likes doing in town, his turn starting at line 10 could go on indefinitely. However, an alternative trajectory in such a case is that one of the participants may initiate a new action, giving rise to a new sequence. This is in fact what happens. After a pause at line 14, Len produces a turn in line 16 that is not semantically transparent. At this point, the therapist initiates a repair sequence. This represents a new action: requesting clarification. The repair takes seven turns (lines 17–23), following which she reverts to a question that follows up on the fourth of the activities that Len likes doing in town: buying things. She thus effectively winds back to line 16, to which her line 24 is a fitted next turn.

In order to initiate the new action, i.e. the request for clarification, the therapist has to display that this is what she is doing, in a way that is recognizable to Len. In this particular case, the therapist starts the turn in line 17 with a word that signals a problem: "sorry" – a lexical device for marking that she is initiating a new action and, furthermore, that the action is likely to involve repair. In the rest of the turn she uses a grammatical and intonational device to indicate more precisely what kind of repair she is seeking: she repeats "some things are", which, discounting "there" which relates back to his prior turn, were the first three words of Len's turn in line 16. She does not reach a syntactic completion point; moreover, she produces these words as an incomplete IP, i.e. without a Tonic. As this is therefore not a complete turn constructional unit (TCU), it invites Len to carry out a repair on his remaining words from line 16: "...mine some things aren't". Len does indeed recognize her turn in line 17 as a new action, and specifically as a repair initiation, as is evident from line 18, where he expands his earlier line 16 by twice inserting "I bought".

If as a new speaker I do not wish to align with the ongoing action sequence, I need as a minimum to display to my co-participants that I am initiating a new sequence. At some point I also need to make the action itself recognizable. In line 17 of (4.1), we saw that the therapist accomplished both these simultaneously: she showed that she was initiating a new action, and that the action was repair. However, in theory and in practice, they are separable. Theoretically, we can envisage that it would be very useful for young children or any other speakers with very limited vocabulary and grammar to have a simple means of signalling that they want to initiate a new action in the talk, even if they do not have the linguistic means to communicate instantaneously what that action is. In practice, it does indeed seem to be the case, and the Tone system provides one resource for achieving this. Gorisch, Wells and Brown (2012) carried out acoustic and interactional analysis of 177 exchanges drawn from spontaneous adult conversation. Their results supported the hypothesis that non-matching of pitch contours is used to initiate a new course of action whereas matching is used by a second speaker for the purposes of interactional alignment. This is evidence that matching of pitch contours is interactionally relevant, as has been proposed by researchers in the phonetics of adult conversation such as Couper-Kuhlen (1996) and Szczepek Reed (2006), as well as by Tarplee (1996) and Wells (2010) in the domain of child–carer interaction. It suggests that one source of phonetic orderliness in naturally occurring talk stems from the requirement upon a next speaker to match the pitch contour of the prior speaker in order to demonstrate alignment with the talk in progress; or else to show disalignment in order to initiate a new action or direction, by demonstrably not matching the pitch contour of the prior speaker.

The existence of a simple system of Tone matching vs. non-matching has important implications for understanding how a conversation can progress even when one participant has little or no recognizable vocabulary and grammar. Such a participant might be an older child with persisting speech difficulties (cf. Chapter 10), an adult with severe aphasia who has very restricted language or a young typically-developing child who has not yet progressed to a stage where he can produce intelligible multi-word utterances. Drawing on the interactions between Robin and his mother, in the next section of this chapter, we show that a child wanting to align with the activity that is underway will choose to match the Tone used by his mother in the previous turn; whereas if the child wants to initiate a new activity, such as querying what his mother just said, then he chooses a contrasting, non-matching Tone: a rise instead of a fall, for example. Such exchanges provide a basis for exploring how the young child gains access to the Tone system of English. Tone matching and Tone non-matching are presented in relation to two phenomena that are key in interaction in general but especially in early carer–child interaction: repetition and repair. Examples are also presented from children who do not operate with the system of Tone matching, giving rise to problems of comprehension for the other participants. The Activities enable the reader to learn to identify matching and non-matching Tones, and to interpret their interactional significance.

Repetition and Tone matching

In interactions between young children and their carers, instances of repetition are common – carer repeating child, and child repeating carer (Keenan, 1983; Tarplee, 1996). A fundamental choice confronts the young child, or indeed any of us as a conversational participant, each time it is our turn to talk: shall I repeat what the previous speaker just said, or shall I say something else?

On many occasions where a second speaker repeats the first speaker's words and also his Tone, repetition of the first speaker's Tone passes off unproblematically. In (4.2), Robin's mother repeats at line 3 the last three of Robin's words from line 2 and uses a rising Tone, as Robin had done. His mother's repetition of his words and Tone accompanies their collaborative play, which continues without any hitch. Thus, mutual matching of Tone across speakers accompanies a joint enterprise with which both participants are aligned.

(4.2)

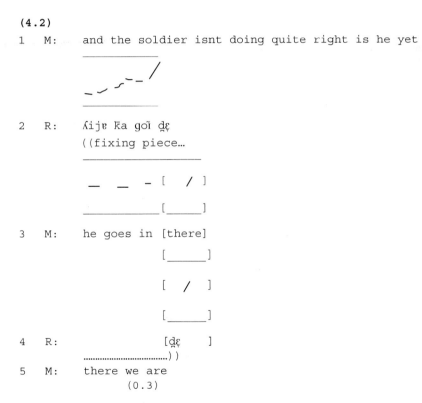

```
1   M:     and the soldier isnt doing quite right is he yet


2   R:     ʌijɐ ꝁa goĭ d̠ɛ̰
           ((fixing piece…


3   M:     he goes in [there]




4   R:                [d̠ɛ̰  ]
           ...........................))
5   M:     there we are
                  (0.3)
```

In Extract (4.3), there is matching of rising Tones across a series of six turns, some but not all of which also involve verbal repetition. Robin is seated on the floor, fitting pieces into a jigsaw puzzle board. He is looking at the board throughout and does not have eye contact with his mother. His mother is sitting on the floor close to the board and to Robin, watching him as he places the pieces on the board.

(4.3)

15 M: whats 'teddy got round his `neck

16 R: a na daɪ a   dɪ di[: :]

          {f} {ff} {f}[_]_____

17 M: [tie(.)tie around teddys neck
                          {p}   {f}   {f}
                (1.7)

18 M: ye[s]

19 R: [da:dɪ di
          {f}

20 M: tie   on teddy
                       {f}

21 R: i   jo ʋe da:: didi
          {f   ff}
22 M: ^yes I think he looks `good ´there
23   So (.) where does the `soldier go
          ((M holds up soldier piece, showing it to R))

In line 15, Robin's mother asks him for some specific information about the teddy piece, which they have been talking about earlier. He responds in line 16. In line 17, his mother ends her turn with a rising Tone. In the absence of an immediate response, following a pause of 1.7 seconds, in line 18 she pursues a confirmation of her interpretation with "yes", again with a rising Tone. This suggests that in line 17 she had been unsure that she had understood him completely.

The pitch pattern in Robin's line 19 echoes not only line 18 but also the final part of his mother's turn in line 17, with its terminal rise. In line 20 she seems to treat Robin's line 19 as a truncated version of line 17: her recast "tie on teddy" is more succinct than her turn in line 17, "tie around teddy's neck". Her Tone in line 20 mirrors the final rise of Robin's line 19. Although his mother's earlier turns in lines 17 and 18 may have been designed as requests for Robin to confirm that she had understood him correctly, there is no evidence that either line 19 or line 20 is being designed or treated as a request: there is no eye contact, and throughout Robin continues to focus on fitting the piece into the puzzle. Rather, the rising Tones appear to be the product of the current speaker (M in 20, R in 21) copying the Tone used by the previous speaker in the preceding turn (R in 19, M in 20).

Why should the participants match each other's Tone? Following the temporary disruptions involving overlap, repair and pause in lines 16–18, Tone matching contributes to a mutual display of alignment between the speakers, who are orienting to a shared understanding and appreciation of the activity in progress. The practice of Tone matching persists over the subsequent turns. In line 21, Robin provides his own expansion, adding [ijo ʋe] prior to [da:: didi], the latter three syllables presumably representing "tie (on) teddy". This latter portion preserves the pitch pattern of the preceding two lines, as does his mother's next turn (line 22): she has been looking at Robin as he places the teddy piece in the board, and offers her confirmation and approval: "yes I think he looks good there". Finally, in line 23, Robin's mother breaks the cycle of Tone matching, with a fall. The change of Tone signals a new action, which is to ask Robin something about a new piece. The shift of Focus onto the new piece is achieved by Tonic placement, as she locates this falling Tone on "soldier".

In this section, we have proposed that Tone matching is used to align with the action in progress, whereas a non-matching Tone can initiate a new course of action, for instance, a repair sequence (Corrin (2010b) gives an extensive account of repair in the talk of Robin and his mother). In Activity 4.1, there is an opportunity to work through the steps involved in this type of analysis. Complete this before reading further.

As we have just seen in Activity 4.1, Robin's turn in line 6 of Extract (4.4) matches the end of the preceding turn: the final words of line 5 and line 6 both have a stepped variant of a falling contour. The step down in line 5 is around seven semitones, and in line 6, also seven semitones. In both versions, the first syllable is louder than the second syllable; the durational ratio of the two syllables appears similar in both versions, at around 2:1, creating a similar rhythmic pattern. Thus, not just the pitch patterns but also the overall prosodic shapes of the two versions of TRACTOR resemble each other. Following Robin's repeat in line 6, his mother closes the topic in line 7, and in line 8 Robin moves to further play. In such cases, both Robin and his mother treat Robin's verbal repeat and Tone match of the word she has just pronounced, as a sequentially fitted move: it serves to close the sequence, without further work. This suggests that his mother is content not only with his comprehension of the word but also with his pronunciation, even though at the segmental level there are considerable phonetic divergences between her version and his (cf. Tarplee, 1996): the initial cluster of

ACTIVITY 4.1

Aims:
- Part 1: to learn how to create a systematic intonation transcription.
- Part 2: to work with the concept of Tone matching.

Part 1

The first part of this activity gives some practice in deriving a systematic intonation transcription from an impressionistic transcript. Study recorded Extract (4.4).

(4.4)

```
1    M:      that's right a duck and what's this one (.)
             what's this (.) Robbie
             ((R looks for tractor)) (2.5)



2    R:      ijɛ                                          here



3    M:      ‖'thats  ´right ‖its a `tractor‖(.)like `that one‖



4    R:      ʋahɛ                                    tractor



5    M:      tractor   can you say tractor
             {f}    {alleg    }  {f}



6    R:      ʔɛː t̞ ɛ                                  tractor
             {f}
7    M:      ‖'thats ´it‖
8    R:      uh ((trying to pull wheel off))
```

First, study line 3 in (4.4). This has been transcribed in two ways. There is an impressionistic transcription of pitch movements, between staves (parallel horizontal lines), which has been made on the basis of careful listening and acoustic analysis of the fundamental frequency (F0) contour. There is also a systematic transcription as demonstrated in the previous chapters, using symbols and diacritics for IP boundaries and Tone, integrated with the orthographic text. The systematic transcription has been derived from the impressionistic transcription following these steps:

1 We needed to decide how many intonation phrases (IPs) there are. Since the defining feature of the IP is a Tonic, realized as a notable pitch movement, the first step was to identify notable pitch movements. In this case, there are three: on "right", "tractor" and "that", marked by underlining, so there will be three IPs.

```
thats right its a tractor(.)like that one
```

2 We notated each Tonic syllable with the appropriate Tone diacritic. In this case, it is a rise on "right", a fall on "tractor" and another fall on "that". We also marked other rhythmically prominent syllables as stressed, e.g. "that's". As explained in Chapter 1, underlining of the Tonic then became redundant, as Tonic is implied by the Tone diacritic.

```
'thats ´right its a `tractor (.) like `that one
```

3 Finally, we could place the IP boundary symbols, ‖. There must be an IP boundary at the beginning and at the end of the turn. Because there are three IPs, we needed to place two further IP boundaries. Each IP boundary must fall between two Tonics, so that there will be just one Tonic per IP. Starting with the boundary between the final two IPs: this must occur after "like" or after "tractor". The pause after tractor suggested that this is the strongest candidate location for an IP break. As for the boundary between the first two IPs, this was more awkward to decide on. It could be after "right" or "its" or "a". There were no strong phonetic reasons to prefer one rather than the other; so we followed the usual convention by placing the IP boundary at the strongest grammatical boundary. Here, that is between "right" and "its":

```
‖ 'thats ´right ‖ its a `tractor‖(.)like `that one ‖
```

Now you carry out the same three steps for line 5:

1 Identify the Tonics, to tell you how many IPs there are. You can temporarily mark them by underlining.
2 On the basis of the impressionistic transcription of pitch provided, decide for each Tonic whether rise or fall is the more accurate description of the Tone. Then notate each Tonic with the appropriate Tone diacritic: ´ (rise) or ` (fall).
3 Insert IP boundary symbols where you consider the boundaries to occur.

Check your answer with the Key to Activity 4.1 at the end of the chapter.

Part 2
In this part of the activity, you apply the concept of Tone matching/non-matching, with reference to lines 5 and 6.

On the basis of your decision about (2) in Part 1, decide whether the relationship between line 6 and the final IP of line 5 is one of Tone matching or Tone non-matching.

Check your answer with the Key to Activity 4.1 at the end of the chapter.

TRACTOR is realized by Robin as a glottal stop, and the vowel of the stressed syllable has a closer quality than the target.

Such examples indicate that repair sequences are a fruitful environment where the child can learn about Tone: here, that matching the Tone of the model is part of producing an acceptable version of the word that caused trouble, which enables the repair sequence to be closed.

Tone non-matching to initiate repair

Extract (4.5) is another labelling sequence, this time based on a picture in a book that Robin and his mother have in front of them. In line 4, Robin's mother initiates a repair on Robin's turn in line 3. Although she already knows what the correct label would be, in line 4 she invites Robin to repair it himself, which he duly attempts to do in line 5. The sequence is similar to earlier extracts as far as line 6, where Robin's mother appears to confirm his attempt at line 5. In line 7, Robin produces a verbal repeat as he did in the TRACTOR example in Extract (4.4); however, this time he does not accompany the repeat with a Tone that matches his mother's. Whereas in the previous turn (line 6) his mother used a rise-fall contour over the phrase, Robin in line 7 produces a rise of five semitones.

(4.5)

```
1    M:     mhm (.) a ´what (.) 'what's `this
2           (4.9)
```

```
3    R:     ma: (.)wiə  dɛ
                   {f}
```

```
4    M:     mhm it's a what
```

```
5    R:      mɛ
            {p p}
```

```
6    M:     t's a man
```

```
7    R:     ma
```

```
8    M:    Yes
           _____
```

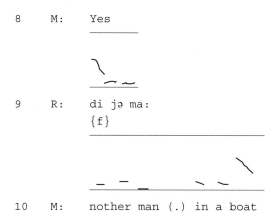

```
9    R:    di jə ma:
           {f}
```

```
10   M:    nother man (.) in a boat
```

His mother's "yes" response in her next turn (line 8) indicates that she is treating Robin's verbal repeat with its non-matching Tone as a request for confirmation. This is different from the turns consisting of verbal repetition plus Tone matching that Robin produced in Extracts (4.2), (4.3) and (4.4). Irrespective of whether Robin's Tone was rising or falling, none of these was treated by his mother as a request for confirmation. Instead, she treated Robin's turns as confirmatory labels that Robin had produced to align with the ongoing action of labelling which she had initiated. The fact that in line 8 of (4.5) she treats Robin's verbal repeat in line 7 differently appears to be due to the non-matching Tone that he produces. This non-matching Tone constitutes his verbal repeat as a new action, i.e. a request for confirmation.

Tone matching in interactions with children who have communication difficulties

To this point, Tone matching and non-matching have been exemplified mainly by reference to interactions between Robin and his mother. It may also be evident when the participants are children with communication difficulties, as is evident in the next two extracts.

Kevin is an 11-year-old boy on the autism spectrum, with severe communication difficulties (Local & Wootton, 1995); see also Chapter 11 of this book. In Extract (4.6), he is playing a board game with his mother.

(4.6)
```
5    M:    ‖'whose `turn is it‖
6    K:    `Kevins turn
           {f}
7    M:    ‖ˇhonest‖
8          ((sound of shaking dice))
9          ‖ 'whatve you `got Kevin ‖
```

In line 5, Kevin's mother asks him to tell her which of them is due to take the next turn in the board game. In line 6, he duly provides an answer that is semantically comprehensible, although atypical in that he refers to himself in the third person: "Kevin's turn", rather than "my turn". In line 7, his mother accepts this as a fitted answer, while querying the honesty of his answer, possibly as a tease. In line 8, Kevin throws the dice and in line 9 his mother asks what the dice shows.

With regard to the participants' use of Tone, the mother's question in line 5 is produced with a falling Tone, which Kevin matches in line 10, thereby aligning his turn with the sequence that his mother has initiated. Thus, it appears that Kevin was able to deploy Tone matching in a way that was fitted to the action in progress in the talk. In line 7, when his mother jokingly asks for a confirmation, she initiates this new action by using a non-matching Tone.

Extract (4.7) is from the conversation between Len, Patrick and their speech and language therapist that was referred to in Extract (4.1). Len and Patrick are 9-year-old boys attending a residential school for children with language and communication difficulties.

(4.7)

```
75   P:   ‖ 'what 'what did it 'look like in the er: `ghost 'train ‖ (0.5)
76   L:   ‖ 'look like in the 'ghost ´train ‖
77   P:   ‖ `yeah ‖
```

In line 75, Patrick asks Len a question, using a falling Tone. In line 76, Len repeats the last five words of Patrick's turn. Apart from not repeating Patrick's dysfluency, the most noticeable difference between his version and Patrick's is that he uses a different Tone: a rise of seven semitones, contrasting with Patrick's fall. Patrick's response in line 77, "yeah", indicates that he treats Len's turn in line 76 as checking that Len has correctly heard Patrick's question in line 75. Thus, Len is able to use a non-matching Tone to initiate a new action, namely to check his hearing or understanding of the prior turn.

These two brief extracts suggest that the system of matching and non-matching Tones may be quite robust in the face of other communication impairments. With this in mind, it is salutary to consider the interaction in Extract (4.6.1). This includes the talk that immediately precedes the exchange between Kevin and his mother presented as (4.6).

(4.6.1)

```
1   M:   ‖ 'whose `turn is it ‖
         (1.5)
2   M:   ‖ 'whose `turn is it ‖
         (1.5)
3   M:   ‖ 'whose `turn is it ‖
         {        lento       }
         (.)
4   K:        `turn is it
           { lento }
5   M:   ‖ 'whose `turn is it ‖
6   K:   `Kevins turn
           {f}
7   M:   ‖ˇhonest ‖
         ((sound of shaking dice))
         ‖ 'what've you `got Kevin ‖
```

Kevin's mother's turn in line 5 is her fourth presentation of exactly the same question to Kevin. Her first two attempts, in lines 1 and 2, elicited no response. Following her third attempt (line 3), Kevin repeats the last three words of his mother's turn in line 4. This turn design - repeating the last three words of the prior speaker's turn - is quite similar to Len's in line 76 of (4.7), which was treated by Patrick as a request for clarification. However, Kevin's mother does not treat his turn in line 4 as a request for clarification: rather than replying with "yes" or "is it my turn or yours?", for example, in line 5 she simply reiterates her original question. The difference between Kevin's response in line 4 and Len's in line 76 is that Len uses a non-matching Tone, whereas Kevin produces a matching Tone. The comparison of these two fragments suggests that the system of Tone matching is important for conversational participants in making sense of the talk. It is also suggests that while Len has command of this system, Kevin does not. Kevin may produce a sequentially fitted Tone on occasion, as in line 6 of (4.6); but the evidence of line 4 suggests that this may be by accident rather than on purpose. Kevin's echolalia is examined further in Chapter 11.

Notation for Tone matching and non-matching

In Chapter 2, the traffic light system of notation was introduced in order to capture the relationship between intonation phrase (IP) structure and turn structure. In this section, we introduce a further notational convention, to capture the relationship between the Tones of adjacent IPs: whether or not they are matching. For any IP, we can state whether its Tone is a match (=) or a non-match (≠) to the preceding IP. The symbol = or ≠ is placed in front of the first IP boundary. Extract (4.7) is presented using this notation in (4.7.1).

(4.7.1)
```
75 P:    ‖ 'what 'what did it 'look like in the er: `ghost 'train ‖ (0.5)
76 L: ≠  ‖ 'look like in the 'ghost ´train ‖
77 P: ≠  ‖ `yeah ‖
```

The notation indicates that Len's Tone in line 76 (a rise) does not match Patrick's Tone in line 75 (a fall). Patrick's Tone (a fall) in line 77 does not match Len's Tone in line 76 (a rise). The notation system is illustrated now from some of the extracts analysed earlier in this chapter.

In Extract (4.2.1), Robin's mother's rising Tone in line 3, matches Robin's rising contour in line 2:

(4.2.1)

```
2    R:        ʌijʊ ka go ĩ dɛ
3    M:    =   ‖ he 'goes in ´there ‖
```

In (4.5.1), Robin's pitch contour in line 7, which is rising, contrasts with his mother's rise-fall Tone in line 6. However, it is then matched by his mother's rise in line 8. This is followed by a non-matching fall from Robin in line 9. In line 10, Robin's mother uses a rise-fall Tone, which matches the high falling contour used by Robin in line 9.

(4.5.1)

```
6      M:          ‖ ts aˆman ‖




                        ⌣


7      R:    ≠      ma                                    man
8      M:    =      ‖ ´yes ‖




                    ⟍
                     ⌢

9      R:    ≠      di jə ma:                          ? man
                    {f}
10     M:    =      ‖ˆnother man ‖ (.) in a `boat ‖
```

In the last three extracts, there is no = or ≠ symbol preceding the first turn in the transcript, because no prior turn is shown with which it can be seen to match or not match. This is an artefact of extracting a short fragment from a longer sequence: as the line numbering suggests, each of these first lines was in reality preceded by other talk. This is true of the vast majority of turns at talk. However, some turns are necessarily produced without reference to a prior turn, such as the very first turn in a conversation; or a turn produced after a lapse in the conversation. In such cases, it is necessary to decide, on the basis of listening to the recording, whether the salient pitch characteristic of this first turn is some kind of fall reaching or approaching the base of the speaker's range, as opposed to a type of rising contour. In our notation, these two contours are respectively symbolized by L (for 'low') and H (for 'high'). It follows that the Tone (located at the Tonic) of any IP will be L or H, as it will either match or not match that first Tone. As will emerge, this is an oversimplification with regard to typical adult talk. However, it is a useful way of viewing and notating talk that involves young children and those with atypical speech and language development.

Having adopted the H/L convention for the first turn, we can dispense with the rise and fall diacritics when presenting a transcript of interaction. Thus, in line 76 of Extract (4.7.2), the ≠ symbol informs us that the Tone of the line is H, because it contrasts with the L of the preceding line 75. In line 77, ≠ tells us that the Tone is L, because it contrasts with Len's H in line 76. The location of the Tonic, and therefore of the Tone, is shown by the light shading, representing a yellow traffic light.

(4.7.2)

```
75  P:  L   ‖ 'what 'what did it 'look like in the er: ghost 'train ‖ (0.5)
76  L:  ≠   ‖ 'look like in the 'ghost train ‖
77  P:  ≠   ‖ yeah ‖
```

In line 3 of Extract (4.2.2), the = symbol indicates an H (rising) Tone, matching the H of Robin's turn.

(4.2.2)

```
2   R:   H    ʌijɐ  ka  go  ĩ  dɛ̰
3   M:   =    ‖ he 'goes in  there ‖
```

How this system plays out over a slightly longer sequence is shown in (4.5.2). In line 7, Robin's Tone is H, contrasting with his mother's L in line 6. His mother matches him with H in line 8. Robin then produces L in line 9, which contrasts with line 8. His mother then matches his L with her own L in line 10. Now complete Activity 4.2 before reading further.

(4.5.2)

```
6    M:   L    ‖ ts a man ‖
7    R:   ≠    ma                              man
8    M:   =    ‖ yes ‖
9    R:   ≠    di jə ma:                     ? man
10   M:   =    ‖ nother man ‖ (.) in a  boat ‖
```

ACTIVITY 4.2

Aim: To learn how to annotate a transcript using the Tone matching notation.

In this activity, we will make use of part of the transcript of Extract (4.4) from Activity 4.1.

(4.4.1)

```
1    M:        ‖its a `tractor‖(.)
2              ‖like `that one‖


              ⌒╲


3    R:        ʋahɛ
4    M:        ‖`tractor‖
5              ‖ can you say `tractor‖


              ⌐
              ⎯╲


6    R:        ʔɛ: t̪ɛ
              {f}
7    M:        ‖'thats ´it‖
```

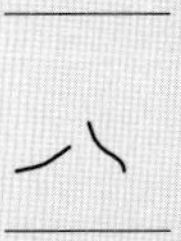

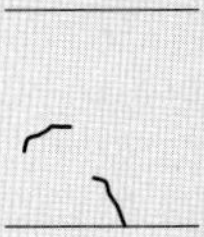

1 For line 1 only: in the blank column, enter either H or L, whichever is appropriate for the Tone in the transcript.

2 For lines 2, 3, 4, 5, 6, 7: decide whether the Tone in each IP matches or contrasts with the Tone of the previous IP. In the blank column, enter = or ≠, as appropriate.

3 Write or type out the complete transcript so that it looks like Extract (4.5.2) presented earlier, including the matching symbols from (1) and (2) above, selected from H, L, =, ≠ . Include Tonic (using underline or shading) but omit the impressionistic pitch transcription between staves. Although they are redundant, you may want to include Tone diacritics, as they can make the transcript easier to read.

Check your answers with the Key to Activity 4.2 at the end of the chapter.

Tones and questions

In this chapter, we have proposed that the speaker's decision to use a rising or falling Tone is primarily determined by the immediately preceding intonational context. This is somewhat at odds with the belief of many English speakers that their choice of a rising vs. a falling pitch pattern is determined by whether or not they are asking a question. This assumption is sometimes reflected in the practice of professionals who work with spoken language, for example, in therapeutic, educational or theatrical contexts. In this section, we will see that the assumption is not well founded.

A humorous allusion to the relationship between Tones and questions occurs in Ian McEwan's novel *Atonement*, where a 13-year-old playwright, Bryony, is rehearsing her cast for an imminent performance of her new play. Nine-year-old Pierrot is an unwilling actor:

> Like his brother, Pierrot had the knack of depriving his lines of any sense. He intoned a roll-call of words. "Do-you-think-you-can-escape-from-my-clutches?" All present and correct.
> "It's a question", Bryony cut in. "Don't you see? It goes up at the end."
> "What do you mean?"
> "There. You just did it. You start low and end high. It's a *question*."
> He swallowed hard, drew a breath and made another attempt, producing this time a roll-call on a rising chromatic scale.
> "At the end. It goes up at the end!"
> Now came a roll-call on the old monotone, with a break of register, a yodel, on the final syllable.
>
> *(McEwan, 2001: 33–34)*

This passage captures nicely the inherent difficulty that children, and indeed adults, have in producing on demand an intonation pattern that comes quite naturally in spontaneous speech. More important for the present context, however, is the fact that Bryony herself has a misconception about the relationship between intonation and questions. Her misconception is that when speakers ask a question, they use a rising pitch pattern.

Before investigating this further, we first need to decide what we mean by "a question". In the written language, the reader recognizes a question by the question mark at the end of the sentence. When producing spoken language that derives from a written text, such as a play or a radio news script, the speaker may reflect the presence of the question mark through intonation. In spontaneous speech, there is no such infallible guide to what is a question. Nevertheless, there is large class of utterances that can be identified fairly reliably as questions, by virtue of their syntactic design. To illustrate this, in (4.8) we present a selection of questions taken from the extracts used in the first four chapters of this book.

(4.8)

(a)

```
9    T:   ‖ 'Len  'what dyou like `doing when you 'go into 'town ‖
10   L:   ‖ er 'seeing the ´[bu]ses ‖ 'seeing the ´trains ‖
11   T:                  [mm]
12   L:   ‖ and 'seeing the `tills ‖ (.)
```

(b)

```
75   P:   ‖ 'what 'what did it 'look like in the er: `ghost 'train ‖ (0.5)
76   L:   ‖ 'look like in the 'ghost ´train ‖
77   P:   ‖ `yeah ‖
```

(c)

```
5    M:   ‖ 'whose `turn is it ‖
6    K:   ‖ `Kevins turn ‖
```

(d)

```
7    M:   ‖ whats `this bit 'called though ‖
8    R:   ‖ çi:j akəlˠ ‖
```

(e)

```
1    M:   mhm (.) a ´what (.) 'whats `this
2         (4.9)
3    R:   ma:(.)wiə  dɛ
```

The first turn in each of these five fragments is designed syntactically as an interrogative: the subject of the sentence follows an auxiliary or copula verb and in addition, each first turn begins with a WH question word: WHAT or WHOSE. The following turn, produced by a different speaker, addresses the content of the first speaker's turn, supplying the information that is sought by the WH-word. In sum, there are good grounds for regarding the first turn of each fragment as a question and the following turn as an answer. The one exception to this is (b), where instead of supplying the requested information, Len checks his hearing of Patrick's turn – a move that may occur following any kind of turn, not only a question.

Having established that each of the first turns in (4.8) is a question, we can now establish whether there is any regularity in the speaker's choice of Tone. A brief examination shows that in each case the Tone is a fall. Although (4.8) presents only a small sample, this observation is in line with what has been found to be generally true for British English: that WH-questions are more likely to have a falling Tone (Couper-Kuhlen, 2012). Such findings contradict Bryony's assumption that questions in English are always done with a rising Tone.

Not all questions start with WH-words, however. Another grammatical class of interrogatives has subject-auxiliary (or copula) inversion, without the initial WH-word. Some examples are given in (4.9):

(4.9)

(a)

5   M: ‖ `tractor ‖ can you say `tractor ‖
     _____

            ⌒
               ⟍
     _____

6   R: ʔɛː t̥ɛ   *tractor*

(b)

2   M: ‖ can you re'member what `this is ‖
     _____

              ─   ─ ─   ⋀
     ─   ─   ⟍
     _____

3   ʔə(.)ʔɛdʒœː ʔɪʒʒ (0.7)pɒkx
4   M: ‖ `top‖ thats `right‖ `top ‖

(c)

     _____

              ⟍
                ⟋
        ─   ─   ⟍
     _____

11   M: (is it) ʔelsa's nose
12   J: hehe

     _____

         ⌐   ─   ─ ⌐
                ─   ⌣
     _____

13   M: can you say ʔelsa's n[ose
14   R: [hehehe
           ((turns head to look at J/camera))
     _____

        ⌐
     _____

15   R: nose ((points at J/camera))

(d)

1   M: ‖ is ꞌthat the Ꞌfunnel ‖
(2.0)

2   R: m̥mok(0.9)   ʔɑ fə   fɑːfɐ
(0.5)

3   M: ‖ ˇthats ꞌright‖⇒the ꞌsmoke Ꞌcomes out of the ˆfunnel ‖

(e)

1   T: ‖ Len‖ can you ꞌsee ꞋPatricks ˇlooking at ꞌyou: ‖ and hes
           ꞋListening to you ‖
2   ⇒ but ꞌyoure [not ꞋLooking at him at ˆall] ‖
3   L: [↑o h   ˆy e s] ‖ ꞋI forꞋgot‖
           ꞋI forꞋgot ‖

In (4.9), the questions in the first turn have a falling Tone, as in (a), (b) and the first question in (c); or a rising Tone of some kind, as in the second question in (c) and in (d). (e) presents a tricky issue of identifying which IP should be considered as the one bearing the Tone associated with the question, the first major IP having a fall-rise ("looking at you") and the second a fall ("listening to you"). This small sample again reflects what has been found in larger studies of question intonation in corpora of British English. In the sample of conversational English studied by Couper-Kuhlen (2012), only 55% of 101 examples of this type of interrogative had a rising Tone, which was not significantly more frequent than a falling Tone.

In studies of the relationship between questions and intonation in English, a third type of question is generally considered: one which has the syntactic form of a declarative, rather than an interrogative. In the written language, the function of such a declarative sentence as a question can be conveyed by a question mark, as in this example from *Atonement*. The first speaker has just arrived back at the family home. The second speaker, his sister, has been living there for some time. "The Old Man" refers to their father.

'And the Old Man's staying in town?'
'He might come later.'

(McEwan, 2001: 48)

This is often thought to be the question-type that is most likely to have a rising Tone, and an actor may choose to read the first line of this exchange in that way. However, when examining corpora of spontaneous talk, it is very difficult to establish a relationship between this type of question and a rising Tone. One difficulty is in deciding whether a syntactically declarative turn is indeed a question, without having recourse to intonation evidence: it is important to avoid the circularity of the argument that runs: "This syntactically declarative turn is a question because it has a rising Tone, therefore a question that has a declarative form will have a rising Tone." Studies that have looked at corpora of spontaneous speech (as opposed to read speech) and have tried to be rigorous about the definition of 'question' have failed to find a strong relationship between rising Tones and declarative questions (Crystal, 1969). Couper-Kuhlen (2012) found that of 14 such 'questions' in her corpus, only one was produced with rising intonation.

In this section we have examined the common belief or assumption that questions are produced with rising intonation. Linguists have refined this assumption to take account of differences between different syntactic forms of question. For teaching purposes, a simplified version is sometimes presented. The claim is that for British English at least, *yes–no* questions, i.e. questions that start with an interrogative form like "do you" or "can you", are made with rising intonation, as are questions that do not have an interrogative form, like "he's ready?" or "no cheese?"; whereas questions that start with WHERE, WHEN, HOW, WHAT, WHO, or WHY, known as WH-questions, are done with a falling pitch contour.

While these claims have not been supported by evidence from recordings of spontaneous conversation, it is possible that they have more validity in relation to the intonation of reading loud. It has been reported that the distribution of Tones is different between reading and conversation, with a greater proportion of rising Tones in reading (Crystal, 1969). Reading aloud is different in its speech processing mechanisms compared to spontaneous speech, an issue that will be considered further in Chapters 8 and 9. However, in their naturally occurring context in spontaneous talk, it appears that questions, statements and other speech acts can all be done with a variety of Tones. While the direction and shape of the terminal pitch contour are often thought to be the determining factor in conveying pragmatic meaning, such as question vs. statement, studies of recorded conversations (Szczepek Reed, 2004; Walker, 2004; Couper-Kuhlen, 2012) indicate that in naturally occurring British English talk-in-interaction, there is no systematic relationship between terminal Tone and pragmatic function.

Because young children and those with communication impairments are exposed primarily to spontaneous conversational speech, our approach is to focus on the importance of the immediately preceding intonational context in determining a speaker's choice of Tone. Rather than select a particular Tone from an intonation lexicon because that Tone is associated with 'question', the child's task is to choose a Tone that contrasts with the Tone used by the previous speaker, if the child wants to initiate a new action. Initiating a new action may sometimes be done with a question; but not all questions initiate new actions.

Tones, words and non-verbal acts: progressing the talk

So far in this chapter we have examined how the Tone system can be used to align with an ongoing action or to initiate a new action. This approach highlights an overwhelming priority for participants in a conversation: to keep the conversation going. Spoken language and written language have commonly been viewed as primarily a means of exchanging information. However, observation of everyday conversation, and particularly of interactions involving young children, demonstrates that much of the time, talk is more concerned with establishing and cementing social relationships. For this to happen, it is of prime importance that the conversation does not fizzle out; so a primary concern of participants is to ensure that the talk progresses. A range of resources are available to participants to achieve this. Obviously there is the choice of words to indicate a new topic or develop the current topic – a theme that was explored in Chapter 3. Then there is the Tone system, which we have been examining in this chapter. A further set of resources is provided by non-verbal acts, including gestures and eye contact. Mature, competent participants in conversations integrate non-verbal acts with spoken language (including intonation) so seamlessly that it is hard for us to become aware of the role being played by each of these three components. This being so, it is a little easier to identify the particular roles of language, intonation and non-verbal acts, and how they can be combined, by studying young children who still have limited verbal resources. For them, as for people with severe communication difficulties, non-verbal acts provide a particularly important resource for progressing the talk.

The aim of this section is to show how the young child can coordinate Tone with words and with non-vocal acts to accomplish social actions and to progress the talk, using examples from the recordings of Robin and his mother. At the start of Extract (4.10), Robin points at a puzzle piece and in line 1 produces a turn which his mother takes to be a label for the piece:

(4.10)

((R pointing & looking at ʙᴀʟʟ jigsaw puzzle piece))

1   R: **L**   ˈd ɛ d ɪ s
                   (0.8)
2   M: ≠   ‖ ts a ˊwhat ‖
                   (0.4)
                   ((R still pointing & looking at ʙᴀʟʟ piece, facing M))

3   R: ≠   ˈʔ æ d ɪ s
                   (0.5)
4   M: ≠   ‖ ˊDaddys ‖
                   (1.0)
5   M: ≠   ‖ ts a ˋball ‖
                   (0.6)
                   ((R turns away towards toy box))

6   R: =   b ɔ ː   ((drops ball piece))

In line 2 of (4.10) Robin's mother initiates a repair from Robin, but he persists with the wrong lexical selection (line 3). His mother corrects it (line 5) and Robin repeats her word, with matching (falling) Tone in line 6. Although Robin's choice of word ("ball") and his choice Tone (matching) in line 6, align with his mother's agenda for the talk, his non-verbal acts tell a different story. When he produces "ball" in line 6, he already has his back to his mother, having turned away from her towards his toy box. As he says the word "ball", he drops the BALL piece. The lexical repeat links his turn to the current topic, the BALL piece. The Tone match aligns his turn in line 6 to the sequence preceding it, and thereby establishes that the referent of BALL has not changed: they are both still talking about the same thing. On the other hand, his non-vocal acts – dropping the ball piece and wandering off – suggest that he is going to initiate a topic shift. Thus, it appears that his non-vocal acts move the interaction on in a new direction, while the verbal components continue on his mother's theme.

In Extract (4.11), first introduced in Chapter 3 as Extract (3.14), the situation is rather more complex than in (4.10), because Robin and his mother are now talking about two different balls. This raises the issue for Robin of how to make clear which ball he is talking about at any given moment. His solution involves the coordination of word, Tone and non-verbal acts.

(4.11)

```
1   M:  L    you got the ˋball
2       =    ‖ ˈwhere does the ˈball ˋgo ‖ (.) from the ˋjigsaw ‖
3            (3.0)
             ((R, holding BALL jigsaw puzzle piece, walks from jigsaw
             to near M))
             _____

             ⋀_
4   R:  =    bɔ ((looking at real ball on floor, drops jigsaw ball))
             {p}
             _____

                 ⋀
             __
5       =    ε jɔ dɔkʰ ((R picks up real ball with lh , transfers it
             to rh))
             _____

                      ↗
             ⌣     ⌣
             _____

6   M:  ≠    ‖ theres  your  ˋball ‖
             _____

             ⋀
             _____
```

```
7   R:  ≠   bɔ ((R picks up jigsaw ball with lh))
            {f}
            _____

              ⌣

                 ⌣
            _____
```

```
8   M:  =   ‖ ` two   balls ‖
9   R:      Heh
            ((R turns round, walks back to jigsaw holding real ball
            and jigsaw ball))
10  R:  =   ʔɛ i (.)  jɛ  ((attempting to put real ball in jigsaw))
11  M:  =   ‖ it doesnt `fit so well ‖ `does [it] ‖
12  R:  =   [jɛ]((fitting jigsaw ball in jigsaw))
13  M:  ≠   ‖ thats ´right ‖(1.3) that one goes in ´there ‖
```

In this sequence, one of the objects in question is a real ball, the other a jigsaw piece depicting a ball. For both participants, there is an issue of clarifying which of the two balls are talking about. In line 2, his mother makes clear that she is talking about the jigsaw piece. In line 4, after a considerable pause, Robin repeats the word "ball" from his mother's previous turn, and matches the Tone by using a falling contour. However, the direction of Robin's gaze, in lines 4–6, makes it clear that his reference is to the real ball, which his mother confirms in line 6. Thus, it appears that his repetition of his mother's word and his choice of matching Tone align his turn with the preceding talk, while his non-verbal act, here his gaze, serves to change the referent of his talk: it is no longer the jigsaw ball that his mother was talking about, but the real ball.

In line 7, Robin repeats his mother's final word from line 6, which again is "ball". However, at line 7, Robin produces a Tone contrast: a high rise-fall, contrasting with his mother's rise. This potentially alerts his mother to a new action or direction in the talk. Robin's non-verbal act clarifies what this is: he picks up the jigsaw piece. This topic shift gets taken up by his mother in line 8, where her Tonic is on "two". By designing her turn in this way, she confirms that the word "ball", which forms Robin's entire turn in both line 4 and line 7, can refer to two different objects in the real world. The topic of two competing balls is then animatedly pursued by Robin, who tries to fit both into the jigsaw. He is not just extending the reference of the label as he did in line 4: he is doing things with each object.

It may be that this interactional occasion provides an opportunity for Robin to appreciate a key fact about language: that a single linguistic sign, like BALL, has multiple referents. We have seen that Robin and his mother are able to make sense of this inter-action by orienting simultaneously to vocabulary, intonation (specifically matching and non-matching Tone) and non-verbal acts. One of the resources drawn on by Robin's mother is the system of Tonic placement for Focus, as in ‖ `two balls ‖ in line 8. We saw in Chapter 3 that this resource for verbal pointing is one that Robin was still in the process of learning at the time of these recordings. In this extract, (4.11), in which he does not produce turns that have more than a single identifiable word, there is no evidence that he can draw on the system of Tonic placement to clarify the topic and referent of his talk in the way that his mother does in line 8. In order to make sense of what Robin is trying to communicate, his mother is therefore all the more dependent on what he conveys through the non-verbal acts that accompany his single word turns.

In this section we have suggested that Tone, words, and non-vocal acts (gaze, gesture, and body movement) are independent but combinable resources. Within a single turn they can be deployed in different combinations to align with the current action; to initiate a new action; or to align and initiate, both at the same time. By drawing on these resources in a coordinated way, the participants can make sense of each other's conversational moves, even when one of the participants, like Robin, has very limited linguistic resources. In Chapter 12, we will return to this theme in relation to interactions involving a 9-year-old boy who has severe hearing and speech production difficulties.

Summary

In Chapter 4 an analytical framework has been presented which allows us to address the following questions about Actions and Tones, in relation to spoken interactions involving a child (C):

Aligning

1 Does C align with the action of the co-participant's prior turn by using Tone matching?
2 If so, what actions does C align with? For example, Assessments; Repairs; Requests; Offers.
3 Does C extend an action to a second TCU in own turn, by using Tone matching within the turn?

Initiating

1 Does C initiate a new action, different from the action underway in the previous speaker's prior turn, by using Tone non-matching?
2 Does C initiate a new action, different from the action underway in C's preceding IP in their own current turn, by using Tone non-matching?
3 If so, what actions does C initiate by Tone non-matching? For example, Repair; Request.
4 Does C recognize that the prior speaker has initiated a new action by use of Tone non-matching, and respond accordingly?

Key to Activity 4.1

Part 1

‖ `tractor ‖ can you say `tractor ‖

1 *Identify the Tonics, to tell you how many IPs there are.* There are two dynamic pitch contours, on the two tokens of the word TRACTOR. The descending contour is distributed over both syllables of the word.

2 *Notate each Tonic with the appropriate Tone diacritic.* The contour is descending in each case so ` is the appropriate diacritic. The pitch on the first syllable is more or less level while on the second syllable it is noticeably falling.

3 *Place the IP boundary symbols.* In theory, the internal IP boundary could be placed after the first "tractor" or after "can" or "you" or "say". However, there is a strong grammatical boundary before "can". The fact that the three syllables "can you say" are delivered at a rapid tempo and at the same (low) pitch level is a further reason not to break them up with an IP boundary.

Part 2

On the basis of your decision about (2) in Part 1, decide whether the relationship between line 6 and the final IP of line 5 is one of Tone matching or Tone non-matching. The Tone of the final IP of line 5 is marked as a fall; Robin's Tone in line 6 is most accurately notated as a fall; so the two Tones are matching.

Key to Activity 4.2

The suggested answers to (1), (2) and (3) are contained in the transcript of (4.4.2):

(4.4.2)

```
3  M:  L    ‖ its a `tractor ‖ (.)
            ‖ like `that one ‖
4  R:  =    ‖ `vahɛ ‖
5  M:  =    ‖ `tractor ‖
            ‖ can you say `tractor ‖
6  R:  =    ‖` ʔɛ: t̠ɛ ‖
7  M:  ≠    ‖'thats ´it ‖
```

CHAPTER 5

The Intonation In Interaction Profile (IIP)

The aim of this chapter is to present an assessment framework that is based on Chapters 1–4. The Intonation in Interaction Profile (IIP) is introduced, with examples from a young typically developing child, Robin, whom we have already met in earlier chapters, followed by extended exemplification from David, a 5-year-old child with unusual intonation, whom we met in Chapter 3. The IIP, as presented in Appendix 3, consists of four pages. The first two pages address the role of intonation in Turn-taking and are based on the questions listed in the summary to Chapter 2. The third page, which is based on the questions listed at the end of Chapter 3, is concerned with intonation and Focus, in relation to the handling of topics. The questions found at the end of Chapter 4, about Tone, with reference to alignment and initiation of Actions, are presented on the final page of the IIP.

The IIP is based on an analysis of children's use of and response to intonation in the context of naturalistic interaction. In his pioneering studies of prosodic disability, David Crystal also based his assessment on naturalistic interaction (Crystal, 1987). Such an approach has the obvious advantage of face validity: if we are interested in finding out more about how children use intonation in real life, then it makes sense to study their intonation in the context of natural conversation, rather than under test conditions. The formal assessment approach adopted by Crystal in the PROP (Prosody Profile), was to profile the client's prosodic behaviour, by tallying the occurrence of different Tones, the variation in Tonic placement and the distribution of IP boundaries, relating this to what was known about normal acquisition of intonation and grammar, as well as their usual distribution in the adult language (Crystal, 1982). Profiling of this type has some important limitations, in that it presents a purely descriptive picture, without leading to hypotheses about the causes of the client's prosodic difficulties, or their functional consequences. Crystal pointed out that this was a consequence of the lack of research, at the time he was writing, into the semantic and social functions of intonation (Crystal, 1982). However, he stressed the importance of identifying meaning and function; for example, when considering the use of pitch range by P, a "severely educationally subnormal teenager", Crystal wrote:

> The problem for the analyst is therefore to decide whether the phonetic contrast between high and low has any phonological significance: does P mean anything by it? The only way to find out, in such a patient, is to scrutinise each context carefully, to see whether there is any evidence to support a systematic interpretation.
>
> *(Crystal, 1987 : 84)*

Children's Intonation: A Framework for Practice and Research, First Edition. Bill Wells and Joy Stackhouse.
© 2016 John Wiley & Sons, Ltd. Published 2016 by John Wiley & Sons, Ltd.
Companion website: www.wiley.com/go/childintonation

Seeking a valid and reliable method for the systematic scrutiny of context in order to identify prosodic meaning, since the 1980s, researchers have drawn on the methods of Conversation Analysis, where claims about a speaker's meaning are derived from careful observation of the speaker's behaviour and of the reactions of the co-participants in the interaction. This approach and the findings about intonation function in English that have resulted from it, underpin Chapters 2, 3 and 4 of this book on which the IIP is based.

The assessment of a child's intonation using the IIP involves a number of steps, listed here:

1 Make a recording of a sample.
2 Prepare a transcription.
3 Carry out intonation analyses of the transcribed data.
4 Complete the IIP profile.
5 Interpret the completed profile as the basis for planning further investigation and/or intervention.

This chapter covers steps 1–4. Step 5, the interpretation of the IIP, is treated at greater length in Chapters 10, 11 and 12.

Recording

Intonation transcription and analysis are time-consuming activities so it is unrealistic in clinical contexts to expect that a large amount of data could be recorded and analysed. On the other hand, as stated at the beginning of the Preface, every time we speak, we have to use intonation, so every utterance recorded can be transcribed and analysed in terms of Turn-taking, Focus and Alignment. Because intonation is particularly sensitive to context, it is valuable to obtain recordings of the child talking to a range of different participants, e.g. parent, peer or teacher. This will be illustrated in Chapter 10. For some children, it may be helpful to record both two-party (one-to-one) interactions and multiparty conversations with at least two other participants, where the opportunities for Turn-taking and participation are different. It is also possible to set up more or less naturalistic game-based interactions that are likely to give rise to particular intonation features. For example, the PEPS-C battery, described in Chapters 8 and 10, uses a lotto type of game to elicit narrow Focus utterances (Peppé & McCann, 2003). A similar approach is taken in the PETAL assessment procedure, described in Chapter 12 (Parker, 1999).

When recording young children or people with communication difficulties, video recordings are desirable, since, as illustrated in Chapter 4, intonation is just one mode of communication, along with gaze, gesture and bodily movement, contributing collectively to the achievement of meaning. That said, the decision whether to use video is one which may be dictated by a number of factors, including availability of equipment and someone to operate it, as well as the level of consent that can be obtained from the participants. In some circumstances, it may be possible for the video recording to be carried out by family members at home, which can enhance the naturalness and spontaneity of the interaction, even if the recording quality is sometimes compromised. Where video is not practical, it is normally possible to make good quality audio recording. For studies where detailed acoustic measurements are needed or where it is important to be able to hear each speaker clearly, even when they are talking in overlap, individual headset-mounted microphones are recommended, though hardly practical for young children in naturalistic settings. However, technological advances in audio recording mean that obtaining clear individual speaker signals may soon be possible using a centrally placed bank of microphones. Rutter and Cunningham (2013) offer valuable guidelines on how to make audio and video recordings of speech for purposes such as this.

Transcription

The transcription format used for the data extracts presented in Chapters 1–4 is recommended when undertaking an IIP. In a word processing program, it is convenient to format the transcript in a table, with line number and speaker identifier in separate columns, then an orthographic transcript of the speaker's words. A further column to the right of the orthographic transcript can be used for notes, including a gloss or translation if needed. If a word is not intelligible, it can be transcribed using IPA symbols. Certain features of speech production are also recorded on the orthographic tier, using conventions derived from Conversation Analysis research: see Appendix 1. These include silent intervals and the start and end points of overlapping talk.

Our approach to intonation transcription was described in Chapter 1. The transcript can be produced on the basis of perceptual observation, in conjunction with acoustic analysis where feasible. Depending on the speaker, one of two types of prosodic transcription should be used. Where the speaker is known to be using the English intonation system, the intonation pattern is usually notated in a *systematic* transcription, as in (5.1) below. A diacritic for the Tone is placed before the first syllable of the Tonic Foot, as for "right", "tractor and "that" in Extract (5.1); the diacritic for primary stress is placed before the first syllable of any other Foot; and the symbols for Intonation Phrase (IP) boundary are placed at the start and end of the IP.

(5.1)

```
1    M:    ‖ 'thats ´right ‖its a `tractor‖(.)like `that one ‖
```

This systematic notation has a practical and a theoretical advantage. From a practical perspective, once the transcriber is comfortable with recognizing the Tones of the English intonation system, it is relatively quick to use. Theoretically, it captures which of the Tones of English the speaker is using, which is important when deciding if the speaker is matching the prior turn or not (see Chapter 4). It shows the location of the Tonic, which indicates the elements that have Focus (see Chapter 3). The location of the Tonic also shows where the Head ends and where the Tail starts, while the IP boundaries show where the Head starts and where the Tail ends, all of which is relevant for Turn-taking (see Chapter 2). This information is invaluable at the interpretation stage.

A systematic notation like this is properly used when the transcriber already knows the speaker's system. In this respect it is like a phonemic notation for vowels and consonants. It can be quite misleading to use a systematic notation where we do not already know the speaker's system, for example, where the speaker is a young child who may not yet have learnt the system, an older child or adult who has never mastered the system or a non-native learner of English. In such cases, where we are unsure of the extent to which the speaker is competent in this particular intonation system, we normally use an impressionistic notation, as described in Chapter 1 and illustrated in Chapters 2–4, particularly with reference to Robin. On the tier above the orthographic transcript, pitch height and pitch movements are presented iconically between parallel horizontal staves, the staves representing the upper and lower limits of the speaker's habitual pitch range. On a tier below the orthographic transcript, loudness, pause and tempo features may be notated using symbols and diacritics of the IPA, including extensions (see Appendix 1). Robin's turn in line 16 of Extract (5.2) is notated in this way, the lowest tier showing variations in loudness.

(5.2)

```
15    M:    ‖ whats  'teddy  got round his `neck ‖
```

```
16    R:    a na daɪ a   dɪ di::
            {f}    {ff}    {f}
```

By using an impressionistic notation at this stage in the process of analysis, we are not claiming that the speaker's use of intonation is unsystematic; rather, that at this point we do not know what the systems are. At the next step, we try to work out the speaker's systems.

It has been argued here that interactional analysis can offer important insights into clinical prosodic research. However, Peppé (2009) suggests that its time-consuming nature is problematic for routine clinical assessment, particularly as it raises difficult practical and theoretical issues about competence and confidence in prosodic transcription. In this section, we offer some suggestions as to how these might be mitigated. Peppé refers to the important distinction between phonological and phonetic transcriptions, and the problems raised by attempting to use a phonological transcription with clinical data, as, for example, is done by (Crystal, 1987). The main problem is that children like David and some of the children to be presented in Chapters 10–12 may produce highly aberrant patterns, in which case it is an oversimplification, if not a distortion, to reduce this unusual prosodic production to a representation in terms of Tone, Tonic and IP boundaries (or an equivalent notation). One alternative which avoids the procrustean issue is to use impressionistic phonetic transcription for all parties to the interaction, supplemented by instrumental (e.g., acoustic) analysis – the latter can be presented separately as spectrograms or pitch tracks or it can be used to verify the impressionistic transcription (Local & Wootton, 1995). While this is the gold standard as far as accurate representation of speech events is concerned, it is demanding in terms of time and expertise and it also shifts the entire job of phonological interpretation onto the accompanying text. This is appropriate for research papers but not practical for everyday clinical work.

The approach that we adopt here combines phonetic and phonological notations. It is suitable for transcribing interactions in which one or more participants (e.g., a SLT client, or a young typically developing child) cannot be assumed to have full access to the prosodic system of the speech community, as represented by the other participants. The child's talk is therefore transcribed impressionistically. Prosodic features of the therapist's or carer's talk, indeed, the talk of any speaker whose system can be assumed to be known, are represented using a phonological notation that is assumed to represent key structures and systems of English intonation.

By carrying out the type of analysis illustrated in Chapter 2 and again later in this chapter, it is possible to establish whether the child already uses intonation features systematically in order to regulate turn exchange, and whether the co-participants respond to his use of intonation features, even if these do not yet coincide with the prosodic system of the adult speech community. Having carried out such an analysis, the traffic light notation can be applied to the talk of child as well as the adult. In this way, the notation used when presenting a transcription can serve to indicate how one important aspect of mutual comprehension, i.e. Turn-taking, is established between child and adult. We have seen in the various transcriptions presented in Chapters 3 and 4 that the same approach can be applied to Focus and to Actions.

Analysis

The IIP itself is completed following a process of analysing the recording and transcript in relation to fundamentals of talk-in-interaction. At this step, we apply to our transcribed data the analytical concepts developed in Chapters 2, 3 and 4. We first identify if the child is using the system of intonation traffic lights (Chapter 2), by examining whether Turn-taking proceeds in an orderly way without excessive overlap or long silence between turns; whether there is intonation prominence close to the end of the child's turns; and whether, in the absence of such prominence, the other participant waits for the child to finish. Thus, the evidence for the existence of the child's system is drawn from the reactions and responses of the other participant. In (5.3), an exchange already discussed in earlier chapters, the pitch prominence on the final word of Robin's turn is followed immediately by his mother's turn.

(5.3)

2   M: ‖ can you re'member what `this is ‖

3   ʔə(.)ʔɛdʒœː ʔɪ33 (0.7)pɒkx
                    {f}
4   M: ‖ `top‖ thats `right‖ `top ‖

If a traffic light system is identified, this can be notated on an orthographic transcript as in (5.3.1), using shading in the way that was explained in Chapter 2:

(5.3.1)

3   R: ʔə(.)ʔɛdʒœː ʔɪ33 (0.7) pɒkx
4   M: ‖ `top‖ thats `right‖ `top ‖

Next we can investigate whether the child is using the Tonic to convey the Focus of the turn. Using the same example, which was analysed in terms of its Focus structure in Chapter 3, it appears that Robin's mother picks up on his final word, interpreting it as TOP. This is evidence that Robin is using Supertonic prominence for narrow Focus. We notate this by **F** in Extract (5.3.2), in the way described in Chapter 3 (cf. Extract (3.12.1).

(5.3.2)

```
3          ?ə(.)?ɛdʒœ: ?ɪʒʒ  (0.7)  ⇑pɒkx
                              {F}
4     M:   ‖ top‖ thats right‖ top ‖
              {F}
```

Finally, we investigate whether the child is using Tone to align with the action of the prior speaker's turn or to initiate a new action. Aligning is accomplished by Tone matching, as described in Chapter 4. In this example, Robin's rise-falling pitch movement reaching the base of his pitch range, matches his mother's fall to the base of her pitch range on "this" in the prior turn, notated as **L**. There is evidence that Robin is using Tone matching to align with his mother's question, by providing an answer. The evidence that his turn is indeed an answer to her first turn is provided by her follow-up turn (line 4), "that's right". On this evidence we can therefore credit Robin with using the system of Tone matching, notated with = in (5.3.3), as described in Chapter 4:

(5.3.3)

```
2    M:   L   ‖ can you reˈmember what `this is ‖
3    R:   =   ?ə(.)?ɛdʒœ: ?ɪʒʒ  (0.7)  pɒkx
                                         F
```

Profiling

The four-page IIP form consists of questions to answer about the child's ability to use intonation to handle Turns, Focus and Actions. It is presented as Appendix 3 for you to copy and use. As we have seen in the Analysis step, answers to these questions are arrived at by reference to the observable behaviour of the participants rather than the intuitions of the profiler. To illustrate how the profile can be completed, we will start by profiling the single turn produced by Robin that was discussed in the Analysis section. It is reproduced as (5.3.4) with phonological notation:

(5.3.4)

```
2    M:   L   ‖ can you reˈmember what `this is ‖

                   ─    ─ ─
                ─      ─         ⋀

3    R:   =   ?ə(.)?ɛdʒœ: ?ɪʒʒ  (0.7)  pɒkx
                                         F
4    M:   =   ‖ `top‖ thats `right‖ `top ‖
```

Just from this fragment, we can start to answer eight of the questions on the profile. These are presented in italics in Figure 5.1. The answers are provisional: more examples from the recorded and transcribed data sample would be needed to confirm them. Although for the other questions on the profile we have no evidence as yet, this example shows how much can be inferred from just a single turn.

TURNS

Gaining the floor

1 Does C refrain from taking a turn until the current speaker has projected the end of her/his own turn? (C observes red light)

Yes: *line 2*	No: line	No evidence:

Comment: *R does not overlap M's Head in line 2*

2 Does C routinely start a turn with minimal pause, following the prior speaker's turn? (C observes yellow and green lights)

Yes: *line 2–3*	No: line	No evidence:

Comment: *R starts his turn in line 3, following M's Tonic + Tail*

Holding the floor

1 Does C produce a turn of more than one word by creating an IP with a Head? (C uses red light)

Yes: *line 3*	No: line	No evidence:

Comment: *R does not produce a Tonic on any of first five syllables of line 3*

Giving up the floor

1 Does C project the end of the turn by using the Tonic? (C uses yellow light)

Yes: *line 3*	No: line	No evidence:

Comment: *R produces biggest pitch movement on final syllable of line 3*

Figure 5.1 Partially completed IIP based on Extract (5.3.4).

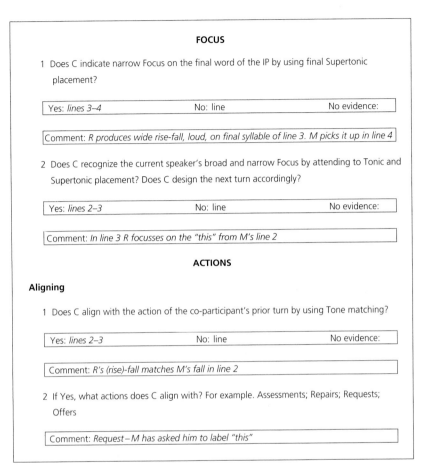

Figure 5.1 (*Continued*)

Using the IIP in a case of atypical intonation

We will now illustrate the use of the IIP with reference to an older child with atypical intonation. In Chapter 3, we met David, a boy with speech and language difficulties from the West Midlands of England, who at the age of 5;4, had an unusual and pervasive prosodic pattern. Because his intonation is atypical, we transcribe it impressionistically, as shown in (5.4). David's words are transcribed using IPA symbols, below which is a gloss.

(5.4)

1   E   ‖'what   dyou think it `is David‖

2   D   **dɛ dɪ gɛ:**
        teddy bear

3   E   ‖yes it ['could be a ˇted]dy bear‖   hh

4   D   [*   *   ]
                      {p   p}

5   E   ‖'whos 'that 'there 'coming up the `path‖
                (1.5)

6   D   **bɔʊsmad̥**
        postman

7   E   ‖'whats he 'going to ´do ‖

8   D   **gɛd ag ə gɛ ta**
        get out a   letter
                        (1.0)

9   E   ‖get 'out a `letter‖

10 D   yes

11 E   ‖and 'whats he 'going to ´do with the   'letter‖
                    (1.0)

12 D   **dʌd ɪt   ɪn   dʌd ɪt   dʊ   gɛ ta   bɒks**
        put it   in (1.7)   put it the letter   box
                    (0.8)

13 E   ‖hes 'going to 'put it 'in the `letter 'box‖

14 D   yes

                (1.0)

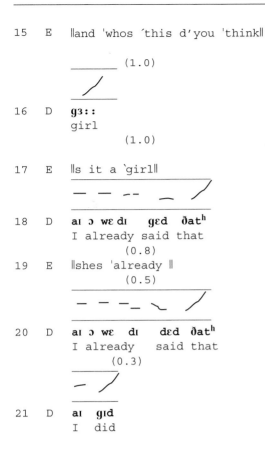

15   E   ‖and 'whos 'this d'you 'think‖

          (1.0)

16   D   **gɜ::**
     girl
          (1.0)

17   E   ‖s it a ˋgirl‖

18   D   **aɪ ɔ wɛ dɪ   gɛd   ðat^h**
     I already said that
          (0.8)

19   E   ‖shes 'already ‖
          (0.5)

20   D   **aɪ ɔ wɛ dɪ   dɛd ðat^h**
     I already   said that
          (0.3)

21   D   **aɪ gɪd**
     I   did

Turn-taking

As explained in Chapter 3, the transcript shows that David invariably locates the main pitch movement on the final syllable of his turn and it invariably has a high rising pitch. Words preceding this final syllable are produced with level pitch around the middle of his pitch range. Following this prosodic pattern, the other speaker, E, starts up. On one occasion where she does not, following line 20, then David repeats the same prosodic pattern. Thus, David's idiosyncratic pattern serves to mark the end of his turns in a clear, consistent and unambiguous way, which is useful for him and his co-participants, given the general unintelligibility of his speech. By clearly signalling the end of his turn at talk, David manages to maintain interactions with others without an unusual amount of pausing, overlap or inter-ruption by co-participants. We can therefore make a phonological transcript of (5.4), presented here as (5.4.1), in which the final syllable of each of his turns is highlighted as the Tonic syllable of the IP, the preceding syllables being highlighted as the Head.

(5.4.1)

1	E	what dyou think it is David
2	D	teddy bear
3	E	yes it [could be a ted]dy bear hh
4	D	[* *]
5	E	whos that there coming up the path
6	D	postman
7	E	whats he going to do
8	D	get out a letter
9	E	get out a letter
10	D	yes
11	E	and whats he going to do with the letter
12	D	put it in put it the letter box
13	E	hes going to put it in the letter box
14	D	yes
15	E	and whos this dyou think
16	D	girl
17	E	s it a girl
18	D	I already said that
19	E	shes already
20	D	I already said that
21	D	I did

On the IIP, we can now complete questions relating to giving up, holding and gaining the floor. Complete Activity 5.1 before reading further.

David has a consistent system for signalling the end of his turn, hence the 'Yes' for the first question under Giving up the Floor, even though his system is non-standard. The fact that he uses a rising pitch, rather than a fall, may be attributable to the local accent: a rising turn-final pitch movement (though of smaller span) is very common

---

ACTIVITY 5.1

Aim: To learn how to complete the 'Turn-taking' questions on the IIP.

1 In the Turns section on page 2 of the IIP, read through the three questions on Giving up the floor. Attempt to answer each question by referring to the phonological transcript of Turn-taking that was presented as Extract (5.4.1), also referring as needed to the phonetic transcript of this interaction that was presented as Extract (5.4). If your answer to a question is *Yes* or *No*, then fill in the line number(s) that provide evidence for your answer. Use the comment box for any further observations relating to the question. As this is a relatively short extract, for some questions it is likely that there will not be evidence either way. When you have attempted each question, check your answer with the Key to Activity 5.1 at the end of the chapter.
2 Repeat this procedure for the four questions relating to Holding the Floor.
3 Repeat this procedure for the four questions relating to Gaining the Floor.
Check your answer with the Key to Activity 5.1 at the end of this chapter.

in the West Midlands variety of English which David is exposed to. However, the fact that the high rise is the *only* Tone evident in David's speech suggests that he lacks the richer set of Tones found in the West Midlands accent. Furthermore, the invariable location of the Tonic on the final syllable of the utterance is atypical of almost all varieties of English, including West Midlands. This has a negative consequence in terms of the word stress system of English: in David's utterance-final words, the stress is always heard to be on the final syllable. It is possible that this aberrant stress pattern contributes to the unintelligibility of his speech output.

On the positive side, there is evidence that David can mark IP boundaries within a longer utterance, as in lines 20–21: "I did" is produced as a separate Tone unit with its own final Tonic, separated from the preceding "I already said that", not only by a pause but also by the final rise on "that". As this example shows, David is able to map IPs onto distinct turn constructional units.

Focus

Having completed questions relating to Turn-taking, we can now move to the section of the profile that deals with Focus. As David's use of Tonic placement and the Supertonic to convey Focus was analysed in detail in the last part of Chapter 3, the analysis itself will be recapitulated only briefly here. In order to do this, we need a phonological transcript that records where the Focus is shown for each speaker in each turn. In the Turn-taking transcript (5.4.1), the Tonic is already marked. In Chapter 3, we saw that usually the Tonic provides a pointer to the listener as to what the speaker is focusing on. This is referred to as Tonic Focus, notated **{TF}**. If the Tonic is very prominent (notated as ⇑ for 'Supertonic'), e.g. a wide pitch movement that is louder and longer than anything in the rest of the IP, then this indicates narrow Focus solely on that word. Where the Tonic is not especially prominent, that is interpreted as signalling broad Focus over the whole of the Head and the Tonic.

As David always produces a Supertonic and it is always on the final word of his turn, in Extract (5.4.3), we assign narrow Tonic Focus, **{TF}**, to the final word of each of David's turns. The bold **{SF}** (for Semantic Focus) beneath the transcript indicates the word or words that could have been expected to be semantically focused, because they represent new information; while information that has already been mentioned is marked with **{-SF}**. In Extract (5.4.2), which was originally presented in Chapter 3 as Extract (3.7.1), Semantic Focus has been assigned without reference to intonation, but solely on the basis of the new information in each turn. Now complete Activity 5.2.

(5.4.2)

```
1   E   what dyou think it  is David

2   D   teddy ⇑bear
              {  TF  }
         {     SF    }
3   E   yes it [could be a  ted]dy bear   hh
         {                  TF              }
         {          SF       }
4   D            [    *      *      ]
```

```
5    E    whos that there  coming up the path
          {                    TF                    }
          {                    SF                    }
6    D    post⇑man
                  { TF }
          {     SF     }
7    E    whats he going to do
          {              TF              }
          { SF}          {-SF}{     SF    }
8    D    get out a lett⇑er
                            {TF }
          {          SF          }
9    E    get out a letter
          {         TF         }
          {         -SF        }
10   D    ⇑yes
          { TF }
          {       }
11   E    and whats he going to ⇑do with the letter
                                {TF }
          {           -SF           } { SF }{     -SF     }
12   D    put it in put it the letter⇑box
                                      {TF }
                    {          SF          }
13   E    hes going to put it in the letterbox
          {                  TF                  }
          {                  -SF                 }
14   D    ⇑yes
15   E    and whos this dyou think
            {      TF      }
            {      SF      }
16   D    ⇑girl
           { TF }
           { SF }
17   E    s it a girl
          {     TF     }
          {     -SF    }
18   D    I already said  ⇑that
                            {TF}
          {       SF       }
19   E    shes already
          {      -TF      }
          {      -SF      }
20   D    I already  said  ⇑ that
                            {TF}
          {         -SF         }
21   D    I ⇑did
            {TF}
          {    -SF}
```

ACTIVITY 5.2

Aim: To learn how to complete the Focus questions on the IIP for a child with atypical intonation.

On the IIP form, read through the five questions on Focus. Attempt to answer each question by referring to the phonological transcript that was presented as Extract (5.4.2), also referring as necessary to the phonetic transcript of this interaction that was presented as Extract (5.4). If your answer to a question is *Yes* or *No*, then fill in the line number(s) that provide evidence for your answer. Use the comment box for any further observations relating to the question. As this is a short extract, for some questions it is likely that there will not be evidence either way. In such cases, place an X next to "No evidence".
Check your answers with the Key to Activity 5.2 at the end of the chapter.

For the adult speaker E, Tonic Focus {**TF**}, and Semantic Focus {**SF**} are sometimes co-extensive, as one might expect. For example, in line 5, the Tonic is on the final word, "path", implying that the whole of the IP is in broad Focus; contextually, the whole of E's turn in line 11 is new, since she has shifted the topic from TEDDY BEAR to POSTMAN. In such cases the Tonic-Focus system is functioning optimally. However, even for typical mature speakers such as E, this is not always the case, as was described in Chapter 3.

For David, this type of discrepancy between semantic Focus and Tonic Focus is the norm rather than the exception. In line 12, for example, he places a Supertonic on the final word, which implies narrow Focus on LETTER BOX, whereas the semantic Focus also includes the action PUT IT IN, since this has not been mentioned before. The same applies in line 8. In line 18, the discrepancy is even more striking: David places a Supertonic, implying narrow Focus, on THAT, a pronoun representing what is already known from line 16 (GIRL); and simultaneously applies no Focus to the new part. I ALREADY SAID. As explained in Chapter 3, these examples show that David is not making use of the usual Tonic-Focus system.

The profile shows that David is inaccurate in the way in which his Tonic placement reflects Focus. The first reason for this inaccuracy is that all his Tonics are Supertonics, implying narrow Focus. As a result, he does not have the means to convey broad Focus (Question 1). The inaccuracy arises, second, from the rigidity with which he always places a Tonic on the final word (in fact, the final syllable) of his IP. This only results in accurate Focus when his turn consists of a single word (Question 2). There is very little evidence that David can highlight a non-final word through Tonic prominence (Question 4), even when this would be expected, as in line 18 of (5.4.2): adult speakers could be expected to place the Tonic on SAID because THAT, in final position, is dispreferred as a location for the Tonic by virtue of being a pronoun. When repeating the same phrase as a repair in line 20, the narrow fall on SAID suggests that he may have some awareness that pitch movement can convey Focus; nevertheless, this pitch movement of about two semitones is overshadowed by the rise of over 15 semitones on THAT. On the other hand, there is some evidence that David responds appropriately to E's use of the Tonic-Focus system (Question 5). The implication of this is that he may understand how the system works but for some reason is unable or unwilling to use it himself. In the discussion of David in Chapter 3 and in the section on Turns in this chapter, it was suggested that it could be a question of unwillingness, because his own idiosyncratic system of final Supertonic placement works very well to mark the end of his turns.

A year after the recording that we have analysed above, David was recorded again at the age of 6;4. His unusual and invariant prosodic pattern had been superseded by the more usual one for the West Midlands variety of British English, whereby the position of the Tonic is determined by considerations of Focus as well as turn completion. A brief illustration is provided in Extract (5.5), taken from a conversation between David and a student speech and language therapist (T), about David's brother:

(5.5)

```
1    T:    ‖so dyou 'play with each 'other at `home‖

                     ╱
           ____

2    D:    ‖yeah‖

3    T:    ‖'what sort of `games dyou 'play‖

                     ╱      ⁻  ⁻  ⁻  ⁻

4    D:    ‖⇑all of the games‖
```

In line 4, the pitch prominence is on "all", rather than on "games". The topic "games" has already been established by the student therapist's question in line 3, and David is contrasting ALL with the interlocutor's expectation of an answer in terms of some specific games. Narrow Focus on ALL is therefore contextually appropriate, leading to the expectation of a non-final Supertonic. David meets this expectation – an achievement that was beyond him a year earlier. Partly as a consequence of such changes, David displayed much greater variety in pitch height and movement in this later recording (see Wells & Local, 1993, for further exemplification). This was accompanied by a marked improvement in his overall intelligibility, suggesting that increased intelligibility allowed a relaxation of his earlier rigid prosodic system for the projection of Turn structure. This analysis led to the hypothesis that David's unusual prosodic behaviour at the age of 5;4 was not a direct consequence of a processing deficit but rather an adaptation to his low level of intelligibility. This idea is discussed further in Chapter 10 in relation to other children with expressive speech and language difficulties.

Actions

As we saw in Chapter 4, the system of Tone in English relates to the social action or actions being performed by the speaker in the turn. We also saw that the type of action (e.g. a request) is not inherent in the Tone; what is key is the speaker's decision whether or not to match the Tone of the speaker of the immediately prior turn. Returning to David at age 5;4, in Extract (5.4.3) we present a systematic transcription of Tone. The transcription of E's turns is as in (5.4). In the case of David, we have placed a rising Tone diacritic ´ on each Tonic syllable, in addition to the Supertonic symbol, to capture the invariant pattern already noted from the impressionistic transcription. A rising pitch movement (though of smaller span) is the most common pattern for the Tonic in the West Midlands variety of English which David is exposed to, as is also the case for several other urban British varieties (e.g. Belfast, Liverpool, Newcastle), which are thus unlike Southern British English in this respect. However, the fact that the high rise is the *only* Tone evident in David's speech suggests that he may lack the richer set of Tones found in the adult West Midlands variety.

Line 1 is notated with **L**, indicating that E starts this extract with a falling Tone reaching the base of her usual pitch range. Each subsequent line is notated to reflect our analysis in terms of Tone matching. Thus, in line 6, for example, David produces a rising Tone; this is followed by a rising Tone from E in line 7, so line 7 is marked as matching, with = ; then in line 8 David produces a rising Tone, so this is also matching. However, in line 9, E produces a falling Tone, which is non-matching, shown by ≠.

(5.4.3)

```
1    E    L    'what dyou think it `is David
2    D    ≠    teddy⇑^bear
3    E    =    yes it ['could be a ˇted]dy bear   hh
4    D    =              [    *      *     ]
5    E    ≠    'whos 'that 'there 'coming up the `path
                    (1.5)
6    D    ≠    post⇑^man
7    E    =    'whats he 'going to ´do
8    D    =    get out a lett⇑´er
                         (1.0)
9    E    ≠    get 'out a `letter
10   D    ≠    ´yes

11   E    =    and 'whats he 'going to ´do with the 'letter
                    (1.0)
12   D    =    put it in (1.7) put it the letter⇑ˇbox
                    (0.8)
13   E    ≠    hes 'going to 'put it 'in the `letter 'box
14   D    ≠    ´yes
                    (1.0)
15   E    =    and 'whos ´this dyou 'think
                    (1.0)
16   D    =    ⇑´girl
                    (1.0)
17   E    ≠    s it a `girl
18   D    ≠    I already said⇑ ´that
                    (0.8)
19   E         she's 'already
                    (0.5)
20   D    =    I already said⇑ ´that
                    (0.3)
21   D    =    I⇑´did
```

In Chapter 4, it was shown that Tone matching is used when the speaker aligns with the action embodied in the prior speaker's turn, continuing on the agenda that has been established. On the other hand, non-matching is used to initiate a new action. In order to complete this section of the profile, it is therefore necessary to decide whether each turn is aligning with or initiating an action. Now complete Activity 5.3.

ACTIVITY 5.3

Aim: To learn how to complete the Actions section on the IIP.

Read through the seven questions in the Actions section. Attempt to answer each question by referring to the phonological transcript that was presented as Extract (5.4.3), also referring as necessary to the phonetic transcript of this interaction that was presented as Extract (5.4). If your answer to a question is *Yes* or *No*, then fill in the line number(s) that provide evidence for your answer. Use the comment box for any further observations relating to the question. As this is a short extract, for some questions it is likely that there will not be evidence either way.
Check your answer with the Key to Activity 5.3 at the end of the chapter.

The Actions section of the IIP shows that David is inconsistent in the way in which he uses matching Tones to align and non-matching Tones to initiate. The inconsistency arises from the consistency with which he always uses a rising Tone. Sometimes this matches E's prior rising Tone, and this conveys his alignment with E's turn, for example, when David is responding to E's question. However, on other occasions where David responds to a question with a rising Tone, this is heard as non-aligning, because E has asked the question with a falling Tone.

In summary, the IIP has shown us that David controls a simple and entirely consistent system for signalling the end of his turn: he uses a rising Tone on the last syllable. However, one consequence is that he is largely inaccurate with regard to the Tonic/Focus system: it works when there should be narrow Focus on the final word, but not otherwise. Another consequence is that he is inconsistent with regard to the Tone matching/Action alignment system. Sometimes David's rising Tone matches E's rising Tone when semantically his response is aligned to E's question. However, on other occasions, this does not happen.

As noted in Chapter 3, the case of David illustrates that what appears to be a disordered prosodic pattern may in fact be an adaptation that improves the individual's chances of participating in conversation. At CA 5;04, David's idiosyncratic prosodic pattern serves to mark the end of his turns at talk in a clear, consistent and unambiguous way, which is useful for him and his co-participants, given the unintelligibility of his speech. By clearly signalling the end of his turn, David manages to maintain interactions without undue overlap or interruption: the Head + Tonic structure provides David with the interactional space to produce turns that consist of several words rather than just a single word. This analysis leads to the hypothesis that David's unusual prosodic behaviour is not a direct result of a processing deficit but rather a compensatory strategy, adapting to his low level of intelligibility. However, it has interactionally problematic consequences for his ability to manage Focus as well as alignment and initiation of Actions. The systematic approach to analysis offered by the IIP enables us to arrive at a balanced picture of David's strengths and weaknesses in respect of the functional use of intonation.

Summary

In this chapter we have introduced the IIP, which is a method for assessing the intonation competences of an individual speaker by examining recordings of their spontaneous speech in naturalistic interaction. While the illustrations in this chapter have been taken from children with atypical intonation, the IIP could also be used to profile the intonation of adult speakers, including speakers who have aphasia or dementia, since the questions in the IIP relate solely to interactional functions, not to developmental factors. In the remaining chapters of this book, we draw on the questions in the IIP to describe patterns of typical and atypical intonation from a developmental perspective. IIPs for a range of children will be presented, enabling the interested reader to become more familiar with this approach.

Key to Activity 5.1

TURNS

Gaining the floor

1 Does C refrain from taking a turn until the current speaker has projected the end of her/his own turn? (C observes red light)

Yes: line *All D's turns*	No: line	No evidence:

Comment: *D only overlaps once (line 4) and that is very quiet*

2 Does C routinely start a turn with minimal pause, following the prior speaker's turn? (C observes yellow and green lights)

Yes: *lines 2, 8, 10, 14, 18*	No: *lines 6, 12, 16*	No evidence:

Comment: *Lines 6, 12, 16 are preceded by silence of c. 1 second*

3 Does C produce an appropriately designed non-competitive turn in overlap, while the current speaker is still talking?

Yes: *line 4*	No: line	No evidence:

Comment: *Unclear what he is saying and so what the function of this turn is*

4 Does C produce an appropriately designed competitive turn in overlap, in a bid to capture the floor while the current speaker is still talking?

Yes: line	No: line	No evidence: *X*

Comment: *D does not produce any competitive overlaps*

Holding the floor

1 Does C produce a turn of more than one word by creating an IP with a Head? (C uses red light)

Yes: *lines 8, 12, 18, 20*	No: line	No evidence:

Comment: *Lines 2, 6, 10, 14, 16 are single-word turns: absence of Head is appropriate to context*

2 Does C produce a turn of more than a single IP by creating a non-final IP before the final IP? (C keeps red light on)

Yes: line	No: line	No evidence: *X*

Comment: *All D's turns of more than 1 word have a single Head + Tonic IP structure*

3 Does C produce a turn of more than a single IP by rushing through a projected TRP at end of the first IP? (C keeps red light on)

Yes: line	No: line	No evidence: *X*

Comment: *D's turns all consist of just 1 IP except lines 20–21, where he waits for a response*

after his first IP

4 Does C resist a turn-competitive incoming by using intonation features? (C keeps red light on)

Yes: line	No: line	No evidence: *X*

Comment: *E never overlaps D, so no evidence of how D would respond to overlap*

Giving up the floor

1 Does C project the end of the turn by using the Tonic? (C uses yellow light)

Yes: line *All*	No: line	No evidence:

Comment: *Tonic is always high rise Tone on final syllable of turn*

2 Does C break off to give way to a turn-competitive incoming? (C uses green light)

Yes: line	No: line	No evidence: *X*

Comment: *E never overlaps D, so there is no evidence*

3 Does C invite collaborative turn completion by producing an incomplete IP as a prompt? (C uses red and green lights)

Yes: line	No: line	No evidence: *X*

Comment: *Line 12 D produces incomplete IP, but no evidence that D expects E to complete*

here. D does respond to E's use of this device in lines 18, 19

Key to Activity 5.2

FOCUS

1 Does C indicate broad Focus over the whole IP by using final Tonic placement?

Yes: line	No: *lines 8, 12*	No evidence:

Comment: *Uses Supertonic on final word, implying narrow rather than broad Focus*

2 Does C indicate narrow Focus on the final word of the IP by using final Supertonic placement?

Yes: *lines 8, 12, 18, 20*	No: line	No evidence:

Comment: *See Q1 above; but there is discrepancy in lines 8, 12, 18, 20, as narrow semantic*

focus is NOT predicted. D also uses Supertonic on single word turns, where narrow vs broad

focus is not an issue.

3 Does C indicate narrow Focus on a non-final word of the IP by using non-final Supertonic placement?

Yes: line	No: line	No evidence:	*X*

Comment: *In this extract, no cases where non-final narrow semantic Focus is predicted. But*

as D always puts Tonic on final syllable of final word, it is unlikely he could do this

4 Does C background non-Focus material, by placing it in the Tail after a non-final Tonic?

Yes: line	No: *lines 18, 20*	No evidence:

Comment: *Tonic is always on final syllable of final word, so no Tails; "old" word may*

receive Supertonic, as in line 18

5 Does C recognize the current speaker's broad and narrow Focus by attending to Tonic and Supertonic placement? Does C design the next turn accordingly?

Yes: *lines 11–12*	No: line	No evidence:

Comment: *D picks up on DO from E's turn, which is the semantic and Tonic Focus and in*

non-final position

Key to Activity 5.3

ACTIONS

Aligning

1 Does C align with the action of the co-participant's prior turn by using Tone matching?

Yes: *lines 8, 12, 16*	No: *lines 2, 10, 14, 18*	No evidence:

Comment: *D always uses Rise; sometimes this matches E's prior turn; but in lines 2, 10, 1 4, Tone*

does not match even though D aligns with E's action by giving responses to her questions. Match not

sensitive to alignment

If so, what actions does C align with? For example, Assessments; Repairs; Requests; Offers

Comment: *request for information about the picture (lines 8, 12, 16)*

2 Does C extend action to a second TCU in own turn, by using Tone matching within the turn?

Yes: *lines 20–21*	No: line	No evidence:

Comment: *D produces 2 x IPs without an intervening turn from E. The second TCU reiterates*

the action of the first; and Tones match

INITIATING

1 Does C initiate a new action, different from the action underway in the previous speaker's prior turn, by using Tone non-matching?

Yes: *line 18 possibly*	No: *lines 2, 10, 14*	No evidence:

Comment: *Unlikely to be intentional non-matching in line 18, as D always uses Rise anyway. Lines*
2, 10, 14: Tone does not match even though D aligns with E's action by giving responses to her
questions. So non-matching not sensitive to alignment and initiation

2 Does C initiate a new action, different from the action underway in C's preceding IP in his own current turn, by using Tone non-matching?

Yes: *line 18*	No: line	No evidence:

Comment: *Tone non-matching in line 18 probably just accidental by-product of always*
using a rise

3 If so, what actions does C initiate by Tone non-matching? For example, Repair; Request.

Comment:	*line 18: D corrects E.*

4 Does C recognize that the prior speaker has initiated a new action by use of Tone non-match, and respond accordingly?

Yes: *lines 9, 13, 17:*	No: line	No evidence:

Comment: *E initiates understanding check, with non-matching Tone .D treats E's turn as*
understanding check: lines 10, 14, 18

CHAPTER 6

Infancy

As our primary focus in this book is on children, it is important to understand how intonation develops in typical children. The aim of Chapters 6–8 is to provide a developmental perspective on the forms and interactional functions of intonation presented in Chapters 1–4, by considering how they emerge as the child matures. Evidence on intonation development is available from studies that researchers have carried out, using a variety of frameworks and methodologies. In order to evaluate these studies in a theoretically consistent way, so that their findings can be compared, we will review them from the perspective of our interactional framework. We present an overview of how the developing child draws on intonation when dealing with progressively more complex interactional and linguistic challenges (cf. Stackhouse & Wells, 1997: 189). One outcome of this review is a model of intonation development, called the Developmental Phase model, presented in Chapter 9 and Appendix 4, incorporating a summary of findings from each of Chapters 6, 7 and 8. This provides a useful comparison when we consider the intonation profiles of children with atypical speech and language development, presented in Chapters 10, 11 and 12.

In this chapter we examine the very first steps in this process, in each of the following four areas:

1 development of relevant perceptual (input) abilities, which are a prerequisite for the development of intonation production;
2 exposure to suitable intonation models by caregivers;
3 deployment of intonation contours in interactionally appropriate ways;
4 production of intonation contours that are phonetically appropriate for the language being learnt.

This chapter covers the period from birth to the point when children are starting to produce utterances that are longer than a single recognizable word. In terms of chronological age, we take this to be around 18 months, though of course there is a good deal of variation among children (Corrin, 2002).

Perception of intonation features

Prior to birth, an infant has already had experience of listening to speech and in the last month or so of normal-term gestation can make use of the experience. One source of evidence for the child's learning of intonation before birth comes from the cries that new-born babies produce. These have been shown to be influenced by the language to which the baby has been exposed (Mampe, Friederici, Christophe, & Wermke, 2009). Summarizing research in this field, Graven and Browne (2008) report that, before birth, infants are able to learn their mother's voice or a melody and to discriminate them from others after birth. They conclude that in the womb the infant can learn to recognize different pitch patterns and rhythms.

There are two features of the environment that affect what the unborn infant can hear. First, the enclosed womb acts as a filter, only allowing certain components of the acoustic signal to penetrate. Second, the womb is a noisy environment, so only sounds above a certain level of loudness will be audible to the foetus.

> The fetus in utero will detect speech, but probably only the low frequency components (below 500Hz) and only when the airborne signal exceeds about 60db. If it is less than that, the signal could be masked by internal noises. It is predicted that the human fetus could detect speech at conversational levels, but only the low frequency components.
>
> *(Gerhardt & Abrams, 2000: S23)*

What kind of speech is the unborn child exposed to? This is not a question that research has addressed to any great extent. It seems to be generally assumed that it will be adult-to-adult speech: the baby can hear the mother as she interacts with other adults. It is possible that in addition the baby will hear a range of other registers of speech, such as the mother's use of infant- or child-directed speech to other children. Parents, carers and siblings may also use infant-directed speech directed toward the unborn child, though to our knowledge this possibility has not been investigated.

To get some idea of the child's experience of speech before birth, it is useful to listen to simulations in which the acoustic signals of normal speech are modified to replicate the ambient noise and filtering properties of the womb. Activity 6.1 makes use of such a simulation.

There has been considerable research interest in young infants' ability to discriminate phonetic cues, including prosodic cues. Sophisticated experimental methodologies have been developed to investigate infants' sensitivity to phonetic changes in stimuli that are played to them. These include measuring changes in the infant's attention by monitoring changes in sucking rate or in head position (Juszczyk, 1997). Nazzi, Floccia, and Bertoncini (1998) demonstrated that even neonates are able to make pitch contour discriminations that are relevant in languages. The participants were

---

ACTIVITY 6.1

Aim: To investigate what aspects of intonation are available to the unborn child.

1 Media File 6.1 simulates the experience of listening in the womb to the voice of a female in her early twenties speaking Southern Standard British English in an informal conversation. Make a note of any features of the woman's speech that you can pick up.
2 In addition to the noise and the filtering properties of the womb demonstrated in the simulation, what other factors may hinder the unborn infant from hearing a clear speech signal?
Check your answer with the Key to Activity 6.1 at the end of this chapter.

French neonates, who in the experiment were able to distinguish between two pitch patterns that are systematically contrasted in Japanese but not in French: a disyllabic low-high pitch pattern vs. a disyllabic high-low pattern. As these French infants had no experience of listening to Japanese, their ability to discriminate this contrast could not have been based on exposure to the pattern before birth.

Related abilities have been demonstrated in slightly older infants (2–3 months) in the discrimination of pitch contours (Karzon & Nicholas, 1989) and other acoustic features relevant to intonation, such as loudness (Bull, Eilers, & Oller, 1984) and duration (Eilers, Bull, Oller, & Lewis, 1984). However, the study by Nazzi *et al.* in 1998 demonstrated that the neonates had the ability not only to discriminate pitch at an acoustic level, but also to extract a common pitch pattern across a list of segmentally diverse words. This ability is a prerequisite for developing representations for the linguistic use of pitch in Tone languages, and also for intonation. The authors concluded that "this sensitivity is part of the universal repertory of infants' innate abilities" (Nazzi *et al.*, 1998: 782). Such studies indicate that from birth, if not before, the basic perceptual mechanisms are in place for intonation development.

As infants get older, there is evidence that perception of linguistic pitch is influenced by the language being spoken around and directly to them. The infant's perception of pitch features seems to be particularly influenced by whether or not the ambient language is a Tone language. Tone languages, which are spoken by the majority of the world's population, are those in which pitch is used systematically to convey differences in lexical (word) and/or grammatical meaning. Examples are Mandarin, Cantonese and Thai, where the function of Tone is primarily lexical. For instance, Standard Thai has five lexical Tones: low, mid, high, rising and falling. Each Thai syllable carries one of these Tones, and Tone alone can differentiate lexical meaning. An example is the syllable /kha/. With mid Tone /kha/ means 'to be stuck'; with low Tone it means 'galangal, a rhizome'; with high Tone it means 'to engage in trade'; with rising Tone it means 'leg' and with falling Tone it means 'to kill' (Kitamura, Thanavishuth, Burnham, & Luksaneeyanawin, 2002). A small number of European languages, including Swedish and Serbo-Croatian, also have a lexical Tone system, though this is much more restricted than in the East Asian languages just mentioned. Grammatical distinctions are conveyed by Tone in many African languages, e.g. Sesotho, Yoruba and Hausa. In non-Tone languages like English, Portuguese and Swahili, pitch is used only for the purposes of intonation, i.e. to convey the types of meaning discussed so far in this book. Sometimes non-Tone languages are referred to as 'intonation languages' though this is misleading, since Tone languages also have intonation systems, in addition to their systems of lexical or grammatical Tone.

Mattock and Burnham, using a head-turn paradigm, showed that at nine months, English-learning infants and Chinese-learning infants already differed in their ability to perceive Tone contrasts as found in language items (Mattock & Burnham, 2006). The stimuli were words from Thai – a Tone language that neither group of children had been exposed to before. At nine months, the children learning Chinese (Mandarin or Cantonese) performed significantly better than the children learning English. However, when the same tasks were given to younger children, aged 6 months, there was no difference between the Chinese-learning and the English-learning groups on this task. On a matched task of pitch perception using a violin rather than a human speaker, there was no difference between Chinese- and English-learning groups at either age point. The authors argue that between 6 and 9 months, children's perception of Tone is reorganized, based on their increased experience of their ambient language. The result is attributed to the fact that the Chinese-learning children, unlike the English-learning children, are themselves learning a Tone language, and thus are having to focus carefully on pitch differences between words.

Children learning a non-Tone language are apparently able to discriminate the relevant prosodic features early in infancy and to maintain that ability. Using disyllabic pseudo-words, Frota, Butler, and Vigário tested infants on a falling vs. rising intonation contrast, which, according to the authors, distinguishes between statements vs. questions in European Portuguese (Frota, Butler, & Vigário, 2014). Infants were able to discriminate this contrast at 5 months and at 8 months. Frota and colleagues argued that the ability to notice pitch distinctions that are relevant in the language being learnt is established early in the first year of life and is maintained. This finding for learners of a non-Tone language thus parallels the conclusion that Mattock and Burnham (2006) came to regarding learners of a Tone language.

In summary, research into early perception suggests that typically-developing infants are sensitive to pitch features of speech from before birth. At birth, they can discriminate pitch contrasts. At the age of 4–6 months, they can demonstrate the ability to make pitch discriminations that have the potential to be linguistically relevant. Subsequently they hold on to that ability but only with specific reference to the type of language they are learning, i.e. a Tone or a non-Tone language. One implication is that prior to cochlear implantation, deaf infants will fall behind their hearing peers on these early pitch-related aspects of phonological development. The communicative impact that this can have is considered in Chapter 12.

Infant-directed speech (IDS)

Having reviewed infants' early pitch perception, we now consider the intonation models that infants are typically exposed to from caregivers, and the ways in which these models may influence intonation development. Given the diversity of intonation systems across languages, and even within dialects of the same language, it is evident that a key factor in intonation development will be the intonation of the language(s) spoken around and to the child. Since intonation conveys meaning, it is important for the child to be able to work out the meaning systems of intonation in the ambient language. Further, for the child who is going to deploy intonation patterns to convey meanings in his own talk, it is the speakers of the ambient language who provide models of those patterns.

In the course of daily life the infant is likely to hear different styles or registers of speech, including adult-to-adult conversation (two-party and multiparty), talk to and between other children, speech from the TV, radio or internet. The most important register to consider here is infant-directed speech (IDS), since it is the register that adult carers typically use when interacting with infants. IDS is distinct from adult-directed speech (ADS) in various ways, some of the most salient of which are prosodic, and it has been proposed that these characteristics of IDS provide assistance to the child in the development of language.

There have been numerous studies of prosodic aspects of IDS, particularly in English. Differences between IDS and ADS include higher pitch, wider pitch range, longer pauses and final lengthening at major constituent boundaries, and a greater tendency to put prosodic focus at the end of constituents (Cruttenden, 1994). There has been a good deal of research attempting to relate such features of IDS to the development of children's ability to segment language input as a basis for recognizing grammatical constituents: the so-called prosodic (or phonetic) bootstrapping hypothesis (Morgan & Demuth, 1996). This hypothesis proposes that, for typically developing children, prosodic factors, particularly the prosodic processing of spoken language input by the infant, may be crucial to the development of other levels of linguistic organization, such as syntax and morphology. However, researchers have not attempted to correlate the prosodic features of IDS with the development of intonation itself. The question that is most relevant to us here has rarely (if at all) been asked: what do the prosodic modifications of IDS mean for the child's learning of intonation? Notwithstanding their different purpose, some of the IDS studies report findings that are relevant to questions that concern us here. First, how does IDS help the infant to find out whether he is learning a Tone language or a non-Tone language? Then, in the case of English, a non-Tone language, how does IDS help the child gain access to the primary functions of intonation: Turn organization (Chapter 2), Focus (Chapter 3) and Action alignment (Chapter 4)?

Tone languages, non-Tone languages and IDS

Some researchers have compared the properties of IDS across different languages, in order to discover to what extent the characteristics of IDS are universal, rather than determined by language and culture. While the prosodic features of IDS described above have been found in several European languages, in some other languages, such prosodic modification is less evident. This has been attributed by some to cultural factors, i.e. attitudes towards and practices of child-rearing, which are known to vary considerably, e.g. in the amount of direct interaction that mothers have with their young children. However, there may also be linguistic factors. This was explored by Kitamura et al. (2002), who compared the IDS of mothers speaking Thai, a Tone language, with that of mothers speaking Australian English. They collected data at different time points, following the mother with her baby from birth to 12 months. They also collected data from each mother talking to adults, so that they could compare IDS with ADS for each language.

In both languages, mothers using IDS would raise the pitch of their voice, as measured by average fundamental frequency; however, the difference between IDS and ADS in Australian English was significantly greater than in Thai. In both languages, mothers used more rising pitch contours in IDS than in ADS; again, the difference was bigger for Australian English than for Thai. Thus, it appears that in their use of pitch in IDS, the Australian mothers deviated more from their ADS norm than did the Thai mothers. The authors attribute these differences to the fact that Thai is a Tone language, and that therefore it is advantageous, in terms of the child's language learning, for the lexical Tones to remain identifiable, even in IDS. If the Thai mothers were to use the wide pitch modifications found in the Australian mothers, there would be a risk of masking the lexical Tone distinctions between, e.g. high vs. mid vs. low, or falling vs. rising. The cross-linguistic differences in IDS are thus a consequence of a particular linguistic driver in Thai as a Tone language, i.e. the need to preserve Tone information for the child's benefit. The results suggest that although there are some prosodic characteristics of IDS that seem to be common to most if not all cultures, IDS can be attuned to specific issues of prosodic learning that are posed by particular languages.

This conclusion is reinforced by longitudinal results from the same study. The last data collection point was when the infants were 12 months old, by which time they would be starting to talk. By this point, the Thai mothers had virtually ceased using the IDS modifications of pitch described above: in terms of prosodic features, they were talking to their infant as if to an adult. This maximized the identifiability of lexical Tones. By contrast, at 12 months, the Australian mothers were using the highest mean pitch of any time point. The authors suggest that this behaviour of the Australian mothers may serve to draw attention to pitch peaks, i.e. Tonics which, as we saw in Chapters 2 and 3, are important in English, both to focus on a new topic or information and also to mark the end of the speaking turn: "Thus, it appears that at 12 months, infant speech development may be facilitated by mothers making language-appropriate modifications to mean F0 [fundamental frequency] which draw infants' attention to specific characteristics of the ambient language" (Kitamura et al., 2002: 387).

In English, a non-Tone language, there are three primary functions of intonation: Focus, Turn construction and Action alignment (see Chapters 2–5). We now consider whether IDS helps the English-learning child gain access to these.

Focus and IDS

Fernald and Mazzie investigated the question of whether, when using IDS, mothers will draw special attention to the function of prosodic prominence in English to highlight focussed words, as described in Chapter 3 (Fernald & Mazzie, 1991). American English mothers told a story to their 14-month-old children from a specially devised picture book about a child getting dressed, where on each new page a new item of clothing was introduced and highlighted pictorially. Each mother also did the same task with another adult as listener, in order to elicit ADS. The mothers routinely used pitch peaks in IDS that were higher compared to ADS. The points of prosodic prominence (i.e. Tonics) were positioned on contextually focussed (new) words more often in IDS than in ADS. The study thus suggests that, in IDS, mothers use the system of Tonic placement in order to highlight important new information, i.e. for narrow Focus; that they do so with greater regularity in their IDS than in their ADS and that they make the Tonics more obvious in IDS than in ADS. This presumably serves to make the system of Tonic placement and Focus more obvious to the infant than would be the case if the infant were only exposed to ADS. IDS should therefore facilitate the infant's learning of this aspect of intonation.

Turn construction and IDS

We saw in Chapters 2 and 3 that the Tonic in English serves a dual function. It may be used to focus on important information, as just discussed. In addition, it is used to project the end of the speaker's turn. We may therefore ask whether IDS can assist the infant in learning about the role of intonation in the construction of turns in conversation. This question has not been directly addressed in IDS research. However, there has been interest in exploring how infants handle intonation phrasing. The preoccupation of that research has mainly been the relation between prosodic (IP) boundaries and syntactic boundaries, particularly clause boundaries. As explained in Chapters 1 and 2, the Intonation Phrase (IP) is the fundamental unit of turn construction. In order to be able to identify potential turn-endings, one skill that the infant therefore needs is the ability to identify IP boundaries. Very often in adult talk, IP boundaries coincide with clause boundaries, so the research that has been conducted into infants' sensitivity to IP boundaries and clause boundaries is relevant to our theme. Much of this work, conducted in the 1980s and 1990s, is summarized by Juszcyk, (1997).

Acoustic studies showed that prosodic markers of clause boundaries are more salient and regular in IDS than in ADS: there are more pitch changes, more instances of segmental lengthening and more pauses (Juszcyk, 1997: 142). This parallels the finding of Fernald and Mazzie (1991) discussed above in relation to Focus. It seems that IDS provides more robust guidance than ADS does to the marking of IP boundaries, and is thus potentially an instructional aid for the infant. Researchers then tried to find out whether infants really do show sensitivity to these major prosodic boundaries. The experiments were based on the idea that in ordinary talk, prosodic (IP) boundaries as described above – marked by features of pitch and lengthening in particular – are often followed by a pause. It was reasoned that, if infants are sensitive to prosodic boundaries, they would prefer to hear a pause when it followed those prosodic boundary features, rather than when it occurred at a random place in the speech stream. To test this out, samples of IDS were recorded and then manipulated experimentally: pauses were inserted either at prosodic (IP) boundaries or at non-boundary places. Infants' preference for one or other of these conditions was assessed using the head-turn procedure. The results suggested that infants as young as 7 months preferred to listen to pauses that coincide with prosodic boundaries. It was then shown that this finding was true for IDS but not for ADS. The finding was replicated with infants as young as 6 months, even when the words in the IDS speech were distorted to make them unintelligible. In sum, this work suggests that the prosodic characteristics of IDS provide a useful model for infants, by helping them to identify IP boundaries (Juszcyk, 1997: 142–144). As explained in Chapter 2, IP boundaries are helpful cues to turn transition, so the ability of identify IP boundaries provides a basis for the child to participate in turn exchange.

Alignment and IDS

In Chapter 4, we proposed that for a speaker of English the major function of Tone choice is to align with the prior speaker, by using a matching Tone, or to initiate a new action, by using a non-matching Tone. We now consider whether there are any features of IDS that potentially have instructional value for the infant in this respect.

Most studies of IDS have been conducted within an experimental paradigm that disregards vocal responses from the infant, focussing instead on other behavioural responses, such as sucking or head turning. This therefore excludes the possibility of finding direct evidence for the interactional effects of Tones in IDS. However, there is some indirect evidence that IDS may help the infant to engage in social interaction. Kitamura et al., reviewing the benefits of IDS for the child as identified by previous research, comment that in addition to providing a direct model for language learning, IDS "engages and maintains attention" and "communicates affect and facilitates social interaction" (2002: 373). They note that infants' preference for IDS over ADS is attributable more to pitch than to other prosodic features such as loudness and duration, although it is not clear what exactly the pitch features are that make IDS more attractive and therefore, presumably which help to engage attention and stimulate social interaction. In their own study, as we saw earlier, Kitamura et al. (2002) found that mothers used more rising pitch contours in IDS than in ADS. This suggests that the

Australian English-speaking mothers may be using more rising Tones at Tonic position. However, without information about the context in which these rising Tones occurred (i.e. following another rising Tone, or following a falling Tone), it is impossible to assess the implications of this finding about IDS with regard to the child's development of the (Australian) English Tone system.

Another proposal is that the action that an adult speaker wishes to accomplish through a turn at talk is communicated more effectively in IDS than in ADS. Having low-pass filtered utterances to render them unintelligible, Fernald (1989) found that listeners were better able to identify the communicative intent of an utterance from IDS than from ADS. This suggests that some of the prosodic modifications that carers make in IDS can enhance the clarity of their utterance in terms of its pragmatic force. It may be that some actions are more susceptible to this enhancement in IDS than others. Bryant and Barrett (2007)found that "prohibition" and "approval" utterances were more easily recognized in IDS than in ADS, whereas for "comfort" and "attention [getting]" utterances there was no difference. However, it is not known whether the relevant modifications are to do with choice of Tone (e.g. more rises) or some other phonetic parameter.

In summary, studies of IDS in non-Tone languages have contributed little to our understanding of whether IDS facilitates the child's learning of how to use Tone matching for interactional and pragmatic purposes. Nevertheless, the results are consistent with the possibility that prosodic characteristics of IDS may facilitate the identification of some social actions in which intonation is implicated.

It seems obvious that the primary factor determining the particular intonation patterns that a child will learn to use will be the intonation patterns that are heard. Our interpretation of the IDS research in this section has been predicated on an assumption – one which appears to underlie virtually all IDS research – that the infant will be exposed to a single accent or dialect of a single language (e.g. Standard Thai or Australian English or American English) and therefore to the IDS register of that accent of that language. However, many young children find themselves in more complex linguistic environments. The effect on intonation development of truly simultaneous bilingual situations, where the child is exposed to two different languages (Gut, 2000) and may be exposed to IDS in both, has hardly been studied. Even where there is a single language, it is quite likely that the child's caregivers speak different varieties of the language to the child. Parents and grandparents may come from different geographical regions; in some situations, the infant may have a child minder who is from a different region or for whom the child's native language is a second language, e.g. an au pair. In the case where the family language is English, it may be that the one parent is a speaker of standard southern British English (SSBE), while another speaks a regional variety, such as Northern Irish, which has a very different inventory and distribution of intonation contours (Wells & Peppé, 1996): in Northern Irish, turn completion is typically accompanied by rising contours whereas in SSBE a fall is most common (cf. Chapters 1 and 2). The infant may have a child minder who speaks a strong Afro-Caribbean variety which does not have the system of Tonic placement found in SSBE and most other British varieties: instead, the main pitch movement is almost invariably located on the final word or even syllable of the utterance, and Focus is done by other means, such as segmental lengthening (Local et al., 1985). Thus, all three of the infant's principal adult interlocutors may speak to the child in the same language (English) but each may be using a more or less different intonation system. Moreover, the proportion of input from these different sources may change over time, due to absence of a parent or change in caring arrangements. If a child's caregivers come from different linguistic or dialect backgrounds, the models of intonation will be mixed, and therefore potentially confusing for the infant trying to establish systems. In some situations, even the Tone language vs. non-Tone language distinction may be obscured. Some varieties of English, e.g. as spoken in Nigeria and by Nigerian families in the UK, retain Tone language features deriving from the African languages spoken in the same area, such as Hausa, Igbo and Yoruba, all of which are Tone languages (Gut, 2000). Dealing with input from a variety of English that has Tone language characteristics, such as Nigerian English, at the same time as a more standard, intonation-only variety such as Southern British English, may pose a challenge for infants who have to work out what kind of prosodic system they needs to learn. Some of the implications for children with language difficulties are discussed in Chapter 10.

Tone or non-Tone language?

From around 9 months, children appear to confront the issue of whether or not the language they are having to learn is a Tone language. As has been mentioned in the section above on IDS, languages can be classified as either Tone languages or non-Tone languages. In Tone languages, pitch is used to distinguish word meaning (lexical Tone) and/or grammatical function (grammatical Tone). An example of the latter is the Bantu language Sesotho, one of the official languages of South Africa. Verbs basically have a Tonal specification of either High or Non-high, but the actual pitch realization, particularly for verbs in the non-high Tone category, varies considerably depending on the context in which it appears. Demuth (1995) reports for a child she studied that the system was only mastered by the age of 3.

It is reported that lexical Tone is acquired earlier by children learning Asian Tone languages such as Thai and Mandarin Chinese, as their lexical Tone systems are more transparent than grammatical Tone systems like that of Sesotho. In her longitudinal study of phonological development in Mandarin (Putonghua), Zhu Hua (2002) analysed the Tonal acquisition of four children (Hua, 2002). She reported that the Tones were mastered by CA 1;10. In terms of the order of acquisition of Tones, the high level and high falling Tones were the first to emerge (CA 1;02) and to stabilize (CA 1;06-1;07). Rising Tones emerged around CA 1;04, and falling-rising Tones between 1;04–1;07, both stabilizing by 1;10. Mandarin is considered to be a relatively simple system, in which individual words tend to retain the same pitch pattern in different phonetic and grammatical contexts. Compared to Mandarin, it takes more time for the child to learn how to produce the appropriate Tone pattern of the Sesotho verb. However, even in Mandarin there are some complications: some Tones take longer to stabilize in the child's inventory because their distribution is more complicated in the adult language (Yip, 2002) and there are combinatorial rules that take up to age 5 to be acquired, according to Li and Thompson (1977).

Given that the acquisition of Tone is well underway in the first half of the second year, an important question for us is: how does the child work out that they are learning a non-Tone language, such as English, rather than a Tone language such as Mandarin, Thai or Sesotho, i.e. that pitch differences in English are *not* associated with lexical or grammatical meaning? For the child learning a Tone language, we saw earlier in this chapter that adults preserved the lexical Tones of the language when using the IDS register, and that this contrasted with the IDS behaviour of adults using a non-Tone language like English, who indulged in a lot more pitch variation. Thus, the ambient linguistic environment may help to steer the child learning the Tone language into making the right choice. However, it is not obvious how this is achieved. It appears that initially, in the first year of life, the infant exposed to a Tone language like Mandarin or Thai may not always reproduce the lexical Tone accurately, and may be using pitch instead for interactional purposes, as in a non-Tone language. The child then progressively comes to appreciate that individual words are associated with a specific pitch contour (Tuaycharoen, 1977). The evidence from the Mandarin studies mentioned above, as well as Tuaycharoen's research on Thai, indicate that the lexical use of pitch is established during the second year of life. Presumably the continued exposure to distinct Tone patterns in IDS that are consistently associated with distinct sets of lexical items helps a child to revise an original hypothesis that pitch primarily has an intonational function rather than a lexical function.

For the child learning a non-Tone language, the evidence from IDS is probably less helpful, sometimes even counter-productive. There is some evidence that in English IDS, certain words are produced with specific pitch patterns, e.g. GOOD with a rise-fall pitch, NO with a low fall or level pitch (Quam, Yuan, & Swingley, 2008). This could be confusing for the child learning a non-Tone language. On the whole, however, words produced by adults in English IDS seem to be characterized by a lot of pitch variation. While this may help the child to discount the possibility that English is a (lexical) Tone language, it provides little positive assistance to the child in working out what the functional role of pitch is in English.

Despite this apparent lack of guidance from the environment, young children learning English learn not to react to pitch as a potential marker of lexical Tone. Quam and Swingley (2010) showed experimentally that children at CA 2;6 were not distracted by changes in pitch when associating a newly learnt segmental string, (i.e. a new 'word') with a particular meaning. The authors conclude by asking how English-learning children come to this understanding, i.e. what the trajectory of development may be up to that point:

> This trajectory could take two forms. Children could start out disregarding pitch variation, and then learn, through exposure to their native language, to attend to pitch at the relevant levels. Alternately, children could start out treating pitch as potentially relevant (e.g., at the lexical level), and then learn to ignore it if their native language does not provide evidence of structure at that level.
>
> *(Quam & Swingley 2010: 147)*

Some evidence to support the second trajectory can be found from the study of Nigel, conducted by (Halliday, 2003). Halliday reports that in the earliest phase of linguistic development, from 9 to 10.5 months, Nigel's first stable and meaningful vocalizations, which do not obviously derive from the ambient language, are associated with a fixed pitch contour. While this is always some kind of fall, the kind of fall, in terms of its starting point and width, may vary depending on the word, as in the examples in Table 6.1 (Halliday, 2003: 36).

A possible interpretation of these data is that Nigel, who is exposed to a non-Tone language (English) is nevertheless entertaining a hypothesis that he needs to learn a

Table 6.1 Nigel's fixed Tone patterns (adapted from Halliday, 2003).

Nigel's utterance	Pitch contour	Assumed meaning
[mnŋ]	high-wide fall	"do that right now"
[bø]	mid fall	"give me my bird"
[ɜ]	mid fall	"do that (again)"
[a]	low fall	"that's nice"
[nŋ]	low fall	"that tastes nice"
[gʷɤy gʷɤy gʷɤy]	low-narrow fall	"I'm sleepy"

Tone language – the hypothesis that children learning Thai or Mandarin subsequently pursue.

Nigel apparently did not pursue this Tone language hypothesis. Instead, according to Halliday, Nigel found out that different Tones come to be associated with different communicative functions. Eventually, by the time of his first word combinations at around 19 months, Nigel began to operate with a simple system whereby he produced utterances requiring some kind of response from an interlocutor, with a rising pitch; whereas utterances that did not require a response were produced with a falling pitch contour. This system, which was maintained for some months, means that the same word or similar phrases can be produced with either a rising or a falling Tone, depending on its communicative function. Thus when Nigel produced chuffa ´stuck with a rising Tone, glossed by Halliday as THE TRAIN'S STUCK, HELP ME TO GET IT OUT, the utterance functions to request an action from the adult; whereas chuffa `stop, with a falling Tone, glossed as THE TRAIN'S STOPPED, does not require a response (Halliday, 2003: 106).

Following Halliday's approach, it can be proposed that children learning a non-Tone language like English are able to dissociate Tone from lexical items once they have realized that Tone can be used contrastively to convey distinct communicative functions. For Nigel, it appears that this process started around 13 months (p. 22), becoming particularly striking at 19 months when he started to produce rising Tones in addition to falling Tones. However, given that adult English lacks transparent associations between distinct pitch patterns and communicative functions, the question remains as to how the child actually manages to arrive at such a system. Indeed, Nigel's use of Tone at this stage was sometimes at variance with what is considered the usual Tone in adult English: Halliday cites the case of imperatives, which Nigel produces with a rise as they are "pragmatic", e.g. squeeze ´orange, directed by Nigel to his carer (p. 106) although in adult English imperatives are "typically falling" (p. 263). We return to this issue later in the chapter.

Intonation in infant interactions

So far in this chapter we have investigated infant perception of intonation-related features and the intonational characteristics of the speech that infants are exposed to. We next consider how infants begin to make use of intonation in interactionally appropriate ways, as active participants in conversations. Cross-cultural studies of language development have pointed to a wide range of variation in how adults, notably parents and other carers, interact with their infant children. Many western parents interact closely and directly with their child, and it is tempting to see their approach as 'teaching' the infant how to do language, including how to do intonation. In other cultures, there appears to be relatively little direct interaction with parents. This has been used to argue that all the children need as input is the ambient language wafting around. However, little research has been reported on precisely what kinds of interactions infants are involved in in such cultures, e.g. with older siblings and other members of the extended family. Here, attention will be given to the potentials of interaction between child and adult (or other older interlocutor) for facilitating the child's development of intonation.

Turn-taking

In Chapter 2 we described how intonation is involved in the construction of turns and the projection of ends of turns. Of course, there is a lot more to turn-taking than intonation. Apart from the linguistic content of turns in terms of grammar and vocabulary, non-verbal aspects such as gesture and, particularly, eye gaze have a key role. Non-verbal behaviour has been a common theme in the considerable body of research on early Turn-taking between infant and carer (for a review, see Filipi, 2009: 2–7). However, in line with the theme of this book, in this section we concentrate specifically on the role of vocalization in early Turn-taking, with a particular focus on intonational aspects. Our question is: how does the Turn-taking function of intonation emerge in early interaction? It has been well documented that infants use vocalizations from birth; that the timing and prosodic design of vocalizations change through the first year of life; and that through the timing and design of their own vocalizations, the mother and other carers actively respond to the infant's production of vocalizations as potential or actual conversational turns. We first consider the timing of vocal turns by the carer and the infant.

In the early months of vocal interaction, it has been reported that a high proportion of the talk by infant and mother is in overlap. In a study of three North American mother–infant dyads, the overlaps peaked when the infants were between 7 and 13 weeks old (Ginsburg & Kilbourne, 1988). This was followed by an increase in non-overlapping alternation between mother and infant vocalizations, suggesting that the infants had become more aware of how the alternation of turns is basic to conversational organization. Subsequent large-scale statistical analysis of Australian English mother–infant interaction confirmed that with even the youngest infants the majority of talk is alternating; thus overlap is less common than alternating turns that do not overlap (Elias & Broerse, 1996). Broerse and Elias (1994) found that mothers typically started talking less than one second following the end of an infant vocalization. In this respect, mothers adhere to the practice in adult conversation of minimizing the gap between turns. Thus, there is already a trend towards a fundamental practice of Turn-taking: to minimize gaps and overlaps (Sacks et al., 1974).

The incidence of overlapping talk changes as the child gets older: the proportion decreases between 3 and 18 months, then increases again until age 2 (Elias & Broerse, 1996). It was suggested that the high incidence of overlap in early infancy may provide conditions that help infants learn that their own vocal behaviour guides the actions of their partner. When the infant is young, the mother produces in overlap many turns that do not add topically relevant information, but simply provide supportive feedback. As the infant gets older, this type of turn is more likely to be produced following the infant's turn, rather than simultaneously with it.

Filipi (2009: 98) presents detailed qualitative analysis of interactions at this stage. In Activity 6.2, we investigate an interaction between one of the mother–child pairs studied by Filipi.

ACTIVITY 6.2

Aim: To investigate Turn-taking between an infant aged 9 months and the primary caregiver.

In Extract (6.2), Rosie (CA 0;9) is sitting in the lap of Kathy, her mother. The transcript is adapted from Filipi (2009: 83). The video recording may be accessed at https://benjamins.com/#catalog/books/pbns.192.05ch3/video/7.

Examine the transcripts of the following lines, watching and listening to the recording if accessible:

1 lines 4–6
2 lines 8–10
3 lines 20–3.

In each case, describe what Kathy does to show that she treats Rosie's vocalization as a conversational turn. First, consider the timing of Kathy's turn. Then note any other features that are relevant in your opinion. Use the traffic light terminology from Chapter 2 as appropriate.

Check your answer with the Key to Activity 6.2 at the end of this chapter.

(6.1)

```
1     K:    ((Holds up a rattle))
2     R:    ((takes it))
3           {( looks at Kathy)
```

```
4     R:    {ʔiʔa::::: ?
            {  ff  }
5           (0.2)
```

```
6     K:    .hh are you happy to ha[{ve it]
7     R:                           { looks away; shakes head
```

```
8     R:                           [(a:]    {əm əm  [  əm  ]
9                                           { looks at Kathy
```

```
10    K:                                             [{ye:s]
11                                                    {nods
12           (0.4)
```

```
13    K:    you {tell me
14              {nods ((Leans forward.))
15    R:    (0.6)
```

```
16    K:    are   {you   {enjoying      that
```

```
17            {((Leans forward.))
18    R:      ((Extends rattle in direction of camera, shakes it.))
              { looks at camera
19            (1.8)
```

```
                    ＼ ─ ─
         ─ ─           ─ ─ ＼
```

```
20    R:      ʔə  ja {ja:  ja  ja  {ja  ja  ja:
                    {ff …  dim  …  f}
21            looks at camera
                          { looks at Kathy
```

```
         ⌒
              ＼ _
```

```
22    K:      {rea:{lly
23            {nods
24    R:      { looks at camera
25            (1.0)
```

In Extract (6.2), Kathy treats the infant's actions as moves in a conversation, minimizing the gap after each of Rosie's vocal turns: she may come in as soon as Rosie has stopped vocalizing (line 22); in overlap with the end of Rosie's turn (line 10); or after only a short pause (line 6). Kathy seems to respond to Rosie having reached a low point in her pitch range, thereby treating Rosie as already using the intonation traffic light system. The extract illustrates how an adult will orient to the alternation of turns with the infant, even though there are no discernible words in the infant's turns.

What do such observations suggest about the development of intonation? It seems that carers are careful about where they place their turn. In general, this reflects the pattern of adult conversation: adults prefer alternating turns with only a short gap between turns. However, adults are also sensitive to the infant's developing skills: they reduce the amount of overlap as the infant gets older. The resurgence of overlap in the latter part of the second year is attributed to changes in the frequency and duration of the partners' talk: at this age the child is starting to produce utterances longer than a single word. Both mother and child are producing longer utterances, and so are more likely to overlap one another.

The suggestion that Rosie and other infants at her stage use pitch to produce a Tonic-like final syllable that signals the end of the turn needs to be treated with caution, however. In a study of children learning American English, David Snow (2002) compared ten infants, aged 10–13 months, to ten 4-year-olds. He measured falling pitch contours produced by the children in a spontaneous free play situation. For the infants, these were monosyllabic utterances – some meaningful, others not (i.e. babble). Snow found that the falling contours produced by the infants had a significantly narrower pitch range than those produced by the 4-year-olds in utterance final position. This suggests that one aspect of intonation that will change and develop with age is the pitch range associated with the Tonic. Because the infants' pitch range is narrow, it is less likely to be perceived by adult listeners as marking the end of the turn. This may be one reason why, when the infant starts producing longer (two-word) turns, the conversational partner is sometimes unsure as to when the infant's turn is complete.

In sum, the evidence suggests that up to around 18 months, mother and infant progressively develop a Turn-taking system rather like the one used in adult conversation. It works fine, though only as long as the infant is producing utterances of not more than a single word. However, it is liable to run into trouble when the child starts to produce longer utterances. Research to be presented in Chapter 7 suggests that by around 18 months, children do not yet have a robust and consistent way of signalling the end of a turn, since they are liable to come to grief when producing turns longer than a single word.

Focus

In Chapter 3 we saw that in multiword utterances speakers of English can use Tonic prominence to focus on a word that represents the important topical element of the turn. As infants at the stage considered in the present chapter do not produce turns of more than a single word, this is not yet an option for them. In spite of this, it is evident, certainly by around one year of age, that the infant and carer are able to participate in interactions about a particular topic. Does intonation have any part to play in this?

It has long been noted by child language researchers that children at the single-word stage may accompany the production of a word by a pointing gesture (Filipi, 2009: 12). This can provide a resource for the child to initiate a sequence and provide a topic, all within a single turn. In line 1 of Extract (6.3) (adapted from Filipi, 2009: 131), Cassandra (CA 1;2) produces a single word, repeated, which seems to be her version of LOOK. This serves to capture the attention of Richard, her father, who is holding her in his arms. She simultaneously points to a piece of furniture.

(6.2)

```
1   C:   ook (.) ook ((points to chest of drawers with middle
         finger right hand.))

2   R:   look wha-.

3                  (0.2)

4   R:   wha-. {((turns in direction of point.))

5   C:   (stops pointing))

6        (0.4)((Rich starts to turn around to face chest of
         drawers))

7   C:   ook ((points to the same object but with her left hand,))

8        (0.4)
```

```
 9   R:   Mm
10   C:   (0.5)   ((stops pointing))
11   C:   ook!
12   R:   reading?
13        (0.8)
14   C:   Ook
15        ((They both turn away.))
```

Richard's response in lines 2 and 4 reveals the limitations of Cassandra's way of nominating a topic: the pointing is not specific enough to identify what it is about the chest of drawers that she wants him to attend to. Even though she stops her original point and points again with her other hand while repeating LOOK (line 7; line 11), Richard still fails to identify what it is that she is indicating. Clearly, the ability to use two words and to highlight one of them as the topic by using Tonic prominence, is going to be an important development, as it will reduce, and often eliminate, the vagueness that is inherent in pointing. This will be discussed in Chapter 7.

Perhaps because of the limitations for the child at this stage in terms of resources for topic nomination, carers are very willing to topicalize any vocal production that the child makes. A vocalization consisting of a short laugh, or an unintelligible syllable or two, is likely to be treated by the adult as a turn at talk from the infant, and the adult will seek a referent for the vocalization. Typically, the adult's response is to ask the child a question in order to identify with greater accuracy what the child's topic is. Interestingly, the same orientation is evident from the carer in an interaction that will be described in Chapter 12, where the child is much older but, as the result of a severe hearing impairment and other difficulties, is unable to produce utterances of more than a word or two. In sum, it is sometimes sufficient for the child merely to create a vocal turn; the carer will then do a lot of work to make sense of that turn, in terms of its topic reference (cf. Filipi, 2009: 85).

Alignment, initiation and matching

In Chapter 4, it was proposed that the main factor determining choice of Tone in the English intonation system is whether or not the speaker wishes to align with the prior speaker's action as embodied in the immediately preceding turn. This gave rise to a series of questions that were incorporated into the Intonation in Interaction Profile (IIP) in Chapter 5. Here we consider the first of these questions from the perspective of the infant: does the infant align with the action of the caregiver's prior turn by using Tone matching?

Infants produce vocalizations from birth. From the outset, researchers distinguish vocalizations that are communicative, where the infant is engaged by or engaging with the mother or other carer, as opposed to ones that apparently are not directed by the infant to any communicative end. There is some evidence that these two classes of vocalization are prosodically distinguishable: for English-learning infants at 10 months, the communicative vocalizations are reportedly characterized by higher pitch and shorter duration than the non-communicative vocalizations (Papaeliou & Trevarthen, 2006). A similar finding has been reported for Catalan infants (Esteve-Gibert & Prieto, 2012). Our focus here is on communicative vocalizations, since interactional situations are the ones in which the infant has to deal with the adult intonation system. However, in Chapter 7, we will consider the role of the non-communicative type of situation in children's intonation development.

We begin by considering studies that have looked at infants' imitation of carers' vocalizations, since evidence of imitation would indicate the infant has a basis for matching another speaker's Tone and therefore for achieving interactional alignment. Careful naturalistic studies of vocal imitation in the first months of life provide insights into the dynamics of intersubjective communication. Papoušek and Papoušek (1989) noted that all the mother–infant pairs in their study exhibited vocal matches at all ages. In a study of French mothers and their babies aged around 3 months, Gratier and Devouche (2011) report that imitation of the mother's pitch contour by the infant was found in 27% of pairs of vocalization where the infant's vocalization followed the mother; almost the same proportion of pitch imitations, 30%, was found in the reverse situation, i.e. where the mother followed the infant. The authors argue that this type of pitch imitation has communicative significance, supporting mutual engagement at the moment where it occurs, and also serves to promote the infant's development of the repertoire of Tones used in the adult language.

Balog (2010) addressed the same question with American English infants, who at 12–13 months were older than those in the French study by Gratier and Devouche (2011). In a similar way, she investigated whether children match the contour direction of the preceding adult utterance. Although the proportion of infant imitations of maternal pitch direction was higher than in the French study, Balog's interpretation of the results was much more negative: according to her, it indicated that the children were not attempting to match their contour direction to that of the immediately preceding adult input: "Children's contour direction was random relative to contour direction in the preceding adult utterance, matching it only 50% of the time" (Balog, 2010: 344). However, this interpretation of 50% imitations as 'random' behaviour does not take account of the communicative role of pitch contour matching, which was recognized by Gratier and Devouche. In Chapter 4, it was proposed that in English, imitation of Tone is a choice that speakers make in order to align with the prior speaker's action. If this is the case, it is to be expected that on many other occasions, as shown in Chapter 4, the speaker will initiate a new action, by *not* matching the prior speaker's contour. Since Balog did not take account of the interactional context or actions being performed in these mother–infant interactions, her data are not readily interpretable, beyond the conclusion that there seems to be *prima facie* evidence that infants at this age do indulge in pitch matching to the mother's prior turn. The 50% proportion of imitations that Balog found may actually represent a developmental increase over the c. 27% reported by Gratier and Devouche for younger infants, although it has to be remembered that the studies did involve different languages.

Unfortunately there have not yet been detailed qualitative studies of specific instances of infant imitation of pitch contour which would throw light on the interactional mechanisms involved in acquiring this intonation system. However, from group studies of the type just reported, it is reasonable to conclude that Tone imitation of the mother by the infant, and vice versa, is a common feature of infant–carer interaction. The results are at least compatible with the proposal that Tone imitation already serves the purpose of aligning with the prior speaker. This position finds indirect support from a body of research proposing that rhythmic synchrony of vocalizations, and accommodation of pitch contours, are core features of early carer–infant interactions (Trevarthen, 2008).

This then leads us to the question of non-imitative turns. Does the infant initiate a new action, different from the action underway in the caregiver's prior turn, by using non-matching Tone? In Chapter 4, it was proposed that a non-matching Tone serves to initiate a new action but does not specify what that action is. However, the hypothesis underlying most research into Tonal development at this stage is that in the adult language, Tone *is* directly related to pragmatic functions, such as 'request' or 'statement', so the infant's job is to learn how Tones map onto these pragmatic functions.

Halliday's study of the intonation development of his son Nigel, referred to earlier in this chapter, is situated squarely within this kind of approach. He identifies six functions which "would serve for the interpretation of the language of a very young child" (Halliday, 1975 :18): Instrumental, Regulatory, Interactional, Personal, Heuristic, and Imaginative. Up to around CA 1;06, Nigel used high level Tones on proper names, and otherwise a variety of falling Tones. Then at CA 1;07, Nigel within a week "introduced a systematic opposition between rising and falling Tone" (Halliday, 1975: 52), which he retained from CA 1;07 to CA 2;0 with complete consistency.

However, there are some difficulties with Halliday's study. First, it is based on field observations without the use of audio or video recordings, which raises the issue of reliability and therefore replicability. Vonwiller (1988) attempted to replicate Halliday's analysis by classifying the audio- recorded vocalizations of six Australian infants at age 9 and age 12 months using Halliday's categories. Her conclusion supports Halliday's analysis: "There is a quite remarkable conformity of tone and pitch height when associated with function as set out by Halliday" (Vonwiller 1988: 125). Her results are summarized in Table 6.2. There seems to be a persuasive mapping from pitch contour to pragmatic function. Rising pitch is associated with questioning (heuristic and regulatory), i.e. directly interacting with a specific person. Level Tones may be used for a variety of functions, including demands. On the other hand, falls and rise-falls are associated with functions other than questions and demands.

However, there is a circularity with this approach, in that the attribution of an infant vocalization to one of these categories is done on the basis not only of accompanying non-verbal and contextual information, but also of the pitch contour itself (Vonwiller 1988: 104).

Studies that have tried to avoid this type of circularity reveal that the approach is conceptually flawed from the outset. The most telling account of the difficulties encountered when approaching the question of Tone acquisition from this perspective is a study of requests by Flax, Lahey, Harris, and Boothroyd (1991). They recorded three American English-speaking mother–child dyads at three time points, between the ages of 0;11 and 1;10 (Child 1) ; 1;2 and 1;8 (Child 2); and 1;0 and 1;6 (Child 3). The aim was to relate pre-selected prosodic variables to communicative functions. Measurements of pitch (F0) direction were made of all utterances, which were then

Table 6.2 Mapping of pitch contour (Tone) and height onto Halliday's functions (adapted from Table 10.3 in Vonwiller, 1988).

Functions	Gloss	Tone	Pitch height
Heuristic	Query; to gain information about environment	rise	high
Regulatory	Control the behaviour of others: challenge; protest; call, request, etc.	rise	mid/high
		level	mid
Instrumental	Satisfy child's needs: demand, want (no specific addressee)	level	mid
Interactional	Interact with others: greetings, naming, agreeing, vocal pointing, etc.	level	mid
		fall	mid
Personal	Express feelings about environment (no specific addressee)	rise-fall	mid
		rise-fall	high

collapsed into two categories: rise vs. non-rise. Measurements of centre, peak and range of F0 were also used. Communicative functions, which were derived from a range of earlier studies, among them Halliday (1975), included four types of request, and three kinds of comment. Utterances were assigned to these communicative categories by the researchers, with provisions for inter-rater reliability.

Three findings are particularly relevant here. First, over time there was no change for any child, in the relation between contextual function and final pitch contour, i.e. rise vs. non-rise. On the face of it, this might be taken as evidence that the intonation system (or at least this aspect of it) is established very early. However, this is thrown into some doubt by the second finding, that there was a considerable difference between the children regarding the proportion of rise vs. non-rise contours used. This between-child variation might still make sense: it may be the case that the basic intonation contrast works in the same way for all the children but that some happen to make more requests than others. However, the third finding was that there was no consistent mapping of intonational form to communicative function: although rises tended to be used for 'requesting' functions rather than for other functions, non-rises too were used for requesting functions as well as for non-requesting functions. As a result, we cannot draw any conclusions about the development of intonation in relation to communicative function. Indeed, the results beg the question of whether even in adult English there is a consistent relationship between rise and request. This possibility was raised in the discussion of questions and intonation in Chapter 4.

Following these inconclusive results, Flax et al. (1991) made a plea for further, more detailed research on the input from caregivers, as this may be a factor in determining how a child uses particular pitch patterns. A further recommendation from Flax et al. was that future research should consider not just the input to the child but also the children's interactions with caregivers. They suggested that in their study the children's use of rise vs. non-rise might have been influenced by quite local factors in the interaction. This is the view taken in Chapter 4, where it is proposed that the main factor influencing a speaker's choice of Tone is the Tone used by the previous speaker.

In sum, it has not proved possible to identify a mapping of infant pitch patterns or Tones onto communicative functions. These potentially negative conclusions do not exclude the possibility, outlined in Chapter 4, that the primary function of Tone choice is to match or not to match the prior speaker's turn, and thereby to demonstrate alignment with the action of that prior turn or else the initiation of a new action. There is some evidence for this in Extract 6.1, which we studied in Activity 6.2 and which is reproduced here:

(6.1)

```
1    K:    ((Holds up a rattle))
2    R:    ((takes it))
3          {( looks at Kathy)
```

```
4    R:    {ʔiʔa::::: ?
            {  ff  }
5          (0.2)
```

```
6    K:    .hh are you happy to ha[{ve it]
7    R:                           { looks away; shakes head
```

```
8    R:                           [(a:] {əm əm [ əm  ]
9                                       { looks at Kathy
```

```
10   K:                                          [{ye:s]
11                                                {nods
12         (0.4)
```

```
13   K:    you {tell me
14             {nods ((Leans forward.))
15   R:    (0.6)
```

```
16   K:    are {you {enjoying that
17         {((Leans forward.))
18   R:    ((Extends rattle in direction of camera, shakes it.))
           { looks at camera
```

```
19          (1.8)
```

```
20    R:    ʔə ja {jaː ja ja {ja ja jaː
            {ff … dim … f}
```

```
21          looks at camera
                          { looks at Kathy
```

```
22    K:    {rea:{lly
23          {nods
24    R:    { looks at camera
25          (1.0)
```

Rosie's turn in line 4 has a falling contour, which is matched by Kathy in line 6. While Kathy's turn takes the form of an interrogative structure, her matching Tone starting on HAPPY suggests that she is responding to and acknowledging Rosie's smile and animated vocalization as an expression of happiness. Starting in overlap over the Tail of Kathy's IP, Rosie produces another, narrower fall, matching the direction of Kathy's Tone. The two participants seem to be aligned on the topic of the rattle and Rosie's pleasure with it. Nevertheless, in line 10, Kathy checks her understanding of Rosie's response in line 8 by producing the potentially confirmatory "yes" but with a non-matching Tone. On not receiving a confirmation from Rosie, Kathy pursues her original question from line 6 with a turn in the form of a syntactic imperative in line 13 and then an interrogative in line 16. Both these turns have a falling Tone, matching each other and the original request in line 6, indicating that despite reformulations of grammar and vocabulary, Kathy is pursuing a single interactional agenda, namely to elicit a vocal response from Rosie, as discussed by Filipi in her analysis of this extract (Filipi, 2009: 85). Finally, in line 20, Rosie produces a vocal turn with a falling pitch contour. Kathy immediately responds using the word "really", which marks Rosie's turn as having been newsworthy, and with a matching falling Tone that shows she aligns with Rosie's turn.

In summary, this extract suggests that in interactions with an infant the carer is able to use Tone matching and non-matching to progress her own agenda. There is also some indication that the infant too may orient to Tone matching as a marker of alignment.

Production of prosodic features

So far in this chapter we have seen that the basics for intonation perception are already in place at birth and that infant-directed speech and interaction between carer and infant may serve to refine both the perception and the production of intonation in the direction of systems that are relevant to the language that the child is learning. There is also a physiological maturational component that may affect intonation production in important ways. Until age 3 months the infant's vocal and respiratory anatomy are quite stable, following which the larynx starts to descend (Kent & Vorperian, 1995). There is an increase in the size of the pharyngeal cavity and by 6 months the laryngeal muscles begin to be used to control pitch (Vonwiller, 1988), leading to noticeable changes in the infant's pitch production. Exploring the effects of such changes on the production of pitch contours, Vonwiller (1988) recorded the vocal development of six Australian infants from 3 to 12 months.

At a phonetic level of description, adult speakers of English can be heard to use a variety of different Tones: simple Tones such as a fall or a rise; and more complex ones such as a fall-rise, a rise-fall or even a rise-fall-rise (Crystal, 1969). The question arises as to whether there is any developmental sequence to the acquisition and mastery of the Tones. It might be assumed that infants start by producing phonetically simple Tones and produce more complex Tones as they get older. Having measured and classified the pitch movements that the children used at 3, 6, 9 and 12 months, Vonwiller (1988) found that the simpler contours (e.g. fall and level) were more common than would be predicted from the adult language in the first six months and but less common in the second six months. Rising pitch and more complex contours showed the opposite developmental pattern. Vonwiller therefore proposed that the more difficult patterns are acquired later than the simpler ones (p. 30).

The dominance of simple falling and level contours in the first few months may be attributable to physiological factors. However, after the age of 6 months, infants produce a wider variety of pitch movements, a higher proportion of which are complex, suggesting that by this age they are starting to overcome earlier anatomical and physiological limitations. Summarizing their extensive review of the literature at this stage, Snow and Balog (2002: 1053) concluded: "Based on the assumption that the reported data are relevant to Tones in well-defined intonation-groups, studies of infant cry and non-cry vocalizations suggest that babies use precursors of intonation from the age of 0;3–0;9." Hypothesizing that here may be further age-related developments and changes in the Tones used, Balog and Snow (2007) compared children aged 12–17 months to a group aged 18–23 months. They examined an inventory comprising 16 different pitch contours (equivalent to Tones) produced by the children. Contrary to their expectations, they did not find a statistically significant difference between the two age groups in terms of the size of Tonal inventory used. Thus, it seems that children as young as 12 months already produce a wide repertoire of pitch contours or Tones, even ones that may appear phonetically complex. The implication of this finding is that the subsequent learning task for the child is not so much to master the phonetic variety of Tone production; rather, it is to deploy the different Tones in meaningful ways, in accordance with the systems of the language being learnt. Nevertheless, there is evidence that some phonetic challenges do still remain in the area of Tone, since Snow (2004) found that 1-year-olds did not control the speed of the falling Tone on monosyllables in the way that 4-year-olds could.

The period from 9–18 months has been characterized by Snow (2006) as a regression, at least with respect to the production of Tones. According to Snow, by 6–8 months, the infant is using quite adult-like falling and rising Tones from a phonetic perspective, i.e. in terms of the pitch range of the fall or the rise. This is also true around the age of 18 months. However, in the intervening period, Snow reports that the pitch range used by infants, for both falls and rises, becomes significantly narrower, and is thus less adult-like. He attributes this to a reorganization that the infants are grappling with, as they work out how pitch contours relate to meaning. This process is provoked by the child's new awareness of intentionality as the basis for communication, along with the onset of the first words.

To infants exposed to a non-Tone language such as English, it will become increasingly apparent that words can be accompanied by a variety of different pitch patterns. As mentioned earlier in this chapter, children have to work out whether each new word they learn has a set pitch pattern and thus that the ambient language is a lexical Tone language. When the infant starts to use words, this may cause him or her some uncertainty as to whether each word should have a Tone. When this happens, it is likely that the child will be uncertain for a while about the role of pitch movement in intonation, for example, as a means of signalling the end of the speaker turn. This may be why children seem to use narrower pitch falls and rises at this stage. As the infant is only really capable of producing one-word turns at this stage, it is not such a problem for Turn-taking, since the carer or other interlocutor will know anyway that after a single 'word', the child has finished the turn. However, as we will see in Chapter 7, it becomes an issue when children move into the two-word or multiword stage. Moreover, because the child's turn consists of a single word, there is no possibility of marking Focus by Tonic placement, so again there is no motivation for the child to produce a particularly prominent pitch movement.

Rather than physiological factors, the main influence on the infant's pitch patterns after the age of 6 months is environmental. In general, observations of children's intonation in this period show the infant reproducing unanalysed gestalts, suggesting that the infant stores an episodic memory of a speech event with its contour. Perhaps as a consequence of the relatively gross phonetic parameters involved, it seems that picking up and reproducing the characteristic prosodic forms of a particular language or dialect may not be particularly hard for children. Studies of infants' production of non-linguistic vocalizations suggest that from 6–12 months infants start to produce vocalizations that reflect the intonation of the ambient language: for example, French infants use a greater proportion of rising contours than English infants (Whalen, Levitt, & Wang, 1991). If there are any universal physiological and maturational tendencies in early intonation development, they soon begin to be overlaid by language-specific features picked up from interactional partners and other speakers in the environment.

It thus appears that from the age of 6–9 months, the infant hears, stores and begins to reproduce language-specific intonation patterns, though without at first relating them to specific meanings. Nevertheless, this is a developmentally important accomplishment from interactional and sociolinguistic perspectives. Pragmatically, we saw in Chapter 4 and have seen in this chapter that Tone matching is a key feature of intonation use, serving to align the current speaker with the previous speaker's action. A production store of contours will therefore form a valuable resource that the child can draw on in order to match another speaker's Tone for interactional purposes. In addition, if the infant has stored accurately the contours heard from more mature speakers of the ambient dialect or accent, then the growing child will be heard as a member of that speech community when using them in future (Local, 1982).

Summary

The main capacities of the infant and behaviours of infant and carer as they relate to intonation are summarized in Table 6.3. The period from birth to 18 months is divided into two phases. The first phase, up to 6 months, is called 'Pre-verbal'. This reflects the fact that in their own vocalizations their use of pitch and loudness is not linked to

Table 6.3 Summary of intonation-related capacities and behaviours evident from 0–18 months.

	TURNS / IP	FOCUS / TONIC	ALIGNMENT / TONE
Pre-verbal **Birth–0;6**			
Internal Maturation Vocal tract; respiratory system	Neonate can hear differences in length of turns he is exposed to Respiratory capacity limits length of vocalization	Neonate can hear changes in loudness and pitch prominence Unable to control loudness locally – only globally	Hearing for pitch discrimination already in place. Limited ability to control own pitch
Input IDS (parent, family)	Carer may respond to vocalization as conveying meaning (e.g. a need, 'request')		Prosodic perception starts to become attuned to ambient language Carer Tone may match infant pitch contour Infant may match carer Tone
Output Non-verbal; cry; cooing	Vocalizations of varying length and phonetic quality		
Paradigmatic **0;6–1;6**			
Internal Maturation	(Reciprocal turn-taking) Increasing respiratory capacity permits longer vocalizations	Non-verbal pointing; gaze Onset of joint attention Increasing local control over production of pitch, loudness and duration	Prosodic perception becomes attuned to ambient language Increasing control over laryngeal actions allows for more precise pitch movements
Input IDS: (family, childcare)	Carer delimits own turns with Tonic Carer responds to infant vocal strings as turns	Carer uses Tonic placement for focus Carers tend to use Supertonic Carers may respond to any child vocalization as topically relevant (Tonic not important)	Carer matches child Tone In non-Tone languages, Carer versions of adult Tones are exaggerated compared to ADS. This is not so in Tone languages
Output Babble; Single word stage	Solo babble play: exploratory extension of IP In interaction: child only produces the Tonic 'word' Child uses 'fall' and 'rise' but not always as distinctly as in the adult language Use of intonation gestalts reflecting adult intonation	Variable 'Tonic' placement in solo babble In interaction: Tonic 'word' only (sometimes combined with babble in IP)	Child works out whether ambient language is Tone or non-Tone language If non-Tone language like English, child works out functional value of Tone matching vs. non-matching Child matches or does not match carer's Tone Child starts to establish Tone inventory for English

words. Equally, while using short strings of words in conjunction with intonation when interacting with the infant, the carer does not expect the words to be understood or the infant to respond with words. The next phase, from 6–18 months, is called the Paradigmatic phase, following a terminological distinction that is made in linguistics research between paradigmatic relations and syntagmatic relations:

> The syntagmatic dimension deals with the sequential characteristics of speech (or writing) seen as a string of units, usually in linear order … The paradigmatic dimension refers to the set of relationships which a linguistic unit has with other units in a specific context.
>
> *(Crystal, 1987: 21)*

The term 'Paradigmatic' underlines that the infant's main task is to make progress in sorting out the Tone paradigms or systems of the language. In the case of a Tone language such as Mandarin or Yoruba, there are more than two contrasting Tones, associated with words or grammatical morphology. In English, a non-Tone language, there is a simple two-Tone system, High (H) vs. Low (L), governed by the requirement to match or not match the prior speaker's Tone in order to align with the prior speaker or to initiate a new action. Adult carers use this system from the outset and there is evidence, as will be seen in the following chapter, that by 18 months the infant is already competent at using this system. The system of Tones, both in English and in Tone languages, may have as its domain a single word and thus is within the capacities of the child at this stage, i.e. before the child is producing turns of two or more words. This contrasts with the next phase, the Syntagmatic phase, described in Chapter 7, where the child's main achievements are to extend the Intonation Phrase to create longer and syntactically more complex turns. This also allows the system of Tonic placement for Focus to come into play.

From the clinical perspective, it is important to consider how intonation development might be arrested at these early phases. This will be illustrated in Chapter 10 in relation to children with severe motor impairments resulting from cerebral palsy and in Chapter 11 with reference to children with severe or profound intellectual disabilities.

Key to Activity 6.1

1 In Media File 6.1, it is possible to hear a woman's voice speaking continuously for just under 2 seconds. There is then a gap of around 1 second, followed by a further vocalization of under 1 second, including a silence of around 0.2 seconds. It is possible to hear the rhythmic grouping of syllables, some being longer in duration than others. The pitch of the final syllable can be heard to rise. Media File 6.1 has been derived from an unfiltered sound file that was originally presented in Chapter 1 as Extract (1.2), as part of Activity 1.1. The fundamental frequency, intensity and temporal features of the utterance were displayed in Figure 1.2. By comparing the two recordings you can gain an impression of what aspects of speech may be accessible to the infant in the womb.
2 Possible obstacles include:
   1 The mother and her interlocutors may speak too quietly. If their voices do not rise above the 60db threshold, they will be inaudible.
   2 The environment in which the mother and interlocutors are located may be so noisy, for example, from traffic, loud music, loud TV or machine noise, that this masks the signal entirely.

3 The development of hearing in the foetus may already be impaired or may be damaged before birth. Exposure to low frequency noise at levels of 70–80db or more will hamper the tuning of the hair-cells to specific frequencies, with consequences for the development of hearing for intonation (Graven & Browne, 2008).

Key to Activity 6.2

Lines (4–6): In line 6, Kathy comes in after a very short gap (0.2 seconds) following the end of Rosie's vocalization in line 4. In line 4, R uses a descending pitch pattern, ending at the lowest point of her 'turn', so K may be responding to this as a yellow traffic light.

Lines (8–10): Rosie's turn in line 8 consists of four syllables. Kathy starts to talk in line 10 following the third of these, hence is in overlap. The first syllable of Rosie's turn has a falling pitch contour to a point low in her pitch range. This is similar to a Tonic fall in English, signalling a yellow light; the second and third syllables are level and low in her pitch range, similar to a Tail in English that signals a green light. Thus, if she is treating Rosie as a user of the English intonation traffic light system, Katie's incoming after the third syllable in overlap is a legitimate one, even though it results in overlap. After her first syllable in line 8, Rosie makes eye contact with Kathy, which in terms of the adult Turn-taking system would be a further invitation to Kathy to take a turn.

Lines (20–23): The first of the final five syllables of Rosie's turn in line 20 is very loud and high in her pitch range; through the remaining four syllables the pitch descends progressively to the base of her presumed range. There is also a progressive reduction in loudness. Following Rosie's last syllable Kathy starts her turn without pause, suggesting that she is responding to the fall in pitch at the end of Rosie's turn as a yellow light. As in line 8, Rosie makes eye contact, here around the antepenultimate syllable of her own turn.

CHAPTER 7

Preschool years

As most children in the UK start school during their fifth year, we take the span of the preschool period to be from CA 1;06 to 4;06, while recognizing that in most countries, including some others where English is the main language, schooling begins later. Precise chronological specification of the endpoint of the period is less relevant than the onset of formal education, since, as will be explained in Chapter 8, school brings new challenges with respect to intonation.

Through the preschool period there are rapid developments in all aspects of spoken language. The child's vocabulary expands massively, and alongside that expansion is the development of vowel and consonant systems, enabling the child to differentiate words from one another in a way that is consistent and intelligible to others (Stackhouse & Wells, 1997). With regard to intonation and the lexicon, for the child learning a non-Tone language such as English, one key step is to learn how to map intonation patterns onto lexical items that have different lengths and shapes, in terms of number of syllables, stress pattern and syllable structure. For a child who is having serious difficulties with segmental phonology, there may be an impact on this aspect of intonation, i.e. with the mapping of an intonation 'tune' onto a segmental 'text'. This will be explored further in Chapter 10.

At the start of this period, there is a key linguistic advance as the child moves from single-word to multiword utterances. Because the child through this period uses longer turns containing progressively more complex grammatical structures, the mapping between tune and text poses important new challenges. It requires physical control over the production of pitch, loudness and duration. It further requires the ability to map these prosodic parameters onto the strings of grammatically organized words and morphemes that make up an utterance. Intonation is now syntagmatically important, functioning to group words together in relation to their grammar.

At least as important, however, are the interactional meanings that the intonation systems convey. In relation to turn construction, intonation may be used to show that the speaker has not yet reached end of the turn (cf. Chapter 2). In relation to Focus and topic, the speaker can highlight one word or phrase through intonational prominence while backgrounding the rest of the turn (cf. Chapter 3). In relation to social Actions, the speaker can match the Tone of the prior speaker in order to align with that prior speaker's Action (cf. Chapter 4). In the early part of this preschool period we will see the child learning to use these systems while interacting with other people.

Children's Intonation: A Framework for Practice and Research, First Edition. Bill Wells and Joy Stackhouse.
© 2016 John Wiley & Sons, Ltd. Published 2016 by John Wiley & Sons, Ltd.
Companion website: www.wiley.com/go/childintonation

By the time they start school, most children will have had the experience of using and responding to intonation as part of successful social interaction. However, disorders in segmental phonology, grammar or pragmatics could interfere in different ways, as would a lack of opportunity for spoken social interaction in the preschool years, as reported in cases of extreme disadvantage.

Tone matching and alignment in the early preschool period

A conception of the function of Tone in English which provides for a transparent account of how the child might acquire the system was outlined in Chapter 4. It was proposed there that Tones are not associated with particular communicative functions or grammatical structures. Instead the speaker's choice of Tone is locally determined: the speaker chooses to match the prior speaker's Tone if continuing the action in progress, or to contrast Tone if initiating a new course of action. In Chapter 6, we saw that this system of Tone matching and contrast was already operative for children below 18 months of age.

There is robust evidence that children at the stage of moving into multiword speech, i.e. towards the end of the second year, make good use of this system, as was illustrated in Chapter 4 from interactions involving Robin at this stage of development. Use of the system is evident in naming or labelling activities, where it is routine for the carer to ask the child to say the name of the picture or toy in front of them. The child's version of the label, provided as a response to the carer's request, may then be followed by an affirmatory repeat by the carer. In a detailed study of such labelling sequences involving children aged 1;7–2;3, Clare Tarplee demonstrated how pitch matching by the adult to the child's labelling attempt serves to construct the adult's turn as an affirmatory repeat rather than as a request for further repair work by the child on his or her attempt (Tarplee, 1993, 1996). Such pitch matching may take the form of a fall or a rise, depending on the pitch contour used by the child. In (7.1), where in line 2 the child names a picture of a BALL in a book, with a rise, the adult matches it with a rise in line 3 (Tarplee, 1996: 418).

(7.1)

1   (1.4)   ((*page is turned*))

2   Child: [bɔbʌˈl]

3   Adult: [bˈɔːəl]
4   (1.8)   ((*page is turned*))

In line 4, adult and child move on to the next page of the picture book. This displays that the adult is not expecting the child to make a new attempt, even though the child's version clearly diverges from the adult's in its segmental content. Thus, the adult's repeat, with its Tone match, is affirmatory rather than repair-initiating.

On the other hand, where the adult uses a repeat to initiate a repair, this is frequently done by *not* matching the child's Tone. In line 1 of Extract (7.2), the child attempts the word TEETH but produces it as two syllables, using a rising Tone over the second syllable; even though it flattens off at the end, it remains high in the child's pitch range (Tarplee, 1996: 420).

(7.2)

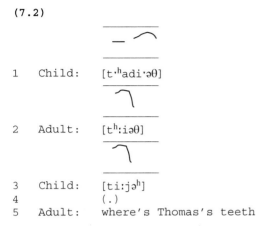

1	Child:	[tˑʰadiˑəθ]
2	Adult:	[tʰːiəθ]
3	Child:	[tiːjəʰ]
4		(.)
5	Adult:	where's Thomas's teeth

In line 2, the adult produces the word "teeth" with a non-matching pitch pattern, i.e. using a falling Tone to the base of the pitch range. This is treated as a model for self-correction by the child, who in line 3 duly makes a second attempt at the word, matching the Tone of the adult model. Thus, we can see that in line 2 the adult uses a non-matching Tone to initiate a new action, namely a repair sequence. In this case the adult's initiation of repair is accomplished with a falling Tone, contrasting with the child's original rising Tone. In line 5, by moving the topic on, the adult displays that the child is not required to make a further attempt at pronouncing TEETH.

Participation in exchanges like these demonstrates to the child very clearly that choice of Tone in English is not determined by the lexicon or the grammar, i.e. that English is not a Tone language, since the same word may be produced with different Tones. Instead, adults and children use rising and falling Tones systematically in order to accomplish interactional (communicative) tasks. In this respect, our approach resembles other functional approaches to intonation, such as Halliday's (see Halliday, 1975). However, the choice of rise or fall is not determined by reference to a set of communicative functions such as requesting or naming, as proposed by Halliday and others. Instead, the choice depends on (1) the Tone used by the other participant in the previous turn; and (2) the speaker's desire to go along with the prior turn or alternatively to initiate repair.

Later developments in the phonetic realization of Tones

There is nothing to suggest further fundamental changes through the preschool years in this functional system of matching and non-matching Tones. However, there may be developments in the phonetic realization of the Tone system. Tones are realized over syllables that make up words, and during the preschool period children's words acquire progressively greater stability with more adult-like segmental and rhythmic properties as they learn to sound more like members of their speech community. One aspect of this relates to the system of lexical stress. In Chapter 1, the relation between lexical stress and intonation was described: in (adult) English the syllable that bears the lexical stress has the potential to become the prominent syllable of a Foot. This includes the Foot where the Tonic is located. Lexically unstressed syllables necessarily carry pitch too, and often contribute to the overall shape of the Tone. Young children's precise phonetic realization of the Tone may diverge from that of adults in various ways. One case is where the child adds an extra syllable to the word, as in (7.1) and (7.2) above, where the child produced TEETH and BALL each with two syllables, the rising Tone being spread out more than in the adult versions. Conversely, it is common for young children to omit unstressed syllables, particularly in words of three or more syllables:

BANANA > [ˈnɑnə], PYJAMAS > [ˈdɑməd], TELEPHONE > [ˈdɛdəʊ], ELEPHANT > [ˈɛfənˌ].

In such cases, the phonetic realization of the Tone will need to be truncated or compressed compared to the adult form, in order to fit onto the reduced number of syllables (Ladd, 2008).

There has been some research into the precise phonetic realization of Tones by preschool children, and how children might differ from adult speakers in this respect. David Snow (1994) carried out a detailed investigation of the phonetic characteristics of (pitch) accent range over utterances of different length, produced by children aged 18–24 months learning American English, and concluded that this aspect of the children's pitch was adult-like, even at the beginning of the period studied. However, the study focussed on falling Tones only and there is some evidence that rising Tones may present a greater challenge. Snow (1998) investigated both rising and falling Tones, this time in a study of 4-year-old children. The children were required to imitate these Tones in non-final and final sentence positions. Acoustic analysis showed that sentence-final rising Tones were harder for the children to imitate than sentence-final falling Tones. However, in non-final position, the opposite was the case: falls were harder than rises. It seems likely that these results derive from the frequency and distribution of rising and falling Tones in different positions in the ambient language, although this can only be confirmed by cross-linguistic studies. Snow also investigated the development of complexity of Tones, in a longitudinal study of children aged 16–25 months (Snow, 1995). There was no clear developmental trend: the children did not use more rise-falls as opposed to simple falls as they got older.

While Snow (1995) reported that the children's pitch range in falling contours was already adult-like, suggesting that this aspect of the phonetic realization of Tone is an early-acquired prosodic feature in American English, his conclusion is not fully supported by subsequent research on British English. Astruc, Payne, Post, Vanrell, and Prieto (2013) investigated falling Tones in utterance final position in an experimental situation, with children aged 2, 4 and 6 years old learning Spanish, Catalan or British English. Results for the nine English children only (three per age group) are summarized here, using the terminology of the present book. The words that were elicited had different lengths (in terms of number of syllables) and stress patterns, e.g. KEY, ˈMONEY, GUIˈTAR, baˈNANA, ˈELEPHANT. It was found that 2-year-olds and 4-year-olds had a wider pitch range than 6-year-olds and adults, and their stressed syllables were longer in duration. This indicates a developmental trajectory in the phonetic realization of

Tones, in the direction of the adult forms. Nevertheless, even the 2-year-old children were able to align the peak of the Tone in relation to the start of the Tonic syllable, and to take account of the differences in length and stress pattern of words in order to achieve an adult-like mapping of the falling pitch contour onto the syllable(s) making up the word. This suggests that young children, at a stage when their segmental phonology is far from complete, demonstrate the ability to realize Tone accurately at a phonetic level, even though children at the younger end of this age spectrum use a wider pitch range.

Turn construction and expansion of the Intonation Phrase

So far, in this chapter we have considered how the young child decides which Tone to use when constructing a turn in conversation, and how that Tone is produced phonetically. We have seen that there is continuity with the infant's use of Tone as described in Chapter 6. One key factor that makes this continuity possible is that, alongside longer turns, the child continues to produce turns consisting of a single word. This was evident in Extracts (7.1) and (7.2), in the single-word turns produced by children from 18–26 months.

Nevertheless, the most obvious change within the preschool period is that the child's turns can get longer. Towards the end of the second year, children typically begin to produce turns of two words, and then move on to produce turns of three and more words. The interest of researchers investigating this key development has mainly been in the child's progressive acquisition of grammar. Grammatical structures emerge as the child develops the ability to produce recognizable words in a stable order so that an utterance can convey more complex meanings than can be done merely by stringing together some single words. Intonation contours, along with other prosodic features such as pauses within the child's turn, are mainly referred to by child language researchers when making analytical decisions about the grammatical status and complexity of the child's utterance. Behrens and Gut (2005), introducing their study of the relationship between prosody and grammatical development in a German-speaking child, pinpoint a key problem with much of the research into grammatical development at this stage:

> However, the attempt to identify syntactic units by their prosody is problematic because of the underlying assumption that all aspects of prosody are already mastered and controlled perfectly at the time of the first word combinations. Several studies on the phonetics and prosody of child speech show that this is not the case … In conclusion, it is very important that one does not simply take prosodic aspects of early combinatorial speech as a reflection of their semantic and/or syntactic status. Rather, it has to be kept in mind that the child is in the process of acquiring the prosody of a language as well as its syntax.
>
> *(Behrens & Gut, 2005: 7)*

In the current section we foreground intonation, since intonation, rather than grammatical development, is the concern of this book. In line with our interactional approach, this means focussing on the role that intonation plays in the child's ability to construct longer and more complex turns. From this perspective, two facts about this stage of the child's linguistic development are particularly relevant.

First, even before producing recognizable combinations of words of the kind that are said to signal grammatical development, children construct longer turns containing elements that are not recognizable. An example we have already seen in previous chapters is Robin's turn in line 3 of Extract (7.3) previously Extract (3.12):

(7.3)

```
2    M:    ‖can you re'member what `this is‖
```

```
3    R:    ʔə(.) ʔɛdʒœ: ʔɪʒ3 (0.7) pɒkx
                                    [f}
4    M:    ‖`top‖ thats `right‖ `top‖
            {f}                 {p}
```

While it is Robin's final syllable that is picked up by his mother as the word TOP, there are five syllables preceding it, which may be meaningful for Robin. Since they are not apparently meaningful to his mother, and certainly not to us as external observers, it is not possible to attribute a grammatical structure to the utterance. Nevertheless, an intonational structure can be identified, as shown in (7.3.1):

(7.3.1)

```
2    M:    L    ‖ can you re'member what `this is ‖
3    R:    =    ‖ ʔə(.)ʔɛdʒœ: ʔɪʒ3 (0.7) `pɒkx ‖
                                          F
4    M:    =    ‖ `top‖ thats `right‖ `top ‖
```

Robin's final syllable has the major pitch movement and is louder than what precedes it, identifying it as the Tonic. This makes the preceding string of four syllables a candidate Head. Thus Robin's turn can be hypothesized to consist of a single IP consisting of Head + Tonic. The placement of the Tonic on the final syllable indicates that the final syllable is the Focus. The matching of that Tone with his mother's Tone from the preceding turn indicates that he aligns with her request, by providing a response. In her next turn in line 4, his mother demonstrates her orientation to all three intonation systems that Robin appears to have used: she responds to his Tonic as a cue to take her turn; she also responds to his Tonic as the semantic Focus of his turn; and she responds to his matching Tone as aligning, by matching it again. Thus, we can see that Robin's mother is able to make sense of Robin's apparently unintelligible turn, because Robin is able to produce his turn with an intonation structure that is meaningful in terms of adult English. Thus, the first key point about this stage of development is that in conversational interaction with a caregiver, a child's unintelligible turns can still make interactional sense.

The second important point is that at this stage, children's talk is not confined to interactions with others. It has often been reported that children also talk to themselves or to imaginary friends. In such situations the child is not interactionally accountable for what they say: no-one is going to ask them what they mean or to correct their pronunciation. Such occasions thus provide a free space for trying things out. We can see this in Extract (7.4), again involving Robin and his mother. At the start, Robin's mother is seated in an armchair directly behind him, drinking a cup of coffee. There is a large box of toys in front of Robin, about a metre away. The shared play and conversation that precede this extract continue in lines 1–4, where they interact on the topic of a toy ball. In line 5, he changes the topic, then his attention moves to the toy box.

(7.4)

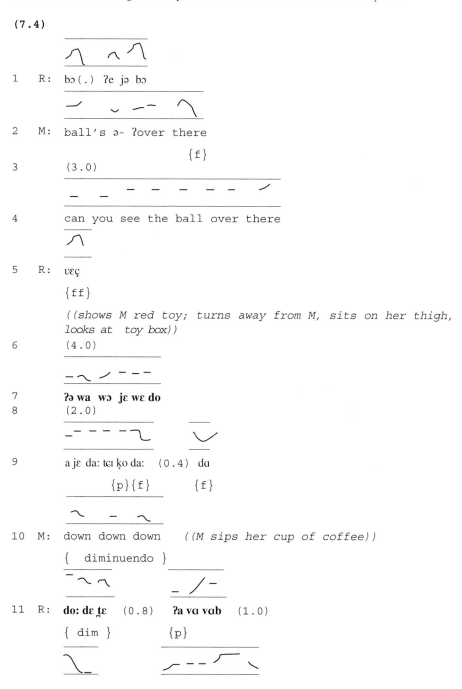

1   R: bɔ(.) ʔe jə bɔ

2   M: ball's ə- ʔover there

3   (3.0)   {f}

4   can you see the ball over there

5   R: ʋɛç

         {ff}

         ((shows M red toy; turns away from M, sits on her thigh,
         looks at toy box))

6   (4.0)

7   **ʔə wa wɔ jɛ wɛ do**

8   (2.0)

9   a jɛ da: tɛɪ k̥o da: (0.4) dɑ

                    {p}{f}   {f}

10 M: down down down   ((M sips her cup of coffee))

         {   diminuendo }

11 R: **do: dɛ t̬ɛ**   (0.8)   **ʔa vɑ vɑb**   (1.0)

         { dim }   {p}

12   **ʤiː jo**   (1.1) ə ja bə ji dja:: dɪ   (1.5)

{f}   {ff}

((through this 'turn', R looks in toy box, with back to M))

13   ə pə tɪ (1.0)

{p p}

14   naː pə tɪ (.) ɪːn (.) ʔaː po

{f} { p   p}

((at end, R takes tractor toy out of toy box))

15   M: wheres the man that goes in the tractor

                      {f}

(4.0)

16   R: **ʔəh**   (0.5)

17   M: where's the man

Following line 5, Robin turns his back on his mother and begins to play on his own, without reference to her. From line 7 to line 14, his mother does not require Robin to interact with her. She does take a turn, in line 10, which is done quietly and without any attempt to make eye contact. There is no evidence that she expects or seeks a response, although Robin does align with her turn in the first part of line 11, repeating the three syllables with the same descending pitch contour. There are thus several lines where Robin is, for all practical purposes, talking to himself: lines 7; 9; 11 (second part); 12; 13; 14. By examining these lines, we can see how the interactionally unconstrained situation that Robin is now in allows him to try out intonation patterns.

In lines 7 and 9, he produces IPs that are six syllables in length. After a brief and quiet turn from his mother in line 10, he goes on to produce a further six utterances, separated by pauses and varying in length from two to six syllables. These utterances display a variety of different pitch patterns, as well as variation in loudness, syllable duration and tempo. On the basis of the recording of this section, as transcribed above, we can apply the phonological notation for IPs that was presented in earlier chapters and which we used for his TOP turn in (7.3.1). This is shown in (7.4.1), where each group of syllables that contains a major pitch movement is notated as an IP, using the symbol for IP boundaries. The syllable with the major pitch movement is notated as the Tonic, by placing a Tone diacritic immediately before it. The Tone is identified on the basis of the pitch contour from the Tonic syllable through any following syllables (the Tail). Where there is extra prominence, as in the second IP of line 12 where the Tonic syllable is very loud and long, this is marked with the Supertonic symbol (⇑). The traffic light shading is applied to the Head and Tonic. For each line, labelling of the intonation structure is provided immediately below the intonation transcript.

(7.4.1)

11   ‖ ʔa ˊvɑ vɑb ‖
            Head + Tonic + Tail

12   IP1: ‖ˋdʑiː jo ‖   IP2: ‖ ə ja bə ji ⇑ˋdjaːː dɪ ‖
            IP1: Tonic + Tail   IP2: Head + Supertonic + Tail

13   ‖ ˊə pə tɪ ‖
            Tonic + Tail

14   IP1: ‖ ˋnaː pə tɪ ‖   IP2: ‖ ɪːn ˋʔạː po ‖
            IP1: Tonic + Tail   IP2:Head + Tonic + Tail

In the four lines of (7.4.1), six potential IPs have been identified, which vary in their structure. Three of the IPs have a Head, the Head varying in length from one syllable to four syllables. All six IPs have a Tail, of one or two syllables, though elsewhere Robin produces IPs without a Tail, for example, the first IP in line 1 of (7.4). These variations in presence and length of Head and Tail give rise to the impression that Robin varies the location of the Tonic. He uses different Tones, i.e. both rise and fall. He also varies the degree of Tonic prominence, using Supertonic (line 12) as well as ordinary Tonics.

In summary, when the interactional pressure is off, Robin seems to produce a rich variety of intonational structures and Tone variation. However, it is important to emphasize this is an externally imposed interpretation, based solely on the perceived resemblance between Robin's prosodic phonetic patterns and the structures and systems that have been identified for adult English. In fact, as Robin is not

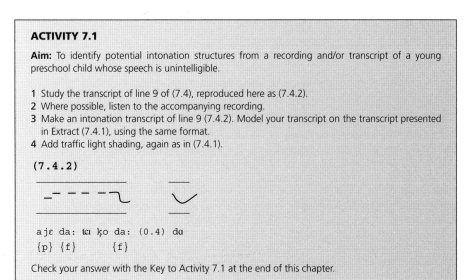

ACTIVITY 7.1

Aim: To identify potential intonation structures from a recording and/or transcript of a young preschool child whose speech is unintelligible.

1 Study the transcript of line 9 of (7.4), reproduced here as (7.4.2).
2 Where possible, listen to the accompanying recording.
3 Make an intonation transcript of line 9 (7.4.2). Model your transcript on the transcript presented in Extract (7.4.1), using the same format.
4 Add traffic light shading, again as in (7.4.1).

(7.4.2)

   aʲɛ daː tɕɪ ḳo daː (0.4) dɑ
   {p} {f}   {f}

Check your answer with the Key to Activity 7.1 at the end of this chapter.

communicating with anyone through these utterances, we cannot infer that he has mastered these systems and structures. Halliday makes this point:

> This is part of the value of the functional approach: it provides a criterion for identifying what is language and what is not. It should be noted that this criterion excludes all instances which are interpreted as linguistic practice. When the child is practising speech sounds, or later on words, phrases, structures, or whatever they are, this is not regarded as language in use; it is not an instance of meaning.
>
> *(Halliday, 2003: 74)*

In such non-interactional situations, Robin displays prosodic resources that he should be able to draw on elsewhere, i.e. in conversational interaction when trying to produce meaningful turns. When talking to himself, it may be that he is actually practising these patterns and variations, getting used to what it feels like both to produce them and to hear himself producing them. One aspect of this practice is an opportunity to associate pitch and other prosodic features with strings of syllables of different shapes in strings of varying lengths, i.e. to practise the details of phonetic realization. In (7.4), there are instances on a single syllable of both simple (e.g. the first IP of line 12) and complex dynamic pitch, e.g. line 1. Conversely, there is distribution of a Tail over more than one syllable, e.g. the rise in line 13, which continues with ascending levels over the two syllables of the Tail.

The structure of this type of play activity, where the child breaks off from interacting with his mother to play on his own, provides the child as turn-occupant with the opportunity to hold the floor for an extended period. Being temporarily disengaged from play that involves talking to his mother thus provides Robin with an opportunity to produce a range of potential IP structures, without the risk of being overlapped and interrupted: his mother is content at this point to sit back and enjoy her cup of coffee. Such opportunities may be important for the young child, who needs to develop the resources that will enable him to secure more extended turns in conversation.

An analogy for the young child talking to himself is the aspiring jazz musician, who at home can practise phrases of varying length, with different rhythmic accents and in different keys, at leisure. This is a necessary preparation for improvising in a performance with a band, where playing is subject to a number of constraints that have the potential to impede fluent performance, particularly while still learning to play jazz, like the child learning to talk. For the jazz soloist, the improvisation will be based on a particular tune, with a particular rhythm, tempo and style, in a particular key and following a set harmonic progression. Furthermore, the improvisation should be responsive to the other members of the band: the player needs to take a turn in a sequence of solos, to initiate and construct a solo in real time within the conventions of a shared jazz idiom, to do so without inappropriate pauses and to display when the solo is coming to an end. Additionally, the solo should be responsive to the topic, i.e. the melody of the tune and to other players' subtopics presented in their solos.

Similarly, the young child learning to talk in interaction needs to be competent in initiating, constructing and ending turns at appropriate points; in identifying, responding to and highlighting topics and subtopics and aligning with other participants. All of this needs to be accomplished in real time, without too much hesitation, since silences are open to different interpretations depending on their length and location. So it needs a lot of practice. The anthropologist Tim Ingold, citing Darwin's characterization in *Origin of Species* of language as an art, proposes that singing, dancing or playing a musical instrument are good analogies with language: each is a skill that is culturally transmitted and requires a great deal o practice (Ingold, 2000).

Treading on your Tail: Post-Tonic expansion of the IP

In the discussion of turn-taking in Chapter 2, an extract was presented (Extract 2.6) that consists of a series of single word turns from Robin alternating with turns from his mother. Such sequences are particularly characteristic of the phase immediately preceding the appearance of multiword utterances that typically occurs towards the end of the second year. For Activity 2.2 in Chapter 2, this extract was used to introduce the system of intonational traffic lights. It shows that Robin and his mother share a simple version of the traffic-light system for turn exchange that is based on the production of the Tonic. Each time that the adult starts a turn after the child has completed an IP with a Tonic, the child receives feedback and reinforcement on the function of the Tonic in delimiting the turn.

However, the continuation of this extract, originally presented as Extract (2.7) in Chapter 2 and reproduced here as Extract (7.5), demonstrates that this simplified traffic light system is vulnerable as soon as the child wishes to produce a turn that consists of more than one meaningful word. How can Robin produce a turn of two or more words without getting interrupted by his mother? To progress to the two-word stage, children need to augment the single-word turns that they have produced hitherto. Those single words have been produced with a Tonic. Thus, the child has two alternatives: to produce the additional word before the Tonic or to produce it after the Tonic. Extract (7.5), originally presented as Extract (2.7) in Chapter 2, demonstrates the risks attached to the second of these alternatives:

(7.5)

In line 6, Robin produces a Tonic (yellow light) on SMOKE, but then immediately produces a further word, which is his version of FUNNEL. He produces this with another Tonic, i.e. a second yellow light. His mother starts her turn after Robin's first Tonic, thus displaying her orientation to the system they have been using up to this point: "Each IP should have one Tonic, so after I hear the Tonic I can start my turn", i.e. only one yellow light per turn. When Robin immediately produces a second Tonic in overlap with his mother's turn-beginning, she breaks off, thereby demonstrating her confusion as to what has happened to the orderly exchange of turns. Although she does not explicitly criticize Robin's behaviour by saying something like "Don't interrupt me when I've started talking", she implicitly provides feedback that something has gone wrong. She then models an alternative way (line 8) to construct the kind of turn that Robin had attempted in line 6.

A little later on, in line 12 of Extract (7.6), Robin redoes his original turn, this time the second word being produced *without* a prominent pitch movement. This turns it into a single IP consisting of Tonic + Tail. After positively evaluating this turn, his mother reproduces in line 13 the same IP structure, with Tonic + Tail, i.e. a yellow light followed by a green light. From this example we can see that the occurrence of overlap potentially offers an important didactic resource for stimulating the development of IP structure and, thus of orderly turn-taking by the young child (Wells & Corrin, 2004).

(7.6)

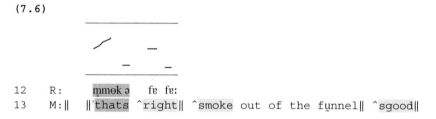

| 12 | R: | mmɵk ɔ   fɐ fʊː |
| 13 | M:‖ | ‖'thats ˆright‖ ˆsmoke out of the funnel‖ ˆsgood‖ |

To summarize, in order to progress to the two-word stage, children need to augment the single-word turn, by producing an additional word either before the Tonic or after it. In line 6 of (7.5), Robin attempted to produce the additional word after the Tonic. As is clear from (7.6), this is a perfectly legitimate way to construct a turn in English. However, the speaker has to produce the post-Tonic word with less pitch and loudness prominence than the Tonic. For this reason the Tail functions as a green light for the next speaker to start talking and so is susceptible to being overlapped.

Getting a Head: Pre-Tonic expansion of the IP

Since a word placed in post-Tonic position (the Tail) is vulnerable to getting obscured, it is not a good place for a speaker to put new and important semantic material. A more promising alternative is to place the additional word or words before the Tonic, i.e. where the traffic light is at red, signalling that other speakers are not allowed to start a turn.

The child's production of multi-element turns is thus ultimately dependent on expanding the number of intonation elements that precede the yellow light that is the Tonic.

As explained in the section, 'Holding the floor' in Chapter 2, there are two ways in which linguistic material can be presented before the final Tonic: either as a Head or as a Non-final IP. In the latter case, they can be combined: the Non-final IP, or the Final IP, or both, can also have a Head. What kind of evidence would indicate that a child is able to create longer IPs in this way? First, if the child's multi-element turn ends with a Tonic and is soon followed by talk from the adult caregiver's turn, this suggests that it is the child's Tonic that marks or contributes to signalling the end of the child's turn to the adult. The complementary piece of evidence is that the adult holds off from starting to talk until the child does produce a Tonic (Corrin et al., 2001). Such evidence would suggest that the child has the ability to expand the IP before the Tonic, i.e. Head; and pre-final IP. Research indicates that at this stage, Robin and other children have this ability (Corrin et al., 2001). This is illustrated in Extract (7.7). Although it is not taken from the same recording session as Extract (7.5), Robin and his mother are again talking about the train piece, the funnel and smoke:

(7.7)

```
1    M:   ‖is 'that the ´funnel‖
          (2.0)
```

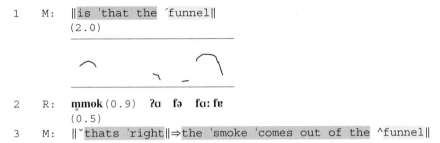

```
2    R:   m̥mok (0.9)   ʔɑ  fə   fɑː fɐ
          (0.5)
3    M:   ‖ˇthats 'right‖⇒the 'smoke 'comes out of the ^funnel‖
```

Following his mother's question in line 1, in line 2, Robin produces five syllables. The first three syllables, which on the basis of the mother's response in line 3, can be glossed as SMOKE OUT OF THE, are located around the middle of his speaking range. The first of these is the most prominent; it stands on its own, and has a falling pitch movement of c. 4 semitones. The fourth and fifth syllables, presumably representing FUNNEL, are louder and carry a large rise-fall pitch movement which reaches the base of Robin's usual pitch range, approximately 14 semitones lower than the end of "smoke". His mother does not start talking until after the fifth and final syllable, even though there was a silence of almost a second following "smoke", his first syllable. This strongly suggests that his mother is responding to Robin's use of pitch as a turn-holding device: she waits until after the fall to the base of Robin's pitch range, on FUNNEL, before she starts her own turn. This kind of example provides evidence that Robin can use intonational resources to create the interactional space to produce a multiword turn. Intonation is thus a powerful resource for children at this stage, not only in securing the floor but also thereby securing a long enough turn to allow them to construct their first multiword utterances (Corrin, Tarplee & Wells, 2001).

What, then, is the intonational structure of Robin's turn? If we consider it in terms of the adult system, there are two alternatives. First, it could be thought of as comprising two IPs, as represented in (7.7.1). This is analogous to his mother's turn in line 3, which is analysed as a single TCU made up of two IPs.

(7.7.1)

```
1    M:   ‖is 'that the funnel‖
          (2.0)
2    R:   ‖ m̥mok ‖ (0.9) ‖ ʔɑ fə   fɑː fɐ ‖
          (0.5)
3    M:   ‖ˇthats 'right‖⇒the 'smoke 'comes out of the funnel‖
```

However, there is one difficulty with analysing Robin's turn in (7.7.1) in this way. The turn in line 3 produced by his mother is analysable as two grammatical sentences, with a major grammatical boundary at the IP boundary. In the case of Robin's turn in (7.17), on the other hand, there seems to be a single sentence, the first IP mapping onto its Subject: ‖ SMOKE ‖ (COMES) OUT OF FUNNEL ‖. The grammar, then, suggests a single sentence, which would mean a single IP with a Head + Tonic structure, as in (7.7.2):

(7.7.2)

1   M: ‖is ˈthat the funnel‖
          (2.0)
2   R: ‖ m̥mok (0.9)ʔɑ fə fɑːfɐ‖
          (0.5)
3   M: ‖ˇthats ˈright‖⇒the ˈsmoke ˈcomes out of the funnel‖

This differs from (7.7.1) in that in line 2 there is just a single IP, with a Head followed by a Tonic. The Head, however, contains a substantial pause.

It is tempting to ask: which of these two alternatives, (7.7.1) or (7.7.2), is the correct analysis of Robin's turn in (7.7)? However, this would not be an appropriate question given Robin's stage of linguistic development. Robin is just beginning to produce multiword utterances and so has not yet established a repertoire of identifiable grammatical structures. We cannot therefore readily identify mappings between grammatical structure and intonation structure. A more useful way of viewing such utterances is that Robin is in the process of sorting out how to construct more elaborate turns. To do this, he has to develop a repertoire of grammatical structures along with a repertoire of intonation structures, and he has to learn how the intonation structures and grammatical structures map onto one another. This is a key point for understanding and assessing intonation in both typical and atypical development. We cannot separate intonation development from the rest of linguistic development: as we have seen in this example, our understanding of the child's mastery of intonation structure depends on our analysis of the grammatical structure of their utterances. The reverse is just as true and possibly even more important: our understanding of what grammatical structures a child is using depends on our understanding and analysis of the child's use of intonation, since we use intonation to identify the unit that we will analyse grammatically. What we have seen in this section is that both grammar and intonation combine in the construction of turns at talk. A turn has to be meaningful, which normally entails being fitted to the context provided by the interlocutor's prior turn. It also has to be identifiable; in particular, the point where the turn ends needs to be marked.

In respect of Extract (7.7), we have already noted that Robin's mother, in her next turn, produces two IPs and that they map onto separate sentences. Her second IP appears to be a recast of Robin's turn and potentially offers him feedback on the grammatical structure. In (7.7.3), we can see that she recasts his string of three or four words as a full sentence of seven words, together with appropriate segmental phonetic changes:

(7.7.3) m̥mok ʔɑ fə fɑːfɐ   → the smoke comes out of the funnel

Additionally, by constructing her second IP as a Head +Tonic IP, where "smoke" is incorporated into the Head, she potentially offers him feedback on what is the appropriate intonation structure for such a grammatical structure: Robin's two IPs are recast as a single IP, mapping onto a single sentence, as shown in (7.7.4).

(7.7.4)   R: ‖ Tonic ‖ (pause) ‖ Head + Tonic ‖ → M: ‖ Head + Tonic ‖

Thus, we can see how in real time a child is presented simultaneously with opportunities to learn about intonation structure and grammatical structure. The key point for the child to learn when creating a multi-element turn is how to produce the non-final element at a pitch level which avoids the two extremes of the pitch range, since reaching the top (H) or base (L) of the range would signal a Tonic. Thus, in line 2 of Extract (7.7), reproduced here as (7.7.5), Robin produces the first element SMOKE, with a narrow rise-fall which is located around the middle of his range.

(7.7.5)

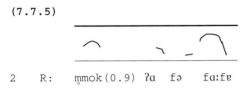

2   R: m̩mok(0.9) ʔɑ   fə   fɑːfɐ

Extract (7.8) and Extract (7.9) present further instances from Robin when 19 months old. In each case, though the transcription of his mother's next turn is not included here, she starts to speak immediately following the end of his turn, i.e. after his Tonic. As she never comes in after the first element, even though in all three examples there is a substantial pause following that first element, she is seen to treat the first element as displaying a red light, i.e. holding the floor.

(7.8)

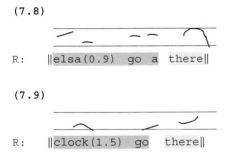

R: ‖elsa(0.9) go a there‖

(7.9)

R: ‖clock(1.5) go   there‖

In (7.8), as in (7.7), the Tonic on the second element is L, whereas in (7.9) it is H. In all three cases, the first element has pitch that does not reach the top (H) or base (L) of Robin's normal pitch range. Though some have more movement than others, the phonetic differences are on a continuum. Clearly mid-pitch is a powerful projector of the red light, i.e. of the status of the first element as the Head of the IP. In all three examples it is powerful enough to override a substantial pause following the first element.

   In Extract (7.10), Robin produces a two-element turn. As in (7.9), the first element has mid-pitch, not followed by a pause on this occasion. The second element is H, creating a Tonic, following which his mother starts to speak.

(7.10)

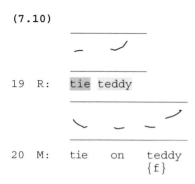

19 R: tie teddy

20 M: tie   on   teddy
{f}

His mother recasts his turn grammatically by adding a preposition, although she still does not create a sentence that is fully grammatical by the criteria of the adult language. She matches his Tone, thereby presenting her turn as a repeat of his turn but not as a repair initiation. In fact, she matches his whole intonation pattern quite closely, with its Head + Tonic structure, as shown in (7.10.1), thereby indicating to Robin that the way in which he composed his turn was legitimate in terms of its intonation structure.

(7.10.1)

19 R: **H** tie teddy
20 M: =   tie on teddy

Children soon begin to produce turns of more than two words or elements. In the next extract, (7.11), originally analysed in Corrin, Tarplee and Wells (2001), Robin at 21 months produces a turn of three distinct elements. The first, "ayaya", cannot readily be glossed as an adult word, but from the hand gesture that accompanies it and the context, it clearly has a deictic function, i.e. to point out something to his mother.

(7.11)

1 R: ə: jə jə ʔ: (0.4)   peːiː (0.4) œədɛ
{f}
2 M: that's where the planes are (.) up in the sky

The first two elements are linked to the child pointing to a picture of a plane: the semantic force is something akin to "this a/ plane/". The pitch movement at the end of the first element [ə: jə jə ʔ:] is clearly at mid-height and held on the level, linking it to the second element [peːiː]. This second non-final element terminates around mid-height, being extended by the prolonged duration of the vowel. The turn is thus left open for the third and final element which adds further syntactic material. It expresses the expanded proposition of planes being located in the sky with an accompanying point gesture. This provides the structure in (7.11.1):

(7.11.1) ‖ ayaya (0.4) plane (0.4) over there ‖

The production of a Head by using mid-pitch would thus appear to be a powerful device to allow the creation of a turn of as many as three elements at this developmental stage.

So far, we have examined turns where the elements preceding the Tonic seem to be lexical. However, Robin also uses the Head + Tonic structure for turns where the words preceding the Tonic appear to be 'grammatical'. An example is Extract (7.3) from earlier in this chapter, reproduced here as (7.12):

(7.12)

```
2   M:   ‖ can you re'member what `this is ‖
```

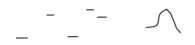

```
3   R:   ʔə(.)ʔɛdʒœ: ʔɪʒʒ (0.7)pɒkx
                                [f}
4   M:   ‖ `top‖ thats `right‖ `top ‖
           {f}                {p}
```

From the context, there is good evidence that the final word is TOP but there is no indication, from anything said or done by either Robin or his mother, that Robin's first syllables refer to another lexical element. It seems more likely that they represent some grammatical material, for example, a repeated ITS'A . Following this suggestion, the transcription would be:

(7.12.1) ‖ er(.)'its a 'its a (0.7) `top ‖

A similar analysis is plausible for (7.13), where on the basis of the context and its phonetic make-up, along with his mother's response, Robin's turn might be glossed "and there's a book" or "another book", i.e.

‖ a'nother `book ‖.

(7.13)

```
1   M:   and what are these
         (2.5)
```

```
2   R:   ə nʌ:: bʊkʰ
3   M:   that's right there's a book
```

These last two extracts share the Head + Tonic structure but in these the 'Head' element is not a major semantic/syntactic element – a situation which is also often the case in adult turns and IPs.

In summary, at his stage Robin and other children learning English are able to produce turns that extend beyond a single word or element. One important device that allows this to happen within talk-in-interaction is that of creating a Head to precede the obligatory Tonic. This Head may contain one or even two additional semantic elements, enabling the child to produce a more complex proposition, e.g. identifying an object and specifying its location, within a single turn. The Head may also house emergent grammatical elements or morphemes. The device works because it serves to hold off other potential speakers: in Robin's case, his mother does not start her turn during his Head but waits until he has produced a Tonic.

How does the child come to learn how to create a Head? Trial and error seem to be one way. If he produces a Tonic on an element (e.g. with a falling pitch to the base of his range) and then tries to continue his turn, he will very likely get overlapped, as we saw in Extract (7.5). The overlap and the subsequent disruption to orderly Turn-taking may provide an incentive for him to produce a first element without a Tonic pitch movement, i.e. with mid-pitch instead. In this way, implicit feedback from conversational partners may help him progress towards the Head + Tonic system.

As for explicit instruction, there are occasions where the IP structure is foregrounded in the interaction. In line 2 of Extract (7.14), his mother invites Robin both to complete the puzzle by fitting in the final piece, and simultaneously to name that piece:

(7.14)

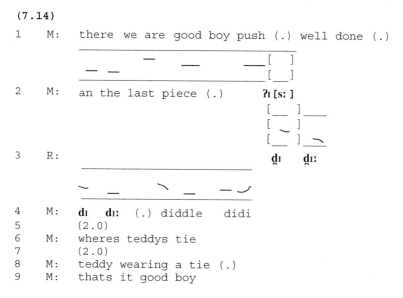

```
1    M:    there  we  are  good  boy  push  (.)  well  done  (.)

2    M:    an  the  last  piece  (.)            ʔɪ [sː ]

3    R:                                          d̪ɪ    d̪ɪː

4    M:    dɪ   d̪ɪː   (.)  diddle     didi
5          (2.0)
6    M:    wheres  teddys  tie
7          (2.0)
8    M:    teddy  wearing  a  tie  (.)
9    M:    thats  it  good  boy
```

In line 2, the mother's turn is intonationally and grammatically incomplete. Moreover, she extends her incomplete IP by lengthening the vowel and consonant of "is" while maintaining level pitch. Although this design could reflect that she herself is conducting a word (or piece) search, it is taken by Robin as fishing for a completion: in line 3, Robin completes it with a noun, TEDDY, which also completes the IP, by providing an L Tonic, with a step to low over the two syllables. In line 4, his mother immediately recycles Robin's word from line 3, matching his pitch and also redoing segmental aspects of Robin's pronunciation, adopting an immature form "didi". From the perspective of intonation, we can see that, in line 2, she produced the Head of an IP without a Tonic. Instead, she invited Robin to produce the Tonic and thereby complete a well-formed IP. The success of this common pedagogical device, used by parents and teachers when trying to elicit a particular word or response, depends on the ability of the child to recognize an incomplete turn, and specifically an incomplete IP.

Overlap and intonation in the preschool period

According to the review that was presented in Chapter 6, there is a decline in the amount of vocal overlap in infant–carer interaction from around 3 months of age, followed by a resurgence from around 18 months until the end of the second year. It has been suggested that this may be due to both child and mother producing longer turns. When overlap occurs, the participants have to take steps to ensure it soon ends, so that one speaker can be heard at a time. In Extract (7.5), we saw that it was Robin's mother who carried the responsibility of sorting out the breakdown of orderly turn exchange that Robin precipitated. There and elsewhere in her conversations with Robin, she does this by making use of practices for overlap resolution that are used by mature speakers of English (Schegloff, 2000; Kurtić et al., 2013), as was described in Chapter 2. At the stage of linguistic and social development that Robin is at, i.e. towards the end of the second year, children do not appear to have the resources to resolve this kind of interactional problem, so this is left to the more mature conversational partner. We encountered the following example in Activity 2.3 in Chapter 2. It is presented here in Extract (7.15) using the traffic light notation, with each IP on a separate line, to highlight what is happening with respect to turn-taking. Robin is trying to fit a piece into the jigsaw.

(7.15)

```
1 R:    L    now push (.)
2 M:    ≠    [mm]
3 R:    ≠    [it] goes there (.)
4 M:         [what go-]
5 R:    =    [it there] (.)
6       =    Push
7 M:    =    what goes in there
```

Each of Robin's first two utterances (lines 1 and 3) is potentially complete, as he produces a perceptible fall in pitch to the base of his usual pitch range. However, after only a micropause, he continues to talk. His mother comes in after Robin's Tonic in line 2 and again in line 4; this displays her expectation that Robin will adhere to the traffic lights system. As a result, they talk in overlap in lines 2 and 3 and again in lines 4 and 5. The second time it happens, his mother breaks off (line 4) before her turn constructional unit (TCU) is grammatically and intonationally complete. She lets him produce another TCU with a Tonic (line 6) before recycling and now completing, in line 7, the turn that she had curtailed in line 4. Thus, in this extract, as in Extract (7.5), it is Robin's mother who has to do the work required to resolve the problem that they are talking in overlap. Yet there is some evidence that Robin may be sensitive to issues around overlap and thus turn-taking: his redoing of line 3 as line 5 suggests that he may be aware of the problem with line 3 (it was overlapped) and that in line 2 his mother was looking for some clarification.

This example shows that Robin's grasp of the traffic light system is not yet firmly established, although his mother acts as if it is. At this stage of development, he shows sensitivity to repair episodes and makes use of them to reformulate his turns, as demonstrated in detail by Corrin (2010b). Corrin points out that this becomes more prevalent as Robin's mean length of utterance approaches two words and that his reformulations result in semantically sharper utterances, i.e. it is clear what he means. These reformulations take the form of an IP made up of Head + Tonic. Thus, not only repair arising from overlap but also repair sequences more widely promote more complex IP and turn structure.

Using intonation to extend a conversational turn is a skill that is already evident in Robin and other young children in the latter part of the second year of life, as they begin to use multiword utterances (Branigan, 1979). This serves to create the interactional space that allows them to develop more complex grammatical structures (Corrin, Tarplee & Wells, 2001). What are the mechanisms that allow these developments to occur? A plausible scenario is that children turn back to holistic intonation patterns heard, stored but not yet used at the Paradigmatic phase described in Chapter 6. In the Syntagmatic phase, they practise the patterns in solo play, as Robin does in Extract (7.4), while in interaction with caregivers they draw on these patterns as prosodic frames within which to express more complex IP structures.

Later developments in Intonation Phrase and turn construction

The construction of longer turns is the key development in the preschool period. We have seen how the transition from single words to multiword utterances depends on creating IPs with a Head and also of turns with more than one IP. However, we saw that it was not always possible to determine whether Robin's extended turn consisted of a Head followed by a Tonic or of separate IPs. As the child begins to create even longer and more complex turns, the distinction becomes more apparent. One type of turn where the child has to be able to combine more than one IP is the list. In Chapter 4, we saw the following example from Len, at the age of 9, reproduced here as (7.16):

(7.16)
```
9    T:    ‖ 'Len  'what dyou like `doing when you 'go into 'town ‖
10   L:    ‖ er 'seeing the ´[bu]ses ‖ 'seeing the ´trains ‖
11   T:                        [mm]
12   L:    and 'seeing the `tills ‖(.)
```

In response to T's question in line 9, Len produces a list consisting of three parts, each part forming its own IP. The two non-final IPs in line 10 have a rising Tone, while the final part in line 12 has a falling Tone. This is a classic intonational design for a list in English. One very common activity where young children soon show this proficiency is in counting aloud. The examples in Extracts (7.17) and (7.18) are from a study by Rachel Arrowsmith of counting sequences involving typically developing children CA 3–4 years and their nursery teachers (Arrowsmith, 2005). The transcripts are reproduced from the original study.

In line 3 of (7.17), the child enumerates the dots on the dice that she has thrown. Each digit is produced as a separate IP, with a rising Tone, until "five", which has a falling Tone. At this point, the teacher starts a turn, matching the child's fall and confirming her correct counting (Arrowsmith, 2005: 73 ff.).

(7.17)

```
1    C    ((throws dice))
2    T    what did you throw? how many?
3    C    ‖ ´one ‖ ´two ‖ ´three ‖ ´four ‖ `five ‖
4    T    `five  there you go you got five didn't you
5         get five get five out then
```

In (7.18), the child produces a similar turn, in line 2 (Arrowsmith, 2005: 122 ff.).

(7.18)

```
1    T    shall we count the spots and see what number it is
2    C    ‖ ´one ‖ ´two ‖ ´three ‖ `four ‖
3    T    ´four and one in the middle makes
4    C    ‖ `eight ‖
5    T    `five doesn't it so that's number
6         ((holds up five fingers))
7    C    ‖ `five ‖
8    T    `five  good girl
9         so you stick that one on the washing line as well
```

Although this time the child has not completed the counting sequence accurately, the teacher again comes in (line 3) following a digit that the child has produced with a falling Tone. However, this time the teacher does not confirm that the child is correct. Instead, by using a non-matching Tone (a rise) in line 3, followed by a grammatically incomplete sentence, the teacher invites the child to continue the counting sequence. Eventually, after further repair work, the child produces the correct final digit in line 7.

The two extracts show that, irrespective of the accuracy of the child's counting, the adult reacts to the IP with the fall as the end of the count or list. Conversely, the adult responds to a rise as non-final. Arrowsmith (2005: 86) reports that the adult came in following the child's rise on less than 25% of occasions, whereas the adult always came in when the child produced a fall following a series of rises. At this stage, it seems that child and adult have a shared system for producing an extended turn that depends critically on the Tone selected by the child for each IP. Thus, shared counting seems to promote the child's ability to produce turns consisting of multiple IPs, with the appropriate intonational design.

This practice of using a rise on a non-final IP provides a basic intonational resource which the child can then apply to the construction of different types of longer turns. Rather surprisingly, there is virtually no published research on this aspect of intonation development. However, a lot of research has been published on grammatical developments at this stage, some of which incidentally provides insights into intonation developments. A case in point is Paul Fletcher's longitudinal study of Sophie, a girl learning British English in a monolingual setting, based on recordings of Sophie with members of her family, mainly her mother (Fletcher, 1985). Fletcher's orthographic transcripts include intonational notation. At CA 2;4, when Sophie had a mean length of utterance (MLU) of 2.5 morphemes, she did not produce any turns that contained complex sentences, i.e. that consisted of more than one clause. These were beginning to appear at CA 3;0, when her MLU had increased to 3.8. Where the clauses were joined by a conjunction like AND, OR or BUT, Sophie used two IPs, as in Extract (7.19) reproduced from Fletcher (1985: 96, line 474):

(7.19)   S: ‖ are those ´small apples ‖ or `big apples ‖

Sophie's IP structure in (7.19) is comparable to the one found in lists and counting sequences as exemplified in (7.16), (7.17) and (7.18), insofar as the Tone of the non-final IP is a rise, while the final IP has a falling Tone. The same is true of the second half of the longer turn produced by Sophie, aged CA 3;0, in (7.20), reproduced from Fletcher (1985: 98, lines 977–978):

(7.20)   S: ‖ ˈwhich one do you like ˋfirst ‖
             ‖ a ˆbig one‖ or a ˋlittle one ‖

On the other hand, where the relation between the two clauses is one of subordination rather than coordination, the first clause is integrated into the Head of a single IP, as in (7.21), reproduced from Fletcher (1985: 91, line 285):

(7.21)   S: ‖ ˈme going to ˈwatch you ˈdoing your ˋriding lesson ‖

In (7.22), the first clause is again integrated into the Head of a single IP, even though Sophie breaks off midway through the Head to repair her grammar (reproduced from Fletcher, 1985: 93, line 372):

(7.22)   S: ‖ ˈwhy did you ˈgive her (.) ˈto her when her been ˆflu ‖

The next recording, involving Sophie and her mother, was made when Sophie was CA 3;5 and had an MLU of 4.5. She produced a wider range of complex sentences and used them more often. While the IP structures noted above continued to appear, the relationship between intonation structure and grammatical structure was not rigid. Fletcher observes: "It is more fruitful for us to consider the prosodic and the grammatical as independent systems which do make intermittent contact; however, neither is wholly determined by the other" (1985: 154).

This indeterminacy is what is found in the adult language, as we saw in Chapter 1. For instance, instead of combining clauses in a single IP, Sophie sometimes produces subordinate clauses + main clause structures with two IPs, as in (7.23), which is reproduced from Fletcher (1985: 144, line 493):

(7.23)   S: ‖ while(.)Hester at ˆschool ‖
             we can buy (.)ˈI can buy some ˋsweets‖

Moreover, in the two-IP structure, it is not always the case that the two Tones are different as in (7.23). In (7.24), reproduced from Fletcher (1985: 144, line 500), the Tone in each IP is a fall:

(7.24)   ‖ and ˈwhen her at ˋcorder   ‖ ˈyou buy some ˋtighties‖

Based on what we have seen of younger children, like Robin at the age of 19–21 months, we might wonder if producing a fall in a non-final IP would lead the adult to start talking before the child can produce the second IP. However, this did not seem to be a big problem for Sophie at CA 3;5. By this age, children are more comprehensible, producing more grammatically well-formed utterances. They are also more intelligible, as segmental phonological immaturities decline. The adult listener is therefore less dependent than previously on intonation cues to the child's turn structure. If Sophie's mother can decode the word WHEN at the start of Sophie's turn in (7.24), she knows, without help from Sophie's intonation, that Sophie is likely to be producing a subordinate clause and so her mother will need to wait for Sophie's main clause before taking a turn. It can be hypothesized that, compared to the stage at which we saw Robin, entering the multiword stage towards the end of his second year, intonation is now less important for the management of Turn-taking, because the child's words and sentences are easier to understand. However, in order to substantiate this, more research is needed on intonation development in relation to grammar and interaction during this important period.

Focus and Tonic placement

In Chapter 3, we saw that Tonic placement is variable and can be used to indicate the focused, new or otherwise topically important element of the utterance.

Developmentally, topics become interactionally relevant from around 12 months, when child and carer relate to and talk about objects 'out there'. Initially the child does this by combining a point with a single word, as we saw in Chapter 7, but once the child begins to produce multiword utterances, there is the possibility of handling this linguistically. In English, this can be done through Tonic placement.

In his review of prosodic development, Crystal indicates that the ability to manipulate Tonic placement (i.e. tonicity), develops very early: "[T]onicity contrasts are early evidenced in jargon sequences (in which sequences of rhythms are built up which resemble the intonational norms of connected speech)" (1987: 69). This was borne out by the passage of solo talk and play transcribed in Extract (7.4), where Robin produced 'jargon' turns with a range of different Tonic placements.

As just mentioned, the functional use of Tonic placement to convey Focus is only possible when the child begins to produce two-word utterances. According to Crystal, the onset of the system of Tonic placement and the onset of the two-word stage are simultaneous: "However it is arrived at, it is plain that around 1;6 in most children, two-element sentences within single prosodic contours are used, and tonic prominence is not random" (Crystal, 1987: 73).

Wieman (1976) attempted to identify the factors that determine Tonic placement at this stage. She examined the placement of the Tonic ("stress" according to her terminology) on the two-word utterances of five children between CA 1;9 and 2;5, with MLU between 1.3 and 2.4. She found first of all that the children were quite consistent in placing the Tonic on some semantic categories rather than others, for instance, locatives and possessives were consistently stressed, agents and attributives consistently unstressed. Thus, according to Wieman, an utterance such as "Blue man" typically has the Tonic on the noun, MAN, rather than the attribute, BLUE. This behaviour is adult-like, to the extent that in adult English, as explained in Chapter 3, different grammatical categories have varying potentials to receive Tonic prominence.

Wieman's second claim was that the location of the Tonic is not random, but influenced by considerations of information Focus: "Children operate with an appreciation of what is new in their utterance, and apply stress accordingly" (Wieman, 1976: 286). Thus, as just mentioned, an utterance such as "Blue man" by default has the Tonic on the noun, MAN, rather than the attribute, BLUE. However, this is not the case when the noun has already been mentioned, as when the child produces the string of words "Man. Blue man." In the latter case, the child would create narrow Focus, on BLUE, by using a Tonic + Tail structure for his second IP: ‖ `man ‖ `blue ˈman‖.

Robin, at the age of 19–21 months, produced turns that fit with Wieman's account. In Extract (7.25), originally presented in Chapter 4, MAN is mentioned by Robin's mother in line 6 and repeated by Robin in line 7.

(7.25)

```
6    M:    L      || ts a  man ||
7    R:    ≠      || ma ||
8    M:    =      || yes ||
9    R:    ≠      || di jↄ ma: ||
10   M:    =      || nother  man ||  (.)  in a   boat ||
```

In line 9, Robin places the Tonic on the first syllable of his IP, not on MAN, which is in final position. He thereby creates a Tonic + Tail structure. His mother responds to his Tonic placement as Robin's way of pointing to the Focus of the talk, by expanding it as ANOTHER MAN. This uses the same Tonic + Tail structure, giving Focus to ANOTHER.

Observations such as these have resulted in a consensus view that the system of Tonic placement and Focus is established very early. Nevertheless, this conclusion was based on only a few studies. Crystal (1987) was sceptical of Wieman's claim that children at the two-word stage manipulate Tonic placement in accordance with the requirements of information focus, pointing to the great methodological difficulties in identifying what is new or old information for the child. In fact, we have already seen in this chapter, in the section on IP expansion, that matters do not always progress as smoothly as Wieman's report suggests. In Chapter 3, we saw Robin making a 'mistake' with regard to Focus and Tonic. The relevant lines of Extract (3.15.1) are reproduced here as (7.26)

(7.26)

```
5    M:   || thats  ´right || n ↑'what comes 'out of the  `funnel||
6    R:   ʔə mɛ ʊ kʰ        [f ɑ f ə ]
               (F)              (F)
7    M:                    [smoke-]
                 (0.5)
8    M:   ||`smoke comes out of the 'funnel|| `doesn't it||
               F
```

In line 6, Robin produces a turn consisting of two elements, SMOKE and FUNNEL. As Robin's mother has mentioned FUNNEL in line 5, the expectation would be that Robin should not place a Tonic on FUNNEL, the already-mentioned topic, but on the new item, SMOKE. In fact, he places a Tonic on both elements, thereby creating two IPs. This leads to a temporary breakdown in the interaction, which entails extensive repair work from Robin's mother. In the course of this, in line 8, she models the preferred intonational form for an utterance where there are two major semantic elements, the second of which has already been mentioned. This preferred form is the Tonic + Tail structure. As can be seen in (7.26.1), which follows on from (7.26), Robin duly produces this structure in line 12, and it is approved by his mother in line 13.

(7.26.1)

```
12   R:    ^m̥mək ə fɐ fɐ:
                F
13   M:||  ||'thats ^right|| ^smoke out of the funnel|| ^sgood||||
                           F
```

Thus, the ability to use Tonic placement to focus on the topic is not necessarily automatic or instinctive for the young child. The child has to work out the system, from their own observations and the feedback they receive.

In the next extract, (7.27), we again find Robin producing two Tonics in a single short turn, causing an interactional problem for his mother. Robin is seated on the floor, fitting pieces into a board. He is looking at the board throughout and does not have eye contact with his mother. His mother is sitting on the floor close to the board and to Robin, watching him as he fits the pieces into the board. Each piece depicts something different; in this extract, a piece depicting a teddy bear is involved.

(7.27)

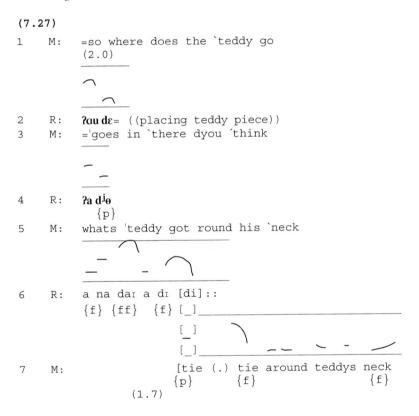

In line 1, Robin's mother introduces the teddy piece, locating the Tonic on the word TEDDY, thereby topicalizing it. After a pause, this topic is taken up by Robin in line 2. It forms the basis for further talk from his mother in line 3, but now there is no direct mention of the teddy, it is implicit as the omitted subject of "goes in there"; and in line 5, where TEDDY is again mentioned, it no longer carries the Tonic. His mother's treatment of the lexical item TEDDY in this sequence conforms to usual descriptions of how new and old (i.e. already mentioned) items are handled in terms of Tonic placement.

In her turn in line 5, TEDDY does not carry the Tonic, which is instead located on NECK. However, Robin's next turn, in line 6, has not one but two clear points of intonation prominence. The first is on [daɪ], TIE, which is the expected focus in response to Mother's preceding question; then there is a further prominence on [dɪdi], TEDDY, at the end. Both Tonics have rising-falling pitch as well as loudness peaks, the first being more prominent on both counts. In line 7, following a brief overlap and self-repair, Robin's mother appears to recast and expand his turn: the Tonic is a rise-fall on TIE, reaching high in her range and mirroring the Tonic on [daɪ] TIE that Robin used. At the lexical level, his mother expands Robin's [dɪdi] (TEDDY) to AROUND TEDDY'S NECK, with a Tonic on "neck" that has rising Tone from low to mid in the range, subordinate to the accent on TIE but nevertheless prominent compared to the two words that precede it. Thus, his mother's turn in line 7 can be seen as a partial recast of Robin's turn from line 6, in intonational terms, involving both copying his Tonic placement (on TIE) and modifying the Tone: instead of Robin's final rise-fall, she produces a low rise. According to standard accounts of English Tonic placement, this reflects the status of TEDDY'S NECK as information that has already been mentioned. Thus, the sequence from line 1 to line 7 illustrates how Tonic placement shifts to reflect the shifting topical status of semantic elements. This is shown by the notation in (7.27.1). The effect is to shift away from Robin's double Supertonics in line 6, to his mother's narrow Focus on TIE in line 7, which is what is required by the context.

(7.27.1)

```
1   M:  =   ‖ so where does the teddy go ‖  ((picking up TEDDY))
                           F
                   (2.0)
2   R:  =   ‖ ʔɑu dɛ ‖  ((placing TEDDY piece))
3   M:  ≠   ‖ goes in there ‖ dyou think ‖
                           F
4   R:  =   ‖ ʔa sʲθ ‖
5   M:  ≠   ‖ whats 'teddy got round his  neck ‖
                               F
6   R:  =   ‖ a  na daɪ  a  dɪ di[: :] ‖
                     F        F
7   M:  ≠                ‖ [tie] (.) tie around teddys neck ‖
                              F                      F
```

Extract (7.27) thus demonstrates how Robin at this stage may produce an IP with two Tonics, as shown in (7.27.2):

(7.27.2) ‖ a na daɪ a   dɪ di: ‖

This was also the case in (7.26), as shown in (7.26.2):

(7.26.2) ‖ ʔə mɛ ʊ kʰ   fɑ fə‖

In both examples, the first Tonic, in a non-final position, marks the (narrow) Focus of his turn, in accordance with the adult system for English. The second Tonic is located on the final word, suggesting that he produces the additional Tonic to display the end of his turn. In this respect, he has not yet mastered the English Tonic placement system, which allows only one Tonic per IP, which needs to be on the Focus even when the Focus is in non-final position. In both extracts, Robin's double Tonic results in overlap and leads to repair, providing opportunities for the child to learn about Tonic placement as a resource for handling Focus.

Later developments in Tonic placement and Focus

There is evidence to suggest that the production of IP-final Tonics, irrespective of Focus considerations, may be common among children learning English, who only later learn to manipulate Tonic placement for Focus purposes. For this, we can refer once more to the transcripts of Sophie presented in Fletcher (1985). The frequency of IP final and non-final Tonics on all transcribed utterances of two or more words at the first three time points studied by Fletcher, is shown in Table 7.1.

From Table 7.1, it may be inferred that at the age of 2;4, Sophie is operating with a strategy of making the final word prominent, with little regard for the requirements of Focus: only 4% of her utterances of two or more words have the Tonic in non-final position. There is a marked difference by CA 3;0, when a third of her utterances have a non-final Tonic and the proportions are very similar at CA 3;5. The data suggest that by the age of 3;0, Sophie has developed the basic system of Tonic placement, but that at CA 2;4 this was not yet established. The persistence of final Tonic placement was illustrated in Chapter 3 by the case of David, a boy with delayed speech and language, who was still using it for every IP at the age of 5;4. The preference for final Tonic placement will be returned to in Chapter 8, with reference to children's performance on intonation tests and when learning to read aloud.

Researchers have investigated the subsequent development of Tonic placement in preschool children by getting children to correct incorrect picture descriptions (Hornby, 1971) or to describe sequences of pictures in which one element has changed, for example, the first might depict a girl riding a bicycle, the second a boy riding a bicycle (Hornby & Hass, 1970). According to these authors, 4-year-old children consistently used emphatic stress (Supertonic placement in our terminology) to correct incorrect statements and to mark contrastive information, i.e. for non-final narrow Focus. MacWhinney and Bates (1978) followed a similar procedure as part of a wider cross-linguistic developmental study involving 3-, 4-, and 5-year-old children. Hornby's finding was replicated, confirming that even 3-year-olds could perform the task and that there was no progression with age. MacWhinney and Bates therefore concluded that this ability was acquired by age 3, although they pointed out that it might be limited to the specific task used in the experiment. The use of such experimental techniques for investigating school-aged children's knowledge of the Tonic–Focus system will be described in Chapter 8.

Table 7.1 Distribution of Sophie's Tonics by position in the IP (based on Fletcher, 1985).

Age	MLU	Number of 2+ word utterances	% non-final Tonics	% final Tonics
2;4	2.53	131	4	96
3;0	3.82	172	34	66
3;5	4.47	199	32	68

Table 7.2 Summary of intonation related capacities and behaviours in the preschool years.

	TURNS / IP	FOCUS / TONIC	ALIGNMENT / TONE
Syntagmatic	**1;6–4;6**		
Internal Maturation	Increase in working memory span (phonological loop) as articulatory skills mature –allows for longer IPs	Greater control over production of pitch, intensity and duration allow for more precise location of Tonic; differentiation of Tonic vs. Supertonic	Greater control over laryngeal actions allows for more precise pitch movements
Input	CDS (family, childcare) -> Peer	Adult provides online feedback re: 'illegal' incomings, illegal overlap by child; Collaborative completions to induct into IP structure	Adult provides online feedback re 'illegal' Tonic placement, by child	Adult models of Tones become less exaggerated and more like ambient ADS
Language	Multiword -> grammar	Dysfluency arises from demands of combining multiple elements within an IP	Turn-final only Tonic 'errors' Double-tonic 'errors'	Tone-matching for interactional alignment is established
	Child extends IP & Turn in interaction: adds non-final IP: use of mid pitch Head: use of level pitch Tail: absence of IP final prominence	Sorts out that (Super)Tonic is used for (narrow) Focus	Tonal inventory established
	Child starts to use overlap functionally Mastery of traffic light system	Sorts out that only one Tonic allowed per IP	Child acquires language-specific phonetic exponents of Tones
	Later: integration of IP structure with grammatical structure, e.g. Lists; subordinate clauses		Later: Tone matching as means of creating alliances etc. in peer interaction
	Turn-taking in multiparty interaction (e.g. peer play)		

Summary

The main features of the preschool years in relation to intonation are summarized in Table 7.2. The most salient developments are Syntagmatic, as children learn how to use intonation to construct turns of more than a single word. The Head, Tonic and Tail are established as different structural elements of the Intonation Phrase. Children come to understand the role that each of these elements plays in talk-in-interaction as part of a system of traffic lights for regulating the orderly exchange of turns. Competence is developed in placing the Tonic on the appropriate word, as required by considerations of Focus. As children progressively use more complex grammatical structures to build semantically more elaborate turns, they master the mapping between Intonation Phrase structures and grammatical structures, such as main and subordinate clauses.

From the clinical perspective, it is important to consider how these syntagmatic intonation developments in intonation might be delayed or arrested. This will be illustrated in Chapter 10 in relation to children with speech and language difficulties, in Chapter 11 with reference to children with autism spectrum disorders, and in Chapter 12 in relation to children with hearing impairments.

Key to Activity 7.1

A suggested intonation transcript is given in (7.4.3):

(7.4.3)

IP1: ‖ a jɛ dɑː tɕɪ ko ˋdɑː ‖   IP2: ‖ ˊdɑ ‖
IP1: Head + Tonic   IP2: Tonic

CHAPTER 8

School years

Most children in the UK start school during their fifth year. School brings new communicative challenges and it is important to recognize the role that intonation may play in dealing with these. With regard to comprehension, the new challenges include having to listen to a wider range of discourse types, media and speakers, including peers and teachers using a range of less familiar accents. As for the production of intonation, challenges may include various kinds of public performance, drama, oral presentations and reading aloud. In this chapter, two questions will be addressed in relation to children who have typically developing speech and language:

1 What intonational competences do children already have by the age of 5?
2 What more does a child have to master during the school years?

Intonation and peer interaction

We will approach the first question through analysis of a short extract taken from six hours of video recorded interactions involving three 5-year-old male friends from the East Midlands of England, referred to here as Johnny, Mick and Fred. The recordings were made in the classroom of their mainstream primary school during free play, over a six-week period. The original focus of the research was on the management of arguments in peer interaction. Detailed analysis revealed that in order to pursue arguments and create alliances, all three children competently deployed a range of lexical and grammatical devices (Tempest & Wells, 2012). An additional resource for accomplishing joint play, including the conduct of arguments and the management of temporary alliances, is provided by intonation. To accomplish their interactional ends, the boys were able to draw on their competence in each of the three basic intonation systems:

• the placement of the Tonic to identify topical focus;
• the use of Tonic to project the upcoming completion of the speaker's turn;
• the use of a matching Tone to align with the prior speaker's agenda; or conversely of a contrasting Tone to initiate a new action.

The interaction reproduced here as Extract (8.1) was originally presented as Episode 1 in Tempest & Wells, (2012). Here it is transcribed using the phonological notation developed in earlier chapters with the addition of Tone diacritics to facilitate reading. The notational conventions are listed in Appendix 1. Prior to this episode, the three

Children's Intonation: A Framework for Practice and Research, First Edition. Bill Wells and Joy Stackhouse.
© 2016 John Wiley & Sons, Ltd. Published 2016 by John Wiley & Sons, Ltd.
Companion website: www.wiley.com/go/childintonation

boys have been discussing what they could play. They stand around a table with an upturned box of plastic connecting model pieces. Johnny (J) is at the top of the table with Fred (F) and Mick (M) standing on either side of Johnny. Mick and Johnny take pieces out of the box while Fred stands and watches.

(8.1)

```
01   J:   L   'no Mick 'Mick let(.) 'lets make a ⇑ `long 'water pipe
              ((attaches green long piece to red cog piece))
02   M:   ≠   'theres ˇgreen 'ones
              ((picks up another long green piece adds it))
03   F:   =   we need ´that
              ((offers a yellow cog to Johnny))
              (2.05)
04   J:       ((looks  at  Freddie,  does  not  take  yellow  cog
              offered))
05   J:   ∅   yeah and we 'nee[::d]
              ((looks at Mick; Mick adds green piece))
06   M:   ∅                    [and] we 'need
07   J:   ≠   'oh ^wait
              ((reaches over and picks up another red cog))
08   M:   ≠   'nother 'one of (.) ´them
              ((gives red cog to Johnny))
09   F:   ≠   need a ` red one Johnny `dont we
              ((holds red piece up))
10   M:   =   mm red ones `on (.)
11   M:   ≠   and a ´green
              ((Mick adds green piece))
12   J:   =   and we 'have ´that 'one::
                 ((adds another red cog))
13   M:   =   'and we need a ˇbendy 'one
              ((adds a green long piece))
14   J:   ∅   yeah 'Mick [Mi::ck
15   F:   =   then we 'need a ˇyellow 'one
              ((offers short yellow piece to Johnny))
16   J:   ∅   yeah and we 'nee::d
                 ((does not take piece from Fred))
17   M:   =   and we need an ˇorange 'one
              ((holds orange long piece up, looks at Johnny))
18   J:   =   and 'then we need ´this 'one
19   F:   ≠   no(.)[no       no     no       `n o :]
              ((starts to attach yellow piece to model))
20   J:   =       ['Freddie we 'dont need a `small] one
              ((moves  to  block  Freddie  from  putting  piece  on
              model))
21   F:   ≠   'yeah we ´do
              ((adds yellow short piece to model))
22   J:       'Freddie
              ((attaches a red long piece))
```

```
23   F:   ≠   'it- 'its a^long bit
                 ((steps back to observe))
24   J:   =   'Freddie 'that bit isnt `long
25   M:   ≠   and 'next we need and 'next we need 'other one of
                 ´these
                 ((offers a red cog and then puts it on model)
26   J:       yeah thats it Mick
```

ACTIVITY 8.1

Aim: To identify from spontaneous conversational interaction some of the intonation competences of a typically developing child in the first year of school.

Study Johnny's contributions to the interaction transcribed as Extract (8.1), then answer the following three questions taken from the IIP (Appendix 3), referring to at least one line from the transcript as evidence for each answer.
1 Does Johnny indicate narrow Focus on a non-final word of the IP by using non-final Supertonic placement?
2 Does Johnny project the end of the turn by using the Tonic?
3 Does Johnny align with the action of the co-participant's prior turn by using Tone Matching?
Check your answers with the Key at the end of the chapter.

Focus

There is evidence from this extract that the boys effectively deploy Tonic placement for the purposes of Focus. A striking use is found in Johnny's turn in line 1. Although the preceding context is not provided in (8.1), the boys have in fact been engaged in making 'water pipes' with connecting pieces. The new shift of topic and activity is to make one that is long. Johnny conveys this by means of a Supertonic, signalling narrow Focus on "long". That this is effective is clear from Mick's next action in line 2: he joins in the construction of the long water pipe.

Throughout the ensuing interaction, each of the boys has cause to produce turns that end with the word ONE, where ONE refers to a connecting piece. In each of these turns, in lines 2, 9, 12, 13, 14 and 20, the Focus is on an attribute of the new piece, either its colour or its size. In all cases, the boys place the Tonic on this attribute, rather than on ONE, showing that they can use the system of Tonic placement to indicate Focus and that they are not limited to placing the Tonic on the final word, as David was in Chapter 4, for example.

There is further evidence that the boys can take account of old and new information when placing the Tonic. In line 10, Mick places the Tonic on the final syllable "on" rather than on the attribute "red", because RED has just been mentioned by Fred in the previous turn. In sum, the boys appear to be fully in command of the system of Focus and Tonic placement.

Turns

As the interaction involves three boys performing a joint activity that they enjoy, quite lot of overlapping talk might be anticipated. In fact, there is rather little overlap; Turn-taking proceeds for the most part in an orderly way, with one speaker at a time.

This can be attributed to their use of the intonation traffic lights system. The majority of turns have a clearly identifiable Tonic (or Supertonic) located close to the end of the IP. The Tonic is routinely preceded by a Head, which does not get overlapped. Where there is a Tail, it is mostly just one syllable. There are some occasions where Johnny and Mick produce an incomplete IP, as in lines 5, 6 and 16. On each occasion it accompanies the grammatically incomplete string "and we need", indicating that they are aware of the relationship between grammatical structure and IP structure. In sum, the boys seem to have command of intonation as a traffic light system for Turn-taking.

Actions

A striking feature of the interaction transcribed as (8.1) is the way in which two of the boys, Johnny and Mick, create a temporary alliance to pursue the building of the long water pipe while excluding Fred from this activity. As described by Tempest and Wells (2012), this is accomplished in part through physical actions, twice by not taking a connecting piece that Fred offers (lines 4 and 16) and once by trying to block Fred from adding his piece to the construction (line 20). In addition, Fred's exclusion is accomplished linguistically. Johnny and Mick align with each other's turns through using a shared linguistic formula, made up of elements from the phrase AND WE NEED, as can be seen in lines 3, 5, 6, 11, 12, 13, 16, 17, 18 and 25. Just as striking is the matching of Tone in their spoken turns. They use a recurrent pattern of a level Head followed by a rising or fall-rise Tone for the Tonic. This serves to align across adjacent turns, as in lines 11, 12 and 13; and again in lines 17 and 18. It also functions to link those turns to other non-adjacent turns (lines 8, 25).

The overall effect is similar to the use of rise or fall-rise Tones to create a list, as discussed in relation to preschool children in Chapter 7. Here, the list, which comprises pieces needed to create the long water pipe, is constructed jointly by two of the participants in such a way as to exclude the other participant. In the sequence starting at line 9, shown below as (8.1.1), Fred tries to join in the shared activity, though he does not match the rising Tone from line 8 that the others are using. In line 10, Mick responds to Fred with a matching falling Tone, showing that his words "red one's on", which imply a rejection of Fred's offer of a red piece, are indeed designed as a reply to Fred. In line 11, Mick again reverts to the listing pattern, indicating that he is re-engaging with Johnny and their joint activity.

(8.1.1)

```
08   M:   ≠   'nother 'one of (.) ´them
                ((gives red cog to Johnny))
09   F:   ≠   need a ` red one Johnny `dont we
                ((holds red piece up))
10   M:   =   mm red ones `on (.)
11   M:   ≠   and a ´green
                ((Mick adds green piece))
```

A little later, from line 19, Fred provokes an argument by trying to impose his view of how the construction should proceed. At this point, there is overlap and also a shift from the rising Tone pattern to an exchange where the Tones are almost all falls (lines

19–24). In the end, Mick re-establishes the rising Tone pattern and, with it, the construction activity, in line 25, reproduced here as (8.1.2):

(8.1.2)

```
25  M:  ≠   and 'next we need and 'next we need 'other one of  ´these
            ((offers a red cog and then puts it on model))
```

In sum, this extract from peer interaction provides some answers to our first question, as it demonstrates intonational competences that these children already have by the age of 5. They are able to deploy the system of Tonic placement for Focus and to use the traffic light system that regulates Turn-taking. Perhaps the most striking intonation accomplishment evident in this extract is their use of matching and non-matching Tones to regulate the alignment of actions across speakers in order to handle the shifting alliances that characterize peer play at this age. From a theoretical point of view, the important feature that the systems have in common is that each is locally managed as the interaction unfolds on a moment-by-moment basis. The current speaker chooses which Tone to use and where to place the Tonic by referring to the prior speaker's Tone and Tonic placement, rather than by accessing a stored lexicon of intonational meanings. Thus, the intonational design of a speaker's turn is shaped principally by its relation to the previous speaker's immediately prior turn, and itself displays an analysis of that prior turn.

In the remainder of this chapter, we consider the new challenges facing children during the school years, from the perspective of intonation. These involve establishing one's social identity in a wider arena, as well as handling the demands of school and education.

Intonation, growth and identity

Children develop physically during the school years and become further acculturated to their local community, both factors impacting on their speech, including intonation. Through the school years, there are changes in children's voices for physiological and sociocultural reasons. One strand of research has investigated age- and gender-related changes in pitch range. In a study of American children aged 3–6 years vs. 7–10 years, Ferrand and Bloom (1996) analysed spontaneous speech along a number of intonational parameters, including mean, range and standard deviation of F0 and also proportion of types of pitch movement ("shift"). Significant differences found on all these measures were attributable to differences between the two male groups: the older boys had lower mean F0, narrower F0 range, smaller standard deviation of F0 and a greater proportion of 'flat' (i.e. level) pitch shifts as opposed to rises and falls. The authors suggest that both physiological maturation and sociocultural factors are involved in the age-related changes in F0 that they found.

Whiteside and Hodgson (2000) carried out a cross-sectional study of the fundamental frequency of 6-, 8- and 10-year-old children, compared to adults, using experimentally elicited material: measurements were taken on the final vowel of phrases like "The red car" uttered in response to a picture-naming task. Participants were from Tyneside, in the North-East of England. A progressive decrease in mean F0 with age was found, though with somewhat different rates of decrease for males as opposed to females. They also measured standard deviation of F0, and found that this measure too decreased with age, indicating a reduction in variability that "could be interpreted as evidence for increased motor control over the larynx with increasing age and maturation" (Whiteside & Hodgson, 2000: 25).

In a study of the spontaneous speech of six children, again from Tyneside, in the course of their sixth year of life, John Local (1982) examined changes in the occurrence of nuclear tone types over this period. In Tyneside English, there is a much greater occurrence of level Tones (c. 20% of all nuclear tones) compared to around 2% in Standard Southern British English (SSBE); conversely, the proportion of falls in Tyneside English is lower (29%) compared to SSBE (52%). During the course of the children's sixth year, there were significant changes in the relative occurrence of Tones, with a decrease in the number of falls and an increase in the number of levels (for both boys and girls) and rises (for girls only). Local concluded that these changes demonstrate how the children's intonation system is becoming more complex, and at the same time closer to the particular adult variety to which the children are exposed. The gender differences suggest that intonation production, in particular, of Tone, might be an aspect of speech where gender can be marked. A plausible explanation for such developmental shifts in Tone use is that, as they get older, children come to interact with a wider range of older local speakers and in the course of these interactions accommodate to the more mature speakers' use of Tones. At the micro-interactional level, this may result from the process of Tonal matching in the service of interactional alignment (cf. Chapter 4).

Testing intonation in the school years

Most published research that has specifically investigated intonation in the school-aged children has made use of specially devised tests or test batteries. In this section, the main findings of English language test-based studies will be presented under headings based on the major functions of intonation outlined in Chapters 2, 3, and 4. While a number of different tests will be described, the presentation is organized in relation to studies that have used the PEPS-C test battery. PEPS-C, an acronym for Profiling Elements of Prosodic Systems – Child version, was developed as an assessment tool that could be used by professionals working with children with communication difficulties (Wells & Peppé, 2001, 2003). In its original paper-based version and the revised, computerized version, it has been used in a number of clinical studies, some of which are described in Chapter 10 and Chapter 11. The largest study to date of typically developing children was conducted using the original version of PEPS-C (Wells, Peppé, & Goulandris, 2004). The revised version is described in Peppé & McCann, (2003).

The full PEPS-C battery incorporates the following dimensions: Input (perception/comprehension) vs. Output (generation/production); and Form (referring to lower-level phonetic processing, where meaning is not involved) vs. Function (involving higher-level processing, drawing on stored knowledge, relating phonetic form to meaning). PEPS-C covers four communicative areas, referred to as Focus, Chunking, Interaction and Affect, each of which is tested for both input and output. The relationship between these communicative areas and the functions of intonation described in Chapters 2, 3 and 4 of this book will be described below. In total, the original version of PEPS-C comprised 16 subtests, eight for Function and eight for Form.

In their study of typically-developing children, Wells et al. (2004) addressed the question: how does functional prosodic performance change after the age of 5? With that in mind, they selected the eight Function tests from the PEPS-C test battery. Participants were selected by age to form groups of 30 (15 male, 15 female), separated by approximately three years; the average ages of the groups, in years, were 5.5; 8.6; 10.8; 13.8. The children were recruited from state-maintained schools in North London. English was their first language and the language spoken in the home and they had no identified speech, language or general educational problems. Each of the four communicative areas in PEPS-C was tested for both comprehension (Input Function) and production (Output Function), giving a total of eight tasks. Each Input task has 16 items, and each Output task has 12 items. The tasks are described in Table 8.1.

The pre-recorded stimuli for the input tasks were presented to each child in a free field, and their responses on all tasks were audio-recorded. The first session was preceded by a vocabulary-checking phase, in which it was ascertained the child was familiar with the words illustrated in the test material. In addition to the PEPS-C battery, each participant was also tested on independent measures of language ability. These standardized tests were administered in order to ascertain whether each child's language development was within normal limits, and to find out how prosodic skills correlated with other language skills. Language production was measured on one expressive language subtest of the Clinical Evaluation of Language Fundamentals - Revised (CELF-R) (Semel, Wiig, & Secord, 1987). For this Formulated Sentences subtest, the child has to make up a sentence using a given word; the child's response is scored for the lexical appropriateness and grammatical coherence of the sentence produced. Comprehension was measured on the Test for the Reception of Grammar (TROG) (Bishop, 1989). In this test, the child hears a sentence and has to match it to one of four pictures; the other three pictures show scenes and objects that might lead the child to select them if the grammar of the sentence has been misunderstood.

Table 8.1 Brief description of PEPS-C Function tasks.

Task name	Description
Focus Input	Recorded stimuli, e.g. 'I wanted CHOCOLATE AND HONEY'/ 'I wanted CHOCOLATE AND HONEY'. Child decides which food the speaker had not received
Focus Output	Tester offers child a picture saying, e.g. 'How about a green bike?' Child has to respond so as to get the picture they actually need, e.g. "I WANT A WHITE BIKE"
Chunking Input	Identification: recorded voice names two foods (e.g. CREAM-BUNS AND CHOCOLATE) or three foods (e.g. CREAM, BUNS AND CHOCOLATE)
Chunking Output	Naming: picture-strip shows two foods (e.g. CREAM-BUNS, CHOCOLATE) or three foods (e.g. CREAM, BUNS, CHOCOLATE)
Interaction Input	Child names picture (e.g. CUP) which tester repeats either fall with low onset (affirming, i.e. 'go on') or rise with high onset (questioning, i.e. 'repeat'). Child decides whether the tester wants child to go on to the next item or to repeat
Interaction Output	Recorded voice speaks a non-word (e.g. PARGLE) or a real word (e.g. CARROT). Child repeats word, to sound as if questioning in order to check understanding (non-word) or affirming, to confirm understanding (real word)
Affect Input	Identification. Single food item on picture. Recorded voice likes it ([m] with rise-fall) or is not keen ([m] with fall-rise)
Affect Output	Child hears food-item (e.g. BANANAS) and, with [m] only, expresses liking or not keen

On the PEPS-C Input tasks, each of which comprises 16 items, each child has only two choices for each item – the response is either right or wrong. Scores of 12 or more indicate that responses are significantly above chance. On the Output tasks, each of which comprises 12 items, the scorer marks the child's production of each item as right (2 points), wrong (0 points) or ambiguous (1 point), giving a possible maximum of 24. In order to interpret the results, it is useful to have a pass mark, above which one can be reasonably confident that the child is in command of the relevant aspect of intonation. This pass mark was set at 18 (75%), since to obtain a score of 18, the child would have to make an unambiguously correct response for at least six items (50%) and make no outright errors. 'Error' and 'ambiguous response' are useful categories for providing a quantitative indicator of age-related differences in performance. However, it cannot be assumed that the intonation patterns that are counted here as 'error' responses do not occur in the adult population. There is considerable variation in the adult population in this respect (Peppé, Maxim, & Wells, 2000). This being the case, it is likely that some of the variation in children's performance is not due to developmental factors, but rather reflects variation in the population at large. In this study, the aim was not to compare children's performance against an adult 'ideal' performance but to identify differences in performance across groups of children of different ages. The children's responses on the four Output tasks were analysed further in order to see whether there were age-related changes in the distribution of error responses and ambiguous responses.

On three of the four Input tasks, there was significant improvement in scores between the youngest and oldest age groups, pointing to some age-related changes in intonation processing and comprehension between the ages of 5 and 14. Moreover, there were significant positive correlations of 5/8 subtests with the CELF-R subtest – three of these being Input subtests – and of 4/8 subtests with TROG, all four being Input subtests. This suggests that the improvements in intonation performance, particularly in comprehension of intonation, may be related to developments in expressive and receptive language skills. However, there were no significant age-related increases on any of the Output tasks. In the following sections, the results for each of the four communicative areas tested will be discussed.

Focus and Tonic placement

Like many studies of children's intonation and Focus, including some described in Chapter 7, the PEPS-C tasks concentrate on narrow Focus. Each item of the Focus Input task takes the form of a single utterance such as (8.2):

(**8.2**) ‖ ⇑`chocolate and ʹhoney ‖

The child has to identify which of two items of food is highlighted by the speaker, and indicate this by pointing to the appropriate picture. The intonation structure for Non-final narrow Focus is represented in (8.2), while the structure for Final narrow Focus is exemplified in (8.3):

(**8.3**) ‖ ʹchocolate and ⇑`honey ‖

Each stimulus consists of a single Intonation Phrase (IP) made up of two Feet. In the Non-final stimulus, such as (8.2), there is a Supertonic followed by a Tail. In the Final stimulus, such as (8.3), there is a Head followed by a Supertonic. Intonation prominence in the form of a Supertonic serves to give narrow Focus on one item of food.

Five-year-olds scored significantly below the pass mark of 75% on the Input Focus task; they also scored significantly lower than the two oldest groups. Only the 13-year-olds scored significantly above the pass mark. They also scored significantly higher than all the other age groups, which suggests that comprehension of Focus is a skill that improves with age during the school years. This is in line with a study of 10-year-old children by Cruttenden (1985) that used a picture-pointing task. Although they performed above chance level, the children were still significantly worse than adults at pointing to the picture that corresponded to the Focus of the spoken stimulus. In a study of English-speaking children aged from 6 to 10 years, Ito, Bibyk, Wagner, and Speer (2014) used eye tracking to investigate the comprehension of the relation between Tonic placement and Focus. The children in their study, even the older ones, were significantly worse at the task than adults, supporting the findings of the studies by Cruttenden (1985) and Wells et al. (2004) that even by the age of 10, children are not adult-like in their comprehension. Ito et al. (2014) did not find improvement in children's comprehension of the Tonic–Focus relationship between the ages of 6 and 10. This is consistent with the finding of Wells et al. (2004) that it was only the 13-year-olds who demonstrated this understanding.

The PEPS-C Focus Output task taps into the child's ability to use Tonic placement in order to achieve narrow Focus on a specific item in the utterance, for the purposes of correcting the previous speaker. It takes the form of a lotto game, in which the cards represent various items of transport in various colours. The child is offered a picture that does not match the ones he already has. The tester pronounces each item with broad Focus, using an intonation contour that does not highlight either the colour word or the vehicle word. Typically this is a descending contour with a low fall on the final word. The child then asks for a different picture, emphasizing the property that differentiates the picture the child wants from the one that had been offered. Thus, exchanges such as (8.4) and (8.5) occur:

(8.4) Tester: ‖ 'how about a 'green `bike ‖
        Child: ‖ I want a a ⇑`white 'bike ‖

(8.5) Tester: ‖ 'how about a 'black `boat ‖
        Child: ‖ I want a 'black ⇑`bus ‖

The child's response is scored as correct if he conveys narrow Focus on the item of new information by placing a Supertonic on it. All the age groups attained the pass mark and there were no significant differences between groups, suggesting that the production of Focus is a skill already attained by the age of 5. This is therefore at odds with the poorer results for the Input task, which tapped comprehension of Focus.

The distribution of errors and ambiguous responses on the Focus Output task was examined with a view to discovering whether there were any developmental patterns in the ability to communicate Focus that were not evident from the quantitative measures. The error rate was small for all groups, though the 5-year-olds made more errors than the other groups on the Non-final Focus responses, where the colour word was to be emphasized. When such errors occurred, the young children tended to locate the Tonic on the final Foot, as in (8.6), thereby conveying the impression of Focus on the vehicle word rather than on the colour word:

(8.6) Tester: ‖'how about a 'white `car ‖
        Child: ‖ I want a 'green `car ‖

This pattern is in line with research on preschool children reported in Chapter 7, which suggests that where children make errors with Tonic placement, it is by shifting the Tonic to the last word in the utterance. One possibility is that some of the 5-year-old children in this study reverted to a developmentally earlier pattern under pressure of the test situation. The opposite error pattern as in (8.7), using a Non-final Tonic where a Final Tonic is contextually predicted, rarely occurred in any group:

(8.7) `Tester: ‖'how about a 'white `car ‖`
    `Child: ‖ I want a 'white 'bike ‖`

However, the most striking finding from the Focus output task is the high number of ambiguous responses that were produced by all age groups for vehicle word responses, as in (8.5.1):

(8.5.1) `Tester: ‖'how about a 'black `boat ‖`
        `Child: ‖ I want a 'black `bus ‖`

There was a strong tendency for the children not to use a Supertonic in final position in the IP, even when, as in (8.5) there was clear contextual motivation for producing narrow Focus. An ambiguous response is where there is, as in (8.5.1), a final fall on BUS but this is not accompanied either by a step up in pitch or by an increase in loudness or duration. The child thus indicates broad Focus over the whole IP, rather than narrow Focus on the final word. Alternatively, ambiguity sometimes arose because the child used two Tonics or Supertonics in the response, as in (8.7.1):

(8.7.1) `‖ I want a ⇑`white ‖ ⇑`bike ‖`

Even in the oldest group, not all the children performed at ceiling on this Output task, which may indicate that some aspects of intonation remain to be acquired in the teenage years. A further possibility is that some aspects of the intonation system, as described in the classic studies of British English intonation, are never actually acquired, or at least are not used consistently even by adults. Although not predicted by theoretical accounts of English intonation, ambiguity in speakers' expression of final narrow Focus has been reported to be quite common in the speech of adult speakers of Southern British English (Peppé et al., 2000). There is thus a degree of variability in the adult population, even from a single dialect area, which needs to be taken into account when considering children's intonation development.

In conclusion, the input and output results for Focus reported by Wells et al. (2004) indicate that on the whole, children's comprehension of the Tonic-Focus relationship lags behind their ability to use the Tonic functionally in their own speech. This lends some support to the conclusions of Cutler and Swinney (1987) that children may be able to use the Tonic to realize Focus in their own speech, before they can make use of it to interpret other speakers' Focus. While children have some understanding of the system in the late preschool period, children's mastery of the interaction between Tonic and Focus may not be fully established until the early teens.

Intonation Phrases, chunking and turn-construction

Chunking in the PEPS-C battery refers to prosodic delimitation of the utterance into units, including Intonation Phrases (IPs). We saw in Chapter 2 that turns are constructed from elements that can be identified in terms of their grammar and also, in part, their intonation features. Although IP boundary features are primarily associated with interactional rather than grammatical units, there are some instances in English where the marking of prosodic boundaries within a turn can also have a grammatical role. It is this kind of grammatical chunking which has been investigated in developmental studies, not least because these grammatical distinctions are amenable to formal testing.

The Chunking tasks in the PEPS-C battery test a grammatical distinction between compound nouns, such as CREAM-BUNS and strings of two nouns, such as CREAM, BUNS. The test stimuli comprise minimal pairs like CREAM-BUNS AND CHOCOLATE, a list of two food items, vs. CREAM, BUNS AND CHOCOLATE, a list of three food items. In the spoken language this distinction can be realized in more than one way. The less salient way of making the contrast is by varying the number of feet within a single IP, as in (8.8) and (8.9):

(8.8) ‖ ˈcream buns and ˋchocolate ‖ (two foods)

(8.9) ‖ ˈcream ˈbuns and ˋchocolate ‖ (three foods)

A more salient way of making the contrast is to produce the utterance with varying numbers of Intonation Phrases, assigning a separate IP to each listed food item:

(8.10) ‖ ˇcream buns ‖ and ˋchocolate ‖ (two foods)

(8.11) ‖ ˇcream ‖ ˇbuns ‖ and ˋchocolate ‖ (three foods)

In (8.11), there are three IPs, whereas in (8.10) there is no separate IP for BUNS. In these examples, the non-final IPs are shown with a fall-rise Tone, which, as shown in Chapter 7, is often used in lists. The marking of IP boundaries may be evident not only by the number of Tones, but also by an audible pause between IPs and the lengthening of the final syllable of the IP. The latter features are frequently used by speakers when drawing attention to this type of contrast (Dankovičová, Pigott, Wells, & Peppé, 2004).

In the Chunking Input task, the child hears a pre-recorded single utterance such as (8.10) or (8.11) and is required to say whether the utterance sounds like two items of food or three. Wells et al. (2004) reported the mean score for all four age groups was above the pass mark of 75%, suggesting that this skill is already established by the time that children begin school. There was age-related improvement, the 10-year-olds scoring significantly higher than the 5-year-olds. Moreover, the children's scores on this task correlated significantly with receptive and expressive language measures. Despite these group trends, the range of scores for each of the four age groups shows that the task is sensitive to individual variability. For example, among the group of 10-year-olds, some children scored at ceiling while others responded at chance level.

A similar experiment was conducted by Atkinson-King (1973) investigating children's ability to comprehend and produce the distinction between compound nouns, such as BLACKBOARD, a board used for writing in a classroom, as opposed to adjective-noun phrases like BLACK BOARD, meaning any board that is coloured black. In terms of intonation structure, these can be represented as in (8.12) and (8.13):

(8.12) ‖ ˋblackboard ‖ (compound noun)

(8.13) ‖ ˈblack ˋboard ‖ (phrase)

Atkinson-King tested 25 American children, ranging in age from 5;10 to 8;10. Following familiarization with the picture stimuli, an Identification test was administered. The child had to choose the correct picture to go with the experimenter's production of e.g. (8.12) or (8.13). Ten of the 25 children scored above chance on this task, the youngest being CA 7;3. Thus, compared to the PEPS-C task administered by Wells et al. (2004), Atkinson-King's task seems to have been harder for children aged 5 and 6.

Another type of intonation chunking was investigated by Beach, Katz, and Skowronski (1996) . Their stimuli were coordinated adjectival phrases differentiated by prosodic phrasing, as in (8.14) and (8.15):

(8.14) ‖ pink and green ‖ and white ‖

(8.15) ‖ pink and ‖ green and white ‖

The participants were adults, and groups of 7- and 5-year-old American children. In an identification task, both groups of children behaved like adults in drawing on pitch and duration features to decide between the two alternatives. Similar to the results of Wells et al. (2004), this suggests that children as young as 5 can use intonation to guide their grammatical interpretation of an utterance they hear.

Cruttenden (1985) investigated children's comprehension of yet another coordinate structure involving intonation phrasing. The two alternative grammatical structures are for a sentence that would be written: "She dressed and fed the baby." In one reading, DRESSED is intransitive, with reflexive meaning, i.e. she dressed herself. This is assumed to require two IPs, as in (8.16):

(8.16) ‖ she ˇdressed ‖ and ˈfed the ˋbaby ‖

In the alternative reading, DRESSED is transitive, with BABY as its direct object. In the test stimuli, this is produced with a single Intonation Phrase, as in (8.17):

(8.17) ‖ she ˈdressed and ˈfed the ˋbaby ‖

The results showed a significant difference between adults and 10-year-old children, suggesting that the ability of the latter to comprehend intonation phrasing is not yet adult-like. However, this result has to be treated with caution since some of the stimuli used are rare in contemporary spoken English: "she dressed" in the meaning of "she dressed herself" is uncommon, "she got dressed" being the more usual form.

We now turn to children's ability to chunk turns in this way in their own speech. In the PEPS-C Chunking Output task, the child is presented with picture-strips, each of which depicts either two items of food (e.g. CREAM-BUNS, CHOCOLATE) or three items (e.g. CREAM, BUNS, CHOCOLATE). The child looks at one picture-strip, unseen by the tester, and tells the tester what is shown there. The tester notes down whether the child sounded as though they were talking about two items of food or three, and then checks by looking at the picture strip. When scoring, the tester compares what the response sounded like with the contents of the picture-strip itself; thus the child is assessed on the ability to realize their communicative intention by signalling the correct number of Intonation Phrases, as in (8.10) vs. (8.11) above, or Feet, as in (8.8) vs. (8.9), aligned appropriately to word boundaries. Wells et al. (2004) reported mean scores above the 75% pass mark for all groups, starting with 82.2% for the 5-year-olds, with no significant further progression with age. This suggests that by the age of 5, many children have acquired the skill of placing IP or Foot boundaries in order to convey the desired meaning. Even so, a quarter of the children tested (31/120), distributed across the age range, scored below the 75% pass mark.

More detailed analysis of the children's responses showed that there was little age-related difference in the rates of ambiguous responses for two-item lists and three-item lists or in the error rate for the three-item lists. However, there were more differences in errors on the two-item lists: the three younger groups performed less well than the 13-year-olds. Children in these younger age groups were more likely to make two-item lists sound like three-item lists, by segmenting the first noun as if it had been a picture on its own. For example, the child is expected to describe the picture depicting CREAM-BUNS, CHOCOLATE (a two-item list) with the structure of (8.8) or (8.10):

(8.8) ‖ ˈcream buns and ˋchocolate ‖

(8.10) ‖ ˇcream buns ‖ and ˋchocolate ‖

The younger children, when making an error, would produce it in a way that was interpreted by the listener as having a structure like (8.9) or (8.11):

(8.9) ‖ ˈcream ˈbuns and ˋchocolate ‖

(8.11) ‖ ˇcream ‖ ˇbuns ‖ and ˋchocolate ‖

The children were thus failing to subordinate BUNS to CREAM as part of the same Intonation Phrase (or Foot). It is possible that the error patterns among some of the younger children, i.e. those in the 5- and 8-year-old groups, reflect immature knowledge of the English intonation system – an interpretation lent some support by the results of the Input task, presumed to tap competence in this aspect of intonation, where significant improvement was found between 5- and 10-year-old groups. An alternative possibility, not controlled for by Wells et al. (2004), is that the tendency of the youngest children to produce more Intonation Phrases is a by-product of a generally slower speech rate that is characteristic of younger children.

The children in the oldest age group made fewer errors overall, and the situation had reversed: they make proportionately more errors by producing three-item lists like two-item lists. CREAM, BUNS, CHOCOLATE, a three-item food list, would be realized with a structure like (8.9) or (8.11). Thus, it appears that sometimes, for some 13-year-olds, the demands of fluency, possibly resulting in a faster speech rate, override the requirements of accurate delimitation of Intonation Phrases.

In all age groups, some children scored at ceiling while others scored around half marks, indicating a lot of variability. In order to discover what features of the children's speech production accounted for these differences, Dankovičová et al. (2004) analysed acoustically the responses of ten children selected at random from the 8-year-old group tested by Wells et al. (2004). Two candidate prosodic boundary features, pause duration and phrase-final lengthening, were analysed in order to establish whether their occurrence was determined by the target. They found that 8-year-old children are not all the same in the use of these prosodic features across individual utterances, and that some children are more consistently accurate than others. Thus, there is variability both across children in the same age band and within speech of the individual child on different occasions.

In a similar study, Katz, Beach, Jenouri, and Verma (1996) investigated children's production of the kind of phrases they had earlier tested for comprehension: [(pink and green) and white] vs. [pink and (green and white)]. Participants were 5-year-olds, 7-year-olds and adults. Contrary to expectations, the children did not manipulate either the length of 'pink' and 'green' or the pauses following them or their pitch patterns, in order to indicate the grouping of the blocks. Thus, in spite of the apparent ability of children of this age to interpret adults' use of prosodic boundaries in an adult-like way (Beach et al., 1996), in their own speech, the children appeared to use neither pitch nor duration features in an adult-like way to convey grouping of objects.

Atkinson-King (1973), as part of the study referred to earlier, investigated children's ability to produce in their own speech the distinction between compound nouns (e.g. BLACKBOARD) and adjective-noun phrases (e.g. BLACK BOARD) that she had tested for comprehension. Output tests of production and imitation were administered, the children's responses being classified as 'compound' or 'phrase' by two judges. In the production test, the children had to name pictures, e.g. of a blackboard or of a black board, using the appropriate prosodic phrasing. Just five children performed above chance level on this task, the youngest of these being CA 7;4. All five were among the ten children who had scored above chance on the Identification task, which suggests that in order to produce the contrast correctly in an appropriate context, it is necessary to understand it. On the Imitation test, where the child had to imitate the experimenter's production of the same items, all 25 children scored above chance. This suggests that young children as young as CA 5;10 do have the phonetic ability to convey this distinction by prosodic phrasing, although most of them do not yet know when to do so.

In summary, the chunking (intonation phrasing) abilities of English and American school-aged children have been tested with regard to both comprehension and production. The results suggest that comprehension has to be established before children are able to produce accurate intonation phrasing, although accurate comprehension does not appear to guarantee accurate production. Another important variable affecting children's performance appears to be the type of linguistic structure, since across the studies described above, which targeted different structures, there were variable results for similar age groups. The apparent variability related to grammatical structure suggests that the mastery of intonation phrasing is closely linked to the child's developing lexical, morphological and grammatical knowledge.

Tone and Interaction

The functions of Tone matching for the purposes of interactional alignment and non-matching for the initiation of new actions, as described in Chapter 4, are tested in the PEPS-C battery, under the communicative area called 'Interaction'. In the Interaction Input task, the distinction is between a low falling Tone, with affirmative meaning, which can be glossed as 'yes I understood'; or a high rising Tone, initiating a repair, which can be glossed as: 'no, I didn't understand, please repeat'. This distinction is thus one of Tone. The child is given a set of pictures, each depicting a single object, e.g. CUP or KEY. The child names what is on one of the pictures. The tester then repeats the name. The tester may repeat with a rising Tone, designed to initiate a repair or request clarification from the child, in which case the child is expected to then say the word again. If the child responds correctly, this should result in a sequence such as (8.18):

(8.18)

```
1   Child:     ‖ ` key ‖ (looking at picture of key)
2   Tester:    ‖ ´ key ‖
3   Child:     ‖ key ‖
```

Alternatively the tester may repeat the child's initial naming with a falling Tone. This is designed to display the tester's accurate hearing and understanding of the child's turn, in which case the child is then expected to go on to the next picture, as in (8.19):

(8.19)

```
1   Child:     ‖ ` key ‖ (looking at picture of key)
2   Tester:    ‖ ` key ‖
3   Child:     (moves on to next picture)
```

Wells et al. (2004) reported that on this Input Interaction task, the means of their three older groups were significantly above the pass mark of 75%. However, the mean for the 5-year-old group was below the pass mark.

The PEPS-C Interaction Output task tests children's use of Tone in their own speech production, again with reference to the functions of aligning and initiating. The child is given one card with a tick on it and another with a question mark. The child hears a list of words one at a time, each being produced with a falling Tone, and is required to repeat each word with an appropriate Tone. In order to prevent the tester picking up visual cues, the child's facial expression is hidden from the tester. After giving the spoken response, the child indicates what had been intended, by pointing to the tick or the question mark as appropriate. The word may be familiar, e.g. CARROT, in which case the child repeats the word in such a way as to confirm that it has been understood, i.e. with a (matching) falling Tone. If the child responds correctly, this should result in a sequence such as (8.20):

(8.20)

```
1   Tester:    ‖ ` carrot ‖
2   Child:     ‖ ` carrot ‖ (spoken from behind screen)
3   Child:     (points to tick symbol)
```

Alternatively, the word may be unfamiliar, e.g. PARGLE, in which case the child is expected to initiate a repair or request clarification, by using a non-matching Tone, i.e. a rise. If the child responds correctly, this should result in a sequence such as (8.21):

(8.21)

```
1   Tester:    ‖ ` pargle ‖
2   Child:     ‖ ´ pargle ‖ (spoken from behind screen)
3   Child:     (points to question mark symbol)
```

In the study by Wells et al. (2004), the three older groups reached the pass mark on this output task, but as with the Input task, the 5-year-olds did not. The distribution of errors and ambiguous responses on the Interaction Output task was then analysed, to see whether there was any developmental change in children's ability to express alignment through Tone matching or initiation through Tone contrast. On the affirming (i.e. matching/aligning) responses, there were relatively few errors in all groups, and these declined gradually with age. On the repair-initiating responses, the 5-year-olds made more than 40% errors. When they made an error response, there was a strong tendency for their 'questioning' (repair-initiating) response to sound affirming, i.e. they matched the tester's Tone, instead of using a non-matching Tone. While it is possible that the younger children have more trouble producing final rising Tones than final falling Tones at a physical level, the fact that on the corresponding Input task, the 5-year-old group had not yet reached the pass mark suggests that their performance on the Output task may be due to a lack of awareness of the functional distinction between matching and non-matching Tones.

The sequences illustrated above in Extracts (8.18) to (8.21) are in fact very similar to sequences that pass off successfully between children and caregivers towards the end of the child's second year of life. Such sequences were illustrated from interactions between Robin and his mother in Chapter 4 and also at the beginning of Chapter 7, with examples from Tarplee (1996). This observation raises the important question, which will be returned to later in this chapter, of why a 5-year-old child may be unable to respond appropriately to an adult intonation pattern in a test situation, when 2-year-old children have no problems doing so in spontaneous interaction.

Patel and Grigos (2006) conducted a similar production study with 4-, 7- and 11-year-old English-speaking children in the USA. The children were required to produce turns such as "Show Bob a bot" (BOT referring to a ROBOT), as a command or as a clarification request, in a play situation. They found that the youngest group did not consistently use pitch height or pitch movement to distinguish between these two functions, though this use of pitch became progressively established across the two older groups. As a result, adult listeners found it difficult to decide whether the utterances produced by the 4-year-olds were statements or questions (Patel & Brayton, 2009). The authors suggest that the children's failure to mark this distinction results from a difficulty in producing final rising Tones, which supports results reported by Snow (1998) for 4-year-olds, summarized in Chapter 7. However, given the evidence that preschool children routinely produce rising tones in spontaneous conversation without apparent difficulty (see Chapter 7), it seems equally likely that the children's difficulty is with understanding the requirements of the task and of taking on board, in a test situation, the notion that clarification requests should be produced with rising intonation.

In summary, the findings of Wells et al. (2004) and of Patel and Grigos (2006) that there are significant improvements between age 4 or 5 and age 10 or 11 suggest that the skills measured by their tasks are acquired in the early school-age period and continue to develop. These skills involve the understanding and production of Tones to confirm or check and understanding. However, the question remains as to why children who are 4 or 5 years old seem unable in a test situation to reproduce uses of Tone that are attested from the spontaneous talk of children who are not yet 2 years old.

Intonation and emotion

There is a commonly held belief that speakers use intonation to express their feelings and that listeners use intonation cues to interpret the feelings of others. So far in this book we have not discussed how emotion might impact on children's intonation. However, an assumed relationship between intonation and attitudes or emotions, such as surprise, reservation, sarcasm and happiness, has underpinned experimental research into intonation with school-aged children. In this section we review some of these studies before considering more broadly the links between intonation and affect.

The PEPS-C battery, as used by Wells, Peppé and Goulandris (2004) in their study of children between the ages of 5 and 13, includes Affect as one of the four communicative areas conveyed by intonation. The PEPS-C Affect tasks test the distinction between strong liking as opposed to reservation, mainly as expressed by use of a rise-fall Tone vs. a fall-rise Tone respectively. In the Affect Input task, the child has two pictures: a smiley face represents 'liking' and a doubtful face represents reservation, explained to the children as being 'not keen'. The child has to indicate the picture corresponding to a recorded stimulus. Each stimulus takes the form of a single syllable consisting of a long bilabial nasal consonant ("mmm") produced with either a rise-fall Tone for liking, as in (8.22) or a fall-rise Tone for reservation, as in (8.23).

(8.22) ‖ ˆmː ‖

(8.23) ‖ ˇmː ‖

Wells et al. (2004) reported that the mean score for all the age groups of children was above the pass mark of 75% and that there was no significant difference between age groups. This suggests that even 5-year-old children are able to understand the use of Tone to distinguish between liking and reservation. However, there was a good deal of variation in the 5-year-old group, with a much higher standard deviation and greater range of scores, suggesting that some 5-year-olds did have problems with the task.

The PEPS-C Affect Output task mirrors the Input task. The child again has the two cards depicting a smiley face and a doubtful face. The tester explains that she wants to know what food the child likes and what food the child is not too keen on. The tester names an item of food, e.g. BANANAS. If the child likes it, they are instructed to say [mː] with an appropriately enthusiastic intonation. This intonation could be a rise-fall Tone as in the Input stimulus shown in (8.22), but other intonation patterns may also be scored as correct if deemed by the tester to convey 'liking', e.g. a fall Tone starting high in the pitch range with a wide span. If the child is not too keen, they should pronounce [mː] with an appropriately unenthusiastic intonation such as the fall-rise Tone used in the Input tasks, shown in (8.23), or a narrow pitch movement low in the pitch range, e.g. a low fall or low rise Tone. While the child is responding, their face is hidden from the tester by a screen, so that only vocal production can signal emotion to the tester. The scorer has access to the child's intention because after uttering each response the child has to point to either a smiley face or a doubtful face. In this way the child's ability to realize the communicative intention phonetically can be assessed.

In the case of both 'like' and 'not keen' responses, 5-year-olds made significantly more errors than the three older age groups, who made few errors. Thus, 5-year-olds appear to have difficulty in expressing both options. In the case of the 'not keen/ reservation' option, when indicating that they were doubtful about a food item, their intonation did not convey this. Similarly, in the case of the 'like' option, they could not use intonation consistently to convey this emotion. One possibility is that the 5-year-olds have less physical control than older children over the production of complex Tones such as the rise-fall and the fall-rise when these need to be mapped onto a single syllable, as required in the Affect Output task. This would then be a difficulty with 'tune' to 'text' association.

Alternatively, the youngest children's difficulties with the Affect Output task could reflect an immature level of understanding of how intonation is used to convey affective meaning. As the 5-year-old group exceeded the pass mark on the corresponding Input task, this would seem unlikely, although earlier research by Cruttenden (1985) suggested that the distinction may not be understood by children as old as 10. Cruttenden compared a group of 10-year-old English children to adults, using a picture-pointing method similar to the one in the PEPS-C input task. The contrasting stimuli were the sentences shown in (8.24) and (8.25):

(8.24) ‖ its a very nice ˇgarden ‖

(8.25) ‖ its a very nice ˆgarden ‖

Cruttenden's results indicate that the adults and children both performed equally well on stimuli like (8.25) but the adults were much better than the children at identifying the affective meaning of 'reservation' in stimuli like (8.24). The implication that this ability is not acquired by age 10 is at odds with the results of Wells et al. (2004) who found that the meaning of 'reservation' associated with the fall-rise Tone was already understood by 5-year-olds. The discrepancy may be due to the difference in the lexical content of the stimuli: in the PEPS-C task, it was a single syllable while in Cruttenden's study, the stimuli were associated with a full sentence, requiring a higher level of semantic and inferential processing. This points to a recurrent theme when examining intonation competence in the school years: that one of the main challenges for children is to associate relatively simple intonation contrasts with different kinds of grammatical and lexical 'text' of varying degrees of complexity.

Such discrepant results raise the possibility that this type of investigation may be based on a false premise, namely that there is a relationship between a speaker's intonation and that speaker's affect, emotion or attitude. There are two grounds for doubting the existence of such a link: first, it is not supported by evidence from the analysis of everyday speech; and, second, apparent relationships can be better explained in terms of other, better-attested intonation systems. The association between the fall-rise Tone and reservation is a case in point. We saw in Chapter 2 and again in Chapter 7 that the fall-rise, which normally does not end at the top of the speaker's range is routinely used on IPs that are not turn-final, where it serves to project another IP in the same turn. That next IP may be the final IP in the turn, in which case it will end L or H, i.e. at the bottom or the top of the speaker's range. Since the fall-rise normally projects an incomplete turn, in cases where the current speaker does stop talking after an IP with a fall-rise Tone, the listener may make the inference that the speaker is holding something back, i.e. expressing 'reservation'. Thus, the expression of 'reservation' through intonation is achieved not through a direct association between a particular Tone and a specific emotion or attitude. Instead, it derives from the speaker's exploitation of the systematic link between intonation and turn-taking.

Moreover, there is little empirical support from research into intonation in everyday talk for a direct relationship between intonation and emotion. A 'direct' relationship would be one where particular intonation features are associated with specific emotions in a context-free way. A striking case is the claim that there are particular prosodic features associated with irony or sarcasm. Researchers have attempted to track age-related changes in children's understanding of the intonation component of irony and sarcasm. Studies by Capelli, Nakagawa, and Madden (1990) and Winner and Leekam (1991) failed to find differences between different age-groups of children. A comparison of these two studies shows that agreement on the intonation correlates of specific emotions is hard to find. The descriptions of sarcastic intonation are quite different for the two experiments: when presenting the stimuli, Winner and Leekam's speaker used a "flat tone" whereas Capelli and colleagues report that their speaker "greatly exaggerated the modulation of pitch". In fact, there is little evidence for any specific prosodic correlate of irony and sarcasm in English (Bryant & Fox Tree, 2005). What listeners seem to respond to as ironic or sarcastic is a noticeable differentiation of the ironic utterance from its non-ironic context, e.g. by a marked reduction in pitch range. Glenwright, Parackel, Cheung, and Nilsen (2014) found that for Anglophone Canadian children aged 5 to 6, as for adults, the bigger the phonetic difference was, the easier it was for the children to detect sarcasm.

Differentiating one's speaking turn from its prior context seems to be the most important phonetic means of displaying attitude or affect. In a prosodic and interactional analysis of spontaneous English conversations between adults, Elizabeth Couper-Kuhlen (2009) demonstrates how speakers can display emotions such as disappointment and irritation in this way. While there is some evidence that the same emotion will be displayed in similar ways on different occasions, for instance, disappointment is displayed with 'subdued' prosody that includes reduced pitch range and loudness, Couper-Kuhlen is careful to point out the same 'subdued' features are also used to convey other emotions, such as sympathy. This point is also evident from conversations analysed by Local and Walker (2008). In one of these, the listener comments explicitly on how the speaker just sounded, "you sound sleepy", following which the original speaker explicitly corrects the listener's interpretation: "I'm not sleepy I'm just kind of sad..." (Local & Walker, 2008: 732–733). Such examples show that vocal features are likely to prove an unreliable guide to a speaker's affective state.

Where affect is displayed by some kind of phonetic differentiation from the prior context, it usually involves global parameters present across the IP, such as pitch range, loudness, tempo and voice quality – parameters that are traditionally labelled as paralinguistic. These do not necessarily impinge on the intonation systems of Tone and Tonic that have been highlighted in this book. One exception to this may be the case of the Supertonic, which has been shown to have a particular role in conveying narrow Focus (see Chapter 3). Ogden (2006) shows how what we have called a Supertonic is also used in environments where two speakers make successive evaluations or assessments. In one of Ogden's examples, reproduced here as (8.26), two English students are talking about a castle they want to visit in Germany:

(8.26) B: ‖ its supposed to be really `pretty ‖
        A: ‖ oh its supposed to be ⇑^gorgeous ‖

By using "gorgeous" compared to B's "pretty", A upgrades her evaluation of the castle compared to B's evaluation, which it follows. A's use of the Supertonic supplements this lexical upgrade. As Ogden shows, the Supertonic works in this context of a second assessment because it contrasts with the less prominent Tonic that was used by B in the first assessment. Here, the system of Tonic vs. Supertonic, which is routinely used to make the distinction between broad and narrow Focus, is exploited by B in her second assessment. It might well be heard as 'enthusiastic'.

In summary, analysis of conversations indicates that there is no simple correspondence between specific emotions and particular intonation features. Where intonation contributes to the display of affect, it is often parasitic upon established intonation systems, the primary function of which is to manage interaction, and it mainly depends on phonetic differentiation from the prior context rather than reference to a dictionary of the affective meanings of prosodic features.

Testing intonation in the school years: what does it tell us?

The results of testing children's intonation suggest that within each of the three functional areas of Focus, Turns and Action, the ability to produce intonation functionally is largely established by the age of 5;0. Chunking and Focus production skills were evident in most of the 5-year-old group studied by Wells et al. (2004). This tallies with the conclusion from Chapter 7 that intonation resources are already used effectively by preschool young children to convey communicative intent. It also tallies with the intonation behaviours of the three 5-year-old boys, Johnny, Fred and Mick, as they negotiated their construction game in Extract (8.1). Consequently, not all intonation skills are likely to show a clear pattern of development through the school years.

There is evidence that some 5-year-olds still have difficulties with certain aspects of the intonation system. However, this seems likely to result from a problem with understanding the demands of the task and how specific intonation features are supposed to relate to concepts such as 'question', or being 'not keen' on something. It is less likely to result from difficulty with the physical production of rising or complex Tones, since there is ample evidence that young children produce these without apparent difficulty in their everyday talk. The conversation presented in Extract (8.1) at the start of this chapter between the three 5-year-old boys illustrates that point repeatedly.

As for intonation comprehension, there is more evidence that this continues to develop after age 5. Wells et al. (2004) found that the children's performance on the PEPS-C input function tasks correlated strongly with measures of receptive and expressive language development, suggesting that during the school years, intonation comprehension as measured by the PEPS-C tasks, develops in line with other aspects of grammatical comprehension and production. This finding contributes to the conclusion that the main problem for school-aged children is how to work out relationships between intonation and grammatical structures. This requires meta-intonation awareness: an ability to reflect on intonation as a component of speech.

At the same time, there may be considerable variation in test performance among children of the same age. This was true of all age groups in the PEPS-C study. However, it is also true of adults as Peppé, Maxim and Wells (2000) found when using an early version of the PEPS-C battery. Although some variation was attributable to education level, a large amount remained which could not be attributed to any of the other factors they investigated, suggesting that even among adults, there are considerable individual differences.

For intonation, as for other areas of language development, questions remain about the relationship between children's ability as demonstrated by performance on tests and their ability as demonstrated by their competence in naturally occurring interactions. Test paradigms that try to force the child to use particular words or structures run the risk that the child will respond in ways that correspond only very indirectly to their behaviour in the language learning contexts of naturalistic conversation. For example, in intonation experiments, stimuli are often devised which seem to ignore the fact that ellipsis is closely related to Focus, i.e. that in responding to a question the person answering will routinely omit 'given' parts of the question. Getting children either to provide unnaturally full answers or to make judgements about dialogues which contain such unnatural sequences is likely to undermine the usefulness and generalizability of the results.

Intonation and reading aloud

In this chapter, discrepancies have been noted between the intonation competence displayed by children in spontaneous interaction and their performance in a test situation. A possible explanation is that rather than accessing intonation competence, tests of intonation such as those in the PEPS-C battery tap into the child's meta-intonation awareness and the ability to demonstrate that awareness in a performance, such as a test situation. Interpreted in this way, the results of test-based studies may be of particular relevance when considering a major challenge that faces school children: learning to read. It is usually quite easy to tell whether a person is talking spontaneously or is reading aloud and it is likely that in part this is signalled by differences in their intonation. As listeners, we make value judgements not only about the accuracy and fluency of a person's reading aloud but also on the aesthetic qualities of their reading. Researchers and educationalists have been interested in identifying what contributes to this perceived expressiveness in reading aloud, which can be viewed as one desirable outcome of reading attainment. According to Cowie, Douglas-Cowie, and Wichmann (2002):

> It is plausible to suggest that fluency depends on the exercise of skills concerned with recognizing and signalling groupings required by the syntax of the text: whereas the skills relating to expression involve recognizing opportunities to signal semantically richer relationships involving, for instance, communicative function, topic significance, or emotional colour.
>
> *(Cowie et al., 2002: 49)*

Studies have drawn on listeners' intuitions of what is 'expressive' and 'fluent', correlating listener ratings of these qualities with speech measures, mainly of pitch and timing. Perera (1989), who relied on auditory analysis of intonation, was surprised not to find a relationship between expressiveness and intonation features. This led her to suggest that there could be other features such as juncture or voice quality that are more relevant for expressiveness. Some acoustic studies have found correlations of expressiveness with some global pitch features, e.g. number and width of pitch movements (Cowie et al., 2002; Benjamin et al., 2013). While, on the whole, these studies have not adopted a functional approach, Benjamin et al. (2013) included as measures of expressiveness the extent of a final pitch fall at the end of declaratives and also the location of pauses within the read sentence. These prosodic features contribute to the division of speech into IPs, i.e. 'chunking'. There is some evidence that the ability to read expressively, as judged by listeners and as characterized by these prosodic features, correlates with reading comprehension (Benjamin & Schwanenflugel, 2010). With this in mind, measures of reading fluency and expressiveness have been devised by educationalists (e.g. Benjamin et al., 2013).

   In the context of this book, the following questions about the relationship between reading and intonation are of special interest:
1 How do children become expressive users of intonation when reading aloud?
2 How does the development of this skill build on the intonation competences that children have developed in the preschool years?
3 How does the development of this skill relate to the development of meta-intonation awareness?

How do children use intonation when reading aloud?

The development of children's use of intonation for reading aloud has been comprehensively investigated by Katharine Perera in a longitudinal study of six children in the North-West of England, between the ages of approximately 5;06 and 8;06 (Perera, 1989). Each child was recorded every three months. In each recording session, the child was asked to read aloud from a book that they were currently using as part of classroom reading instruction. In the final session, all the children read the same, specially prepared passages, designed to target specific features of English intonation, the aim being to compare the children and investigate the degree of variability in reading aloud among children of the same age. In the first and the last sessions, each child was also asked to tell a story, based on some pictures provided by the researcher. The aim was to provide a sample of non-read speech, so that the intonation of the child's reading could be compared with the intonation of the same child's habitual talk. Perera transcribed all the recordings with an intonation notation that largely followed that devised by O'Connor and Arnold (1973) for their text book for foreign learners of British English. While it is more elaborate than the notation provided in Chapter 1 of this book, they share the same basic features. In the remainder of this section we will discuss some of Perera's findings in relation to the main functions of intonation.

Turn-construction and chunking

As would be expected, there was a massive improvement in children's reading speed between the first and last recording sessions: the mean increased from 27.3 to 128 words per minute (Perera 1989: 219). This increase in reading fluency had an impact on the intonation patterns used: the younger children used shorter Intonation Phrases (IPs) and more rising Tones, reflecting that in the earlier sessions they would read a sentence in short chunks, sometimes word by word or else in short phrases, often using a rising tone on the non-final IPs. This is evident in (8.27), from child SB in Session 3 (Perera, 1989: 300):

(8.27) ‖ ´Im ‖ (.) ´going ‖ (.) ´to (3.0) ‖ ´try ‖ (2.0) ʹthat aˋgain ‖

Children at this stage "often reach a full stop or line end with audible relief, marking closure with a falling tone and a sigh" (p. 369).

A key difference between conversation and reading aloud is that when reading aloud, the child is typically given the floor for an extended period. Occupancy of the floor is not constantly under threat in the way that it is, for instance, for the three boys playing together in Extract (8.1). In that kind of peer interaction, the current speaker has to display that he has not yet finished his turn until such time as he is ready to relinquish the floor, drawing on the traffic light system of intonation. When, as in reading aloud, the speaker's turn is not under threat, the main function of intonation is to help the listener to make sense of what is being read. Thus, intonation chunking is used by the speaker to enhance comprehensibility. In the early sessions of Perera's study, the children appeared to use rising tones to show that they had not yet reached the end. Thus, when starting to read, the children recapitulated the start of the multiword stage in spoken language development, where each spoken element that the child produces has its own IP, as was the case for Robin at the onset of the multiword stage described in Chapter 7.

However, the children soon learnt that, when reading, this is not necessary. The fact that there was a higher proportion of low-rise Tones in their oral story telling than in their reading suggests that in oral story-telling they were aware of the need to project that they have more to say (p. 363).

Even in the first session, at the age of 5, the children took account of grammatical structure, often reading the text in small chunks that coincide with grammatical phrases rather than random strings of two or three adjacent words (p. 474). By age 6;05 they were using IP boundaries to mark major grammatical boundaries in the text (p. 473). This suggests that they appreciated an equivalence between the sentence in the written language and the turn-constructional unit in conversation. At the mean age of 8;05, there was over 80% agreement about where to place IP boundaries, indicating that the children shared a convention about how IPs should be mapped onto the written text.

The division of written text into IPs when reading aloud is aided by the English punctuation system. Commas can serve to indicate IP boundaries, as in examples (8.11) and (8.12) from the PEPS-C Chunking tasks, reproduced here as (8.28) and (8.29). The comma following < Cream> in (8.29) shows that there is likely to be an IP boundary when the sentence is read aloud:

(8.28) Spoken: ‖ˇcream buns ‖ and ˋchocolate ‖ (two foods)
   Written: < Cream-buns and chocolate >

(8.29) Spoken: ‖ˇcream ‖ˇbuns ‖ and ˋchocolate ‖ (three foods)
   Written: < Cream, buns and chocolate. >

However, commas can be fallible as a guide to sentence-internal IP boundaries. For example, the rules of English punctuation forbid the use of a comma between < buns > and <and> in (8.28) and (8.29), even though an IP boundary is likely to occur there. Children have to learn about such mismatches between spoken and written language. The same problem does not arise with the sentence-final IP boundary, since at the end of a sentence it is obligatory to place either a full stop, a question mark or an exclamation mark.

From the outset, learning to read and write entails learning about punctuation. In the assessment framework guidelines for teachers published in 2009 by the UK Curriculum and Qualifications Authority, some awareness of punctuation and pausing at full-stops is included from the very beginning (Reading Level 1). In addition, Level 1 guidelines for writing make reference to awareness of capital letters and full stops to mark the beginning and end of a sentence. At Level 2, for children aged 6 and 7, the framework states that there should be some fluency and expression in reading, taking account of punctuation and speech marks. In writing, in addition to accurate demarcation of sentences using capital letters and full stops, there should be some accurate use of question marks, exclamation marks and commas in lists. Since in the course of learning both to read and to write, children are asked to read aloud from books and from their own writing, they are very soon confronted with the issue of how to pronounce punctuation marks when they occur in a text. Apart from pausing at full-stops, there is no obvious consensus on how to pronounce other marks such as < ? >, < ! > or < , >. In this respect, the interpretation of punctuation differs from the pronunciation of letters and letter combinations, for which there is usually a consensus, such that when reading <Cream> for example, <C> will be pronounced [k], <ea> will be pronounced [i] and <m> will be pronounced [m], although sometimes variation is found, as for <r>. The lack of an agreed pronunciation for question marks and commas has some interesting consequences for the intonation of children's reading aloud, as will be discussed later in this chapter.

Focus

Focus is not routinely marked in English orthography (Perera, 1984). Although a writer can use underlining, capitalization or italics, this option tends to be used sparingly, only on occasions where there is narrow Focus on an item of special importance for the text. Despite the shortage of guidance from punctuation as to Focus, Perera (1989) reports that at age 8 there was 80–85% agreement across the six children in her study on placement of the Tonic. Over time there was a significant increase in non-final Tonic placements, which seems to be due to the occurrence of longer and lexically more complex IPs, resulting from the more complex texts that the children read as they got older. By the age of 8, the distribution of Tonic placement was similar to that found in the children's oral storytelling, which was similar at age 5 and at age 8. This is evidence that in the course of learning to read, children progressively learn to reproduce when reading aloud those features of intonation that they already use in their speech.

Across all sessions, the children produced relatively few examples of Tonic placement that Perera deemed to be errors in terms of the Focus requirements of the text. Over half of these 'errors' (n=55) were cases where the child used a final Tonic, signalling broad Focus, where the prior context predicts narrow Focus on an earlier word in the sentence. Perera gives the example of an error made by all the children in the text *A Trip to the Zoo*, which they all read in the final session. The first 14 lines of this text, which was specially constructed by Perera to elicit intonation features, are reproduced as Figure 8.1. Now complete Activity 8.2 before reading further.

ACTIVITY 8.2

Aim: To identify some of the issues related to intonation that arise when reading aloud.

1 Make a copy of the passage from *A Trip to the Zoo* presented in Figure 8.1.
2 Read the passage aloud. Make an audio recording of your reading.
3 Listen to your recording line by line. Make an intonation transcription on your copy of the following lines: **3** (omit *she said*); **4**; **8** (omit *said Mrs Brown*); **9** (omit *said Jim*); **10**. For each line of these lines, transcribe as follows:
    1 Underline each Tonic word.
    2 Insert a stress mark before other prominent syllables: '.
    3 Insert Intonation Phrase (IP) boundaries at the start and end of each IP: ‖
    4 Insert a Tone diacritic before each Tonic syllable, choosing from: ˋ Fall; ˊ Rise; ˆ Rise-fall; ˇ Fall-rise.
4 Make a note of alternative intonation patterns that you might have used and of any difficulties you experienced.
Check your answers with the Key to Activity 8.2 at the end of this chapter.

1 Jim and Jane went to the zoo with their class.

2 Their teacher, Mrs Brown, was very glad that the weather was good.

3 "It's a lovely day, isn't it?" she said.

4 "What do you want to see first?"

5 "Lions," said Bob.

6 "Monkeys," said Sally.

7 "Elephants," said Peter.

8 "Let's go and see the elephants first," said Mrs Brown.

9 "Oh good," said Jim, "I like elephants."

10 There were three elephants, two big ones and a baby.

11 Jane was amazed that they were so big.

12 "Aren't they enormous," she said.

13 Jane had a bun in her bag.

14 She gave it to Sally and she gave it to the baby elephant.

Figure 8.1 Extract from the reading passage *A Trip to the Zoo*. Source: (Perera, 1989: 125).

All six children read the first part of line 10 with the intonation shown in (8.30):

(8.30) ‖there were 'three `elephants‖

The Tonic is placed on the final word, even though the Focus and therefore the Tonic would have been expected on THREE, since ELEPHANTS has occurred in the immediately preceding lines of the passage, i.e. lines 7–9 (Perera, 1989: 383). The children in Perera's study sometimes used this pattern in the oral story telling session at age 5, though not at age 8 (p. 393). This echoes the common developmental pattern found in spontaneous talk among young typically developing children, described in Chapter 7, as well as some older children with delayed speech development, like David who was described in Chapters 3 and 5. Thus, it appears that when learning to read, children may sometimes recapitulate immature patterns that they may have used in spontaneous speech when younger. The same tendency to place the Tonic at the end of the IP when the context requires an earlier narrow Focus was noted when discussing the PEPS-C results relating to Focus, being particularly common among the youngest age-group, the 5-year-olds in the study by Wells et al. (2004). Taken together, these observations support a developmental interpretation: when children learn to read aloud, they have to reflect consciously on the Focus-Tonic relationship, just as they do in the PEPS-C Focus tests, and in both situations children are liable to revert to a stage of intonation development that they have already moved though in their spontaneous oral language use. This is then relevant to our second question about reading aloud: How does the development of this skill build on the intonation competences that children have developed in the preschool years?

Action and Tone

The proposal that when children learn to read aloud they recapitulate immature patterns of intonation is also supported by the children's use of Tones. Perera (1989: 298) reports that the numerical distribution of Tones in reading at age 8 was similar to the distribution found in the children's oral story telling at age 5, though different from the distribution in the children's reading at age 5. Perera suggests that the child's intonation when learning to read thus catches up with what the child is already able to do with intonation orally.

Of the three core systems of intonation, it is the Tone system that, according to Perera's analysis, displays most variability among children learning to read. One point of particular interest is the choice of Tone for questions, since questions have an invariant marking in the orthography, i.e. the question mark, but are variable in their Tone in spontaneous speech, as explained in Chapter 4. The text, *A Trip to the Zoo*, contains a number of questions, all but one of which have a grammatical interrogative form. There are four yes–no (polar) interrogatives, like (8.31), occurring later in the passage than the extract in Figure 8.1.

(8.31) "Did you like the animals?"

For yes–no questions like this, the children used either a rising Tone or a falling Tone, the split being approximately equal. By contrast, all the children used a falling Tone on the two wh-interrogatives. For example, line 4: "What do you want to see first?" was produced as in (8.32):

(8.32) ‖ what do you want to see `first ‖

There is one question in *A Trip to the Zoo* that is not marked syntactically as an interrogative, its status as a question being indicated solely by a question mark. It is shown here as (8.33):

(8.33) "Yes," said Mrs Brown "but we can come again soon."
"Tomorrow?" asked Jim.

All six children used a falling Tone on Tomorrow, contrary to what is often thought to be the usual choice of a Rise for this type of question (cf. Chapter 4). Two children had used a rise on the preceding line, so the fall on "Tomorrow?" was a non-matching Tone, as might be expected to initiate a new action such as Jim making a request. However, it seems that the children's use of Tone in reading aloud does not necessarily adhere to the spoken interaction system of matching vs. non-matching , since the other four children had produced the preceding line with a fall and so by using a fall on "Tomorrow?" produced a matching Tone.

The six children were all consistent in using a falling Tone on a tag question that expects agreement, as in line 4 of Figure 8.1: "It's a lovely day, isn't it?" Conversely, they all used a rising Tone on a tag question that requests confirmation, when the speaker clearly is uncertain about this knowledge, as in (8.34):

(8.34) Jim wasn't certain. He said, "I think it's a goat, isn't it?"

In summary, there was a high level of agreement among the six children on the choice of Tone for all types of question except the yes–no polar interrogative. A falling Tone was the most common one for the other types of question, except for the question tag that clearly requests confirmation. It seems that these six children were not following the rule that questions should be produced with a rising tone. As mentioned in Chapter 4, this rule is invoked in the novel *Atonement* by 13-year-old Bryony when coaching 8-year-old Pierrot to speak the lines of her play:

> He intoned a roll-call of words. "Do-you-think-you-can-escape-from-my-clutches?" All present and correct.
> "It's a question", Bryony cut in. "Don't you see? It goes up at the end."
> "What do you mean?"
> "There. You just did it. You start low and end high. It's a *question.*"
>
> *(McEwan, 2001: 33–34)*

In this matter (as in other matters central to the plot of the novel), Bryony is convinced that she is right, whereas in reality she is quite mistaken: most of the time, questions in English do not go up at the end.

As we shall see in Chapter 9, intonation in reading aloud draws on quite different psycholinguistic mechanisms from intonation in interaction, being essentially a process of "tune-to-text" mapping. When reading aloud, the speaker is provided with a written text which contains a great deal of information about how to pronounce the consonants and vowels of the words in the text. This comes from two sources. The first is the phonetic information that is encoded in most of the letters and letter combinations of an alphabetic system like that of English. The second is the knowledge of the pronunciation of the whole word that is stored in the reader's mental lexicon along with its meaning and its spelling (cf. Stackhouse and Wells, 1997: Chapter 6), which means that the reader can retrieve the pronunciation of a known word even when, like the word YACHT, its spelling is not phonetically very transparent.

On the other hand, a written text provides very little information as to how to produce its intonation. What information there is relates to the placement of prosodic boundaries. We have seen that the full stops, question marks and exclamation marks are a reliable guide to placing an IP boundary, though the absence of these at a particular place in the text does not mean that there is no IP boundary there. A comma can be a good guide to the presence of an IP or Foot boundary, although again the absence of a comma at a particular place in the text cannot be taken to mean that there is no prosodic boundary at that point. Tonic placement is only rarely marked in the text. Italics are occasionally used to indicate narrow Focus, in which case they imply a Supertonic when reading aloud. Otherwise, the reader has to rely on understanding the text as a whole in order to work out whether the Focus is broad or narrow and where the Tonic should therefore be placed. As for Tone, the punctuation system supplies no reliable information. In English punctuation, the question mark is largely redundant, since questions are already associated with interrogative syntactic structures. If question marks are omitted from a text, in the large majority of cases, it is quite clear from its syntax that a sentence is intended to be a question. This being the case, in order to give a prosodic interpretation to punctuation conventions such as the question mark, it may be necessary for the child, as apprentice reader, to buy into some prevailing intonation stereotypes shared by English speakers and readers. One such stereotype is that at the level of intonation there is a formal distinction between questions, which have a rising Tone, and statements, which have a falling Tone. Despite the stereotype, many teenage and adult readers persist in not conforming to this expectation, as is evident from experiments that attempt to get adults to read questions with a rising intonation (e.g. Grabe, Post, Nolan, & Farrar, 2000).

The third question posed at the start of this section on learning to read aloud was: how does the development of the skill of reading aloud relate to the development of meta-intonation awareness? We have suggested in this chapter that during the school years children develop awareness of intonation, as is evident in the performance of children of different ages on tests of intonation such as the PEPS-C battery. This awareness is necessary in order to learn to read texts aloud with meaning and expression and its development is evident in the kinds of intonation pattern used by beginning readers in Perera's study. However, using the example of question intonation, we have also suggested that being aware of intonation does not necessarily entail an accurate understanding of how intonation functions in everyday conversation; nor does it lead to a consistent approach to intonation when reading aloud, e.g. when reading questions.

Summary

In this chapter on the intonation of school-aged children we have been mainly concerned with the question: what more does a child have to master during the school years? From the perspective of daily spoken interaction, the short answer is: "Not much." We have seen that, at the start of schooling, children are likely already to have a command of the three intonation systems that play a fundamental role in spoken interaction. The contexts in which they come to be used will expand, however. For example, Hellermann (2003), in a study of Grade 11 and Grade 12 classroom interactions in the USA, shows that intonation contour matching in particular is a powerful resource for the management of pedagogical exchanges that is used by teachers and responded to by their teenage students.

The longer answer is that there are important changes and developments in the use and particularly the understanding of intonation in the school years. In test situations, children in the school years do not display adult-like comprehension of all aspects of English intonation. While 5-year-old children can demonstrate important functional intonation skills, there are further developments in prosodic comprehension between the ages of 5;0 and 8;6, some aspects of intonation continuing to develop after that. Non-adult-like performance has been demonstrated in children as old as 10. Furthermore, functional prosodic comprehension correlates significantly with the development of other aspects of language.

In a study of the spontaneous speech of 12 children from Tyneside in the course of their sixth year of life, which coincides with the first year of formal schooling, John Local (1982) showed that there was a highly significant increase in number of words per tone unit (Intonation Phrase) over the period studied: at the beginning of the period under study, the mean was c. 2.2–2.4, while at the end of the sixth year, the mean number of word per tone unit was c. 2.9, at lower end of the range reported for comparable speech style for adults (Local, 1982: 70). The results indicate that extension of the Intonation Phrase, which we have highlighted as the most salient development of the preschool period, continues into the school years.

This increase in IP length indicates that one of the challenges for the school-aged child is to map onto ever more complex grammatical structures the basic intonation systems that emerged in early childhood out of spoken interaction. The child encounters increasingly complex grammar at school, particularly through exposure to the written language. The developing ability to map intonation onto grammatical structures relies on a growing awareness of what intonation can do. As this awareness develops, children can exploit intonation for expressive purposes when reading aloud as well as in other oral activities such as drama, debating and giving presentations.

Paradoxically, as the child's spoken language becomes more intelligible, comprehensible and sophisticated, the original functions of intonation become less important. Once children are able to produce turns consisting of complex grammatical structures, e.g. with subordinate and main clauses, in which all the words are intelligible, the listener is less dependent on intonation traffic lights to know when the turn is coming to an end: this is evident from the meaning of the words as they combine in phrases and clauses. Similarly with Focus, it is possible to use word order and grammatical choices to highlight one element of the turn and to background the rest, so there is less need for Tonic prominence. Alignment and initiation of new actions can also be achieved by lexical and grammatical means, with less reliance on Tone matching and contrast.

However, these systems are still part of the individual's repertoire of resources and are particularly in evidence in adverse conditions for communication. Such conditions may be environmental, e.g. in a noisy situation, words are likely to be less intelligible so speakers and listeners will be more reliant on intonation cues of pitch, loudness and duration , which are more robust perceptually than the cues to vowels and consonants.

The adverse conditions may also be internal, affecting one of the participants in the conversation. In Chapter 6, we saw that the three intonation systems were particularly evident in adult speech when talking to infants, characteristic of the register of infant-directed speech (IDS). A similar register may be used by parents and professionals, such as speech and language therapists, when working with children who have difficulties with hearing, comprehension or social interaction. The child who has speech output difficulties and for that reason has reduced intelligibility, may be more reliant on intonation in order to participate in conversations. This was the case with David, presented in Chapters 3 and 5. As we shall see in the remaining three chapters, this may also be the case for children who have difficulties with expressive language and with social interaction. When considering such children, it is important therefore to have an understanding of the typical course of intonation development. Providing such an understanding has been the aim of this chapter along with the previous two chapters. However, the picture of intonation development presented here highlights variability. It appears that the age of acquisition of a specific ability may vary; levels of ability in a specific skill vary across children; and competence in different modes (comprehension and expression of intonation) may become evident at different ages. As a result, caution is required when attempting to assess the intonation abilities of an individual child from a developmental perspective. With that caveat, the main points from this chapter are summarized in Table 8.2. The summary tables from Chapters 6, 7 and 8 are collated in Appendix 4.

Table 8.2 Summary of intonation-related capacities and behaviours in the school years.

		TURNS/IP	FOCUS/TONIC	ALIGNMENT/TONE
Internal Maturation		General development of meta-awareness enables child to progressively become more aware of intonation chunking, e.g. compound nouns	General development of meta-awareness enables child to progressively become more aware of Tonic/Focus (as in PEPS-C Bingo & other Focus experiments)	Laryngeal changes, including puberty General development of meta-awareness enables child to progressively become more aware of Interactional role of Tone (as in PEPSC)
Input	Adult – Teacher - Peer	Instruction (explicit/ implicit) on Turn-taking in formal situations. e.g. classroom Teaching about punctuation and its relation to sentence structure (full stop, comma, etc.) as equivalent to Intonational chunking of spoken turns Teaching of word-by-word decoding and reading aloud	Adult uses Tonic to signal new/important information in complex spoken input e.g. stories read aloud, and lessons on range of subjects .Child has to follow Topic development	Instruction (explicit/implicit) in classroom re. matching aligning and non-matching/ initiating, around repair & correction sequences Teaching about written language punctuation and its assumed relation to speech acts, e.g. Question, Exclamation
Language	Learning to read (aloud); oral narrative; drama	Needs to work out relationship between spoken Turns / TCUs and written sentences Dysfluency induced by demands of orthographic decoding recapitulates dysfluency of early 'Syntagmatic' phase Can lead to 'error' where child recruits List intonation (non-final IPs) to deal with reading aloud a (non-list) sentence word by word	When reading aloud, child needs to work out how the Focus in a sentence can be identified from the sentence itself in relation to the prior written context (given/new); and then apply Tonic or Supertonic accordingly in the right place When reading aloud, can lead to recapitulation of final Tonic 'error' pattern found in early Syntagmatic phase	Child acquires dialect-specific phonetic exponents of Tones Increasing awareness of indexical sociophonetic dimension of intonation Learns 'adult' conventions about mapping between speech act, as indicated by punctuation, and Tone choice. Establishes a Tone 'lexicon' for reading/ drama/meta tasks Can lead to 'errors' where child uses spoken language/interactional conventions (e.g. Tone matching for alignment) instead of written language conventions (i.e. a Tonal lexicon)

Key to Activity 8.1

Here is one example from the transcript to answer each question. Further instances are mentioned in the text of the chapter.

Line (1): To convey broad Focus, the Tonic would be located on "water pipe" rather than "long". The Supertonic on "long" indicates that water pipes have just been a topic of conversation.

Line (12): Johnny produces an IP with a Tonic on the penultimate word, signalling a yellow traffic light. Mick then immediately takes a turn. This is one of the clearest examples. See text for further discussion.

Line 12 matches Mick's turn in Line 11. Johnny aligns with Mick's action of placing a piece on the model by placing a further piece on the model himself.

Key to Activity 8.2

1 Listen to the recording of this passage (8.35).
2 Note any differences between that reading and your own reading.
3 Study the intonation transcription of the lines presented as Extract (8.35.1), which is based on the corresponding recording:

(8.35.1)

```
3    ‖its a 'lovely `day ‖`isnt it‖
4    ‖'what do you 'want to 'see`first‖
8    ‖'lets go and 'see the`elephants 'first‖
9    ‖'oh^good‖ I ˇ like 'elephants‖
10   ‖there were`three 'elephants‖ 'two ˇ big 'ones‖ and a`baby‖
```

CHAPTER 9

Models

In the preceding chapters we have set out an approach to intonation that is based on how adults and children use intonation in everyday conversation. The Intonation in Interaction Profile (IIP), presented in Chapter 5 and reproduced in Appendix 3, incorporates the three principal functions of intonation in interaction: (1) Turns: gaining, holding and giving up the floor; (2) Focus; and (3) Actions: aligning and initiating. For practical purposes of assessment and intervention planning, on many occasions this theoretical framework may be more than sufficient: it underpins the comprehensive set of questions on the profile, which address comprehension as well as the production of intonation in the conversational context. Once a profile has been made, it can be used to identify weaknesses that may provide a focus for intervention. Importantly, it also identifies strengths which can be exploited to optimize a child's communicative potential. Case studies illustrating how this works are presented in Chapters 10, 11 and 12.

However, our understanding of children's intonation, its development and its atypical manifestations is enhanced by adding a complementary psycholinguistic perspective. In Chapter 6 of Stackhouse and Wells (1997), we proposed that the use of a psycholinguistic processing model could help to formulate with greater clarity the different types of (segmental) speech difficulties and their relationship to literacy difficulties. Complementary to the processing model, in Chapters 7 and 8 of Stackhouse and Wells (1997), we also presented a developmental phase model in order to understand the unfolding trajectory of speech and literacy skills through the course of a child's development. In this book, we adopt a similar approach with regard to intonation, this time beginning with a developmental phase model.

Developmental phase model for intonation

In Chapters 6, 7 and 8 we identified some key features of intonation development from birth through infancy, preschool years and school years. At the end of each chapter the key points were summarized as a table. Those tables are collated here as Table 9.1. From Table 9.1, we can track developments of three kinds, assembled under

Children's Intonation: A Framework for Practice and Research, First Edition. Bill Wells and Joy Stackhouse.
© 2016 John Wiley & Sons, Ltd. Published 2016 by John Wiley & Sons, Ltd.
Companion website: www.wiley.com/go/childintonation

the headings of *maturation, input* and *language,* each of which will be explained further below. At the broadest level we identify four phases of intonation development:

1 Preverbal
2 Paradigmatic
3 Syntagmatic
4 Metalinguistic

The Preverbal phase

At the Preverbal phase, described in Chapter 6, the infant displays competences and behaviours, in terms of both perception and production, that act as precursors to the development of intonation systems. However, as yet, these competences and behaviours are not connected with the ambient language.

The Paradigmatic phase

At the Paradigmatic phase, from approximately 6 to 18 months, the infant works out the contrastive value of pitch movements, primarily over a single syllable or word, though sometimes also over longer gestalts. A key step for the child is to work out whether or not the ambient language is a Tone language, i.e. whether or not pitch contrasts have a lexical (or morphological) function. If not, i.e. if the ambient language is a non-Tone language, then the child has to work out what the function of pitch contrast is. In the case of English, this means that the child has to identify the local function of Tone matching to accomplish alignment in conversation; and of Tone non-matching to accomplish the initiation of new actions. This phase, described in Chapter 6, is termed paradigmatic because the child has to work out the paradigm or system of contrastive forms, in this case Tonal forms, with the meaning that is associated with each Tone. This may be primarily lexical or morphological in a Tone language but primarily interactional in a non-Tone language such as English (cf. Chapter 4).

The Syntagmatic phase

At the Syntagmatic phase, described in Chapter 7, the child learns how to use intonation to help understand and construct turns of more than just one word. It requires competence in locating the Tonic on the appropriate word, as required by considerations of topic and Focus (cf. Chapter 3). It also involves knowledge of the Head, Tonic and Tail as different parts of the Intonation Phrase and the role each plays in talk-in-interaction as part of a system of traffic lights for regulating the orderly exchange of turns (cf. Chapter 2). As children progressively use more complex grammatical structures to build semantically more elaborate turns, they master the mapping between Intonation Phrase structures and grammatical structures, for example, lists of noun phrases or main vs. subordinate clauses. By the end of the Syntagmatic phase the child will be using intonation to participate fully in conversational interaction with adults and with peers, as was illustrated at the start of Chapter 8.

The Metalinguistic phase

The Metalinguistic phase, described in Chapter 8, starts around the age of 5. It is when the child becomes conscious of intonation as a dimension of speech which speakers can manipulate for communicative purposes. Intonation awareness is a skill that

Table 9.1 Developmental phase model of intonation.

	TURNS	FOCUS	ACTIONS
Preverbal	**Birth–0;6**		
Internal Maturation	Vocal tract; respiratory system	Neonate can hear differences in length of turns they are exposed to	Neonate can hear changes in loudness and pitch prominence	Hearing for pitch discrimination already in place
		Respiratory capacity limits length of vocalization	Unable to control loudness locally - only globally	Limited ability to control own pitch
Input	IDS (parent, family)	Carer may respond to vocalization as conveying meaning (e.g. a need, 'request')		Prosodic perception starts to become attuned to ambient language
				Carer Tone may match infant pitch contour
				Infant may match carer Tone.
Output	Nonverbal; cry; cooing	Vocalizations of varying length and phonetic quality		
Paradigmatic	**0;6–1;6**		
Internal Maturation		(Reciprocal turn-taking)	Non-verbal pointing; gaze	Prosodic perception becomes attuned to ambient language
			Onset of joint attention	
		Increasing respiratory capacity permits longer vocalizations	Increasing local control over production of pitch, loudness and duration	Increasing control over laryngeal actions allows for more precise pitch movements)
Input	Infant-directed speech (IDS): family, childcare	Carer delimits own turns with Tonic	Carer uses Tonic placement for focus.	Carer matches child Tone
		Carer responds to infant vocal strings as turns	Carers tend to use Supertonic.	In non-Tone languages, Carer versions of adult Tones are exaggerated compared to adult directed speech (ADS). This is not so in Tone languages.
			Carers may respond to any child vocalization as topically relevant (Tonic not important)	

(Continued)

Table 9.1 (*Continued*)

	TURNS	FOCUS 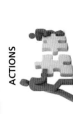	ACTIONS 
Output	Babble; Single-word stage	Solo babble play: exploratory extension of IP In interaction: child only produces the Tonic 'word' Child uses 'fall' and 'rise' but not always as distinctly as in the adult language Use of intonation gestalts reflecting adult intonation.	Variable 'Tonic' placement in solo babble In interaction: Tonic 'word' only, sometimes combined with babble in Intonation Phrase (IP)	Child works out whether ambient language is Tone or non-Tone language If non-Tone language like English, child works out functional value of Tone matching vs. non-matching. Child matches or does not match carer's Tone. Child starts to establish Tone inventory for English.
Syntagmatic	**1;6–4;6**			
Internal Maturation	Increase in working memory span (phonological loop) as articulatory skills mature –allows for longer IPs	Greater control over production of pitch, intensity and duration allow for more precise location of Tonic; differentiation of Tonic vs. Supertonic	Greater control over laryngeal actions allows for more precise pitch movements
Input	Child directed speech (CDS): family, childcare. Peers	Adult provides online feedback re: 'illegal' incomings, illegal overlap by child Collaborative completions to induct into IP structure	Adult provides online feedback re. 'illegal' Tonic placement, by child	Adult models of Tones become less exaggerated and more like ambient adult speech

Language	Multiword -> grammar	Dysfluency arises from demands of combining multiple elements within an IP Child extends IP & Turn in interaction: adds non-final IP: use of mid-pitch Head: use of level pitch Tail: absence of IP final prominence Child starts to use overlap functionally. Mastery of traffic-light system Later: integration of IP structure with grammatical structure, e.g. Lists; subordinate clauses Turn-taking in multiparty interaction, e.g. peer play	Turn-final only Tonic 'errors' Double-tonic 'errors' Sorts out that (Super)Tonic is used for (narrow) Focus Sorts out that only one Tonic allowed per IP	Tone-matching for interactional alignment is established Tonal inventory established Child acquires language-specific phonetic exponents of Tones Later: Tone matching as means of creating alliances, etc. in peer interaction
Metalinguistic	**4;6–14**			
Internal Maturation		General development of meta awareness Enables child to progressively become more aware of intonation Chunking, e.g. compound nouns	General development of meta awareness. Enables child to progressively become more aware of Tonic/Focus	Laryngeal changes, including puberty General development of meta awareness enables child to progressively become more aware of Interactional role of Tone
Input	Adult – Teacher – Peer	Instruction (explicit/implicit) on Turn-taking in formal situations, e.g. classroom Teaching about punctuation and its relation to sentence structure (full stop, comma, etc.) as equivalent to Intonational chunking of spoken turns Teaching of word-by-word decoding and reading aloud	Adult uses Tonic to signal new/important information in complex spoken input, e.g. stories read aloud, and lessons on range of subjects. Child has to follow Topic development.	Instruction (explicit/implicit) in classroom re matching aligning and non-matching/initiating, around repair & correction sequences Teaching about written language punctuation and its assumed relation to speech acts, e.g. Question, Exclamation

(Continued)

Table 9.1 (*Continued*)

	TURNS	FOCUS	ACTIONS
Language	Learning to read (aloud); oral narrative; drama	When reading aloud, child needs to work out how the Focus in a sentence can be identified from the sentence itself in relation to the prior written context (given/ new); and then apply Tonic or Supertonic accordingly in the right place	Child acquires dialect-specific phonetic exponents of Tones
	Needs to work out relationship between spoken Turns/TCUs and written sentences		Increasing awareness of indexical sociophonetic dimension of intonation
	Dysfluency induced by demands of orthographic decoding recapitulates dysfluency of early 'Syntagmatic' phase	When reading aloud, can lead to recapitulation of final Tonic 'error' pattern found in early Syntagmatic phase	Learns 'adult' conventions about mapping between speech act, as indicated by punctuation, and Tone choice. Establishes a Tone 'lexicon' for reading/drama/meta tasks
	Can lead to 'error' where child recruits List intonation (non-final IPs) to deal with reading aloud a (non-list) sentence word by word		Can lead to 'errors' where child uses spoken language/interactional conventions (e.g. Tone matching for alignment) instead of written language conventions (i.e. a Tonal lexicon)

children can then draw on when reading aloud, in order to convey the meaning of the text by the appropriate deployment of IP boundaries, Tonic placement and choice of Tone. There may be side-effects of reading instruction, which result in the child learning some fictions about spoken language. Thus, children seem to pick up the view that questions (in English) are closely associated with rising Tones, which is statistically not the case in conversation. Nevertheless, it does provide the child with a strategy for interpreting the question mark symbol when reading aloud, as discussed in Chapter 8.

With this overview in mind, we can now consider the information presented in Table 9.1. For each Phase, there are rows for Maturation, Input and Language, intersecting with columns for the three functional areas of intonation, i.e. Turns, Focus and Actions. This enables us to track the interaction between these different dimensions.

Maturation

Maturation refers to non-linguistic aspects of developments within the child. Such developments are physiological or cognitive. Physiological developments relevant to intonation are mainly to do with the vocal tract. They involve progressive increase in the child's respiratory capacity, which influences the potential length of an Intonation Phrase, since mostly the IP will be co-extensive with a breath group. Increasing control over respiration enables finer differentiation of intensity and therefore perceived loudness over the syllables that make up the IP, thus allowing for alternating stress, Foot structure and the signalling of the Tonic through relative loudness. The downward movement of the larynx as the infant grows will also affect the production of pitch. Later at puberty the male larynx undergoes major changes that affect the overall pitch of the speaking voice.

Maturation of cognitive capacities is also noted in Table 9.1. While infant perception is already highly attuned for speech (including for vocal pitch) at birth, subsequent refinements involve fine tuning of the perceptual apparatus towards the specific features of the ambient language. Another cognitive capacity that is relevant to intonation development is working memory, since increase in working memory span will allow the child to hold and parse longer IPs. The maturation of more high-level cognitive capacities may impinge on the development of intonation, for example 'theory of mind': this will be explored in the discussion of autism spectrum disorders in Chapter 11.

Input

Input is an important variable when describing the development of intonation. One obvious change is the number and range of others who interact with the growing child. This will lead the child to refine notions about what the possibilities of intonation are and what intonation may signify sociolinguistically as well as communicatively. In the early months and years it is the adult carers, particularly parents, who are likely to provide the most input. We saw in Chapter 6 how the intonation features of adults' talk to children change as the child gets older. This provides not just a phonetic model for the child, but also, in the context of shared talk, a demonstration of how intonation systems like Tone matching are used to accomplish social actions.

Language

The heading of Language encompasses developmental features of intonation as they interface with other levels of language. At the lexical level there is a link between intonation and the child's first words, the words they hear with their different meaning, Tone features and stress patterns, and the growth in vocabulary. Grammatical word classes influence the location of the Tonic, as described in Chapters 3 and 6. The syntactic level is particularly important as the child gets older, since grammatical structures have to be mapped onto IP structures.

Interactional Processing Model for Intonation

The developmental model that we have outlined here helps us to understand how the development of intonation relates to the development of auditory processing, linguistic representations, speech planning and execution, as well as external factors. In turn, this can help us understand the possible impact on a child's intonation comprehension and production, of deficits in one or more of those areas. It also throws light on the relationship between intonation as used in conversation, and the ability to use intonation in other types of speech activity such as reading aloud.

In addition to a developmental phase model, Stackhouse and Wells (1997) presented a single word processing model as a way of exploring the issues involved in typical and atypical development of speech production. Such a model does not aim to account for all aspects of a child's speech, language and communication; it focuses principally on the comprehension and production of single words and on the individual as an autonomous agent. This type of model has been described as an "autonomous transmission model" (Pickering & Garrod, 2004). The model, like others of this type, has been found useful in the assessment and intervention planning for children with developmental speech and literacy difficulties (Baker, Croot, McLeod, & Paul, 2001; Waring & Knight, 2013). While it is restricted to single word processing, that model incorporates both Input (perception and comprehension) and Output (generation and production).

From Chapters 1–5 we have seen that such an autonomous model would be inadequate as a way of describing the processing of intonation, since the intonational design of an utterance is shaped to a large degree by its relation to the previous speaker's immediately prior turn. The model of intonation processing that we present in this chapter therefore explicitly incorporates two participants, using a format that draws on the interactive alignment model of Pickering and Garrod (2004). It is a model of production, which attempts to trace the steps involved when the speaker produces an utterance with its intonation. This intonation processing model does not explicitly incorporate the steps that the individual as listener passes through when making sense of the intonation of a heard utterance. However, at each step, when describing the generation of the current speaker's turn, the model refers to the current speaker's input processing of the previous speaker's turn.

The model is presented in Figure 9.1., where intonation components are shown in italics. The vertical organization of the model, as in standard box-and-arrow processing models, is designed to capture the order of the steps in processing that are involved when a speaker produces an utterance. The first step, shown at the top of Figure 9.1,

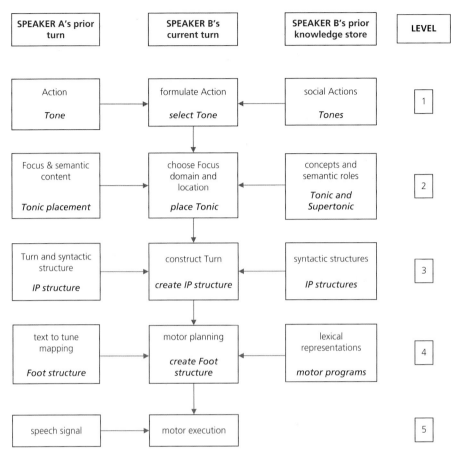

Figure 9.1 Intonation processing model.

is the generation of a social Action, e.g. a request. The second step is to select or formulate the topic that will be the Focus of that action. This is followed by the construction of the speaking Turn in which the speaker will express that action and topic. This third step involves formulating in parallel the semantic, syntactic and the intonation structure of the turn. The fourth step, motor planning, involves access to the lexicon: words and formulaic phrases are chosen to convey the semantic meaning and fill the syntactic slots provided for at the third step. For each word or phrase, there is a motor program (Stackhouse & Wells, 1997) with its own rhythmic structure, determined by the lexical stress pattern that forms part of each lexical representation (see Chapter 1). At this motor planning step, the concatenation of the selected words and phrases provides the Foot structure of the Intonation Phrase, as described in Chapter 1. It is at this motor planning step that the intonation processing model connects with the output side of the single word processing model of Stackhouse and Wells (1997). The fifth and final step is motor execution, where the speaker moves the organs of the vocal tract in order to produce an audible signal.

The *horizontal* organization of the model captures the two main factors that determine the form that Speaker B's turn will take. The boxes to the right of Speaker B's current turn represent the prior knowledge on which Speaker B can draw at each step in the process of generating an utterance. This part of the model reflects a fairly standard approach to sentence and utterance generation (cf. Levelt, 1989). The boxes to the left of Speaker B represent the previous speaker's turn. Each horizontal arrow represents a potential influence from the prior speaker's turn on the current speaker's formulation of his own turn. In the model of Pickering and Garrod (2004), this influence is focussed on lexical selection and selection of syntactic structure: they discuss experimental studies that demonstrate how lexis and grammar used by the prior speaker (A) unconsciously prime Speaker B, whose own grammar and lexis are thus likely to incorporate elements that he or she has just heard. While Pickering and Garrod (2004) are concerned to demonstrate the unconscious and automatic character of this "alignment" of Speaker B to Speaker A, that is not an issue which we will take up here. In our model, we mainly highlight how the *intonation* choices made by Speaker B are responsive to features of Speaker A's turn. As will be discussed and as the model shows, these intonation choices interact with lexical and grammatical choices.

With specific reference to intonation, we will now consider each processing step in turn. To illustrate this, we return to the exchange between Robin and his mother that we have discussed in previous chapters, reproduced here as Extract 9.1:

(9.1)

```
1      M:    ‖now 'whats (.) 'whats `this‖
             ((handing a TOP piece to R))
2      M:    ‖can you re'member what `this is‖
```

```
       ─       ─     ─ ─            ─
   ─         ─       ─           ⌒ \
```

```
3      R:    ʔə(.)  ʔɛdʒœː  ʔɪʒʒ  (0.7)  pɒkx
                            {f}
4      M:    ‖`top‖ thats `right ‖ `top‖
             {f}                   {p}
                    (1.2)
5      M:    and where does that `go
6      M:    does that go in ´there
             ((Robin tries to fit TOP piece into board))
```

In terms of the intonation processing model in Figure 9.1, Robin's mother has the role of Speaker A in lines 1–2; Robin in line 3 has the role of Speaker B, responsive to his mother's turn. We will demonstrate the model in relation to these two turns primarily. However, it is important to bear in mind that Robin's turn in line 3 also functions as a Speaker A turn as it expects a response from his mother, which it duly gets in line 4. Thus, Robin's turn in line 3 illustrates the duality that inheres in almost every turn in conversation: it looks back to the immediate preceding turn, which helps to shape it, while simultaneously it looks forward to the following turn, which it helps to shape.

Action formulation and Tone selection

Psycholinguistic models of communication have tended to be based on a concept of information transfer: the origin of an utterance lies in the speaker's desire to construct a message in order to communicate information to a listener. As researchers have focussed increasingly on 'dialogue' (within psychology), discourse and pragmatics (within linguistics) and conversation analysis (originally within sociology), there has been a growing understanding that in conversation in particular, most of the time, talk is motivated by the desire to perform social actions of various kinds, the communication of information being subservient to this social goal. "First, a speaker selects what action the turn will be designed to perform. Second, he or she selects the details of the verbal constructions through which that action is to be accomplished" (Drew, 2005: 82).

Furthermore, from an interactional perspective, each turn forms part of an unfolding activity that is organized as a sequence of turns. It is evident that both Robin and his mother treat the sequence in Extract (9.1) as part of a labelling activity. The first action of the sequence, in lines 1 and 2, is that Robin's mother requests a label for a piece of the puzzle that they can both see, and which his mother is holding. She produces a form i.e. "what's this" that on other occasions might be used as a genuine request for information about the piece of the puzzle they are looking at. However, on this occasion it is evident that she already knows the answer, that it is a picture of a (spinning) top. Her reformulation in line 2 indirectly displays the status of her initiating action as a test question rather than a genuine request for information: "can you remember what this is" indicates that they have talked about the spinning top before. In line 3, Robin's action is to accede to her request by providing a label.

In terms of the model in Figure 9.1, the mother's action of requesting a label constrains the action that Robin can take as Speaker B: he needs to provide a label. If he were to do something else, e.g. refuse verbally, or walk off without replying, this would be a dispreferred response, likely to initiate a new sequence. As it is, by providing a label in line 3, Robin now constrains what his mother may do next: in line 4, she acknowledges Robin's label , by repeating the word TOP and then assessing his response positively: "that's right".

With regard to the intonation of these turns, the model indicates that it is Tone choice that primarily relates to action selection, as described in Chapter 4. The mother has used a falling Tone in line 1 "what's this"; we have no specific evidence as to why she has made this choice, though as noted in Chapter 4, statistically WH-questions are more likely to carry a falling than a rising Tone in Standard Southern British English. Her use of another fall in line 2, i.e. a matching Tone, indicates that despite the change of wording her second question is performing the same action as the first, namely requesting a label. In line 3, Robin matches his mother's fall, indicating that he aligns with the action that she has initiated. We have already seen that he aligns verbally too, by providing the requested label. He has chosen to align rather than to initiate another action, e.g. to ask for clarification about his mother's question. Because his choice of

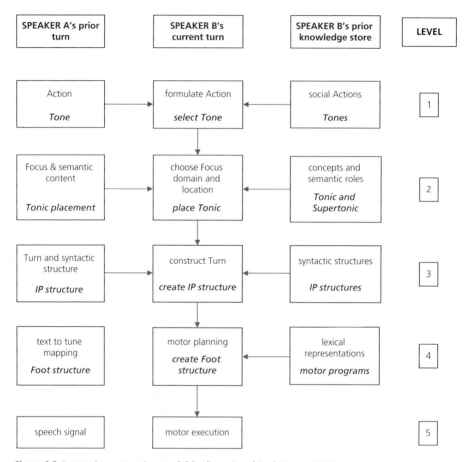

Figure 9.2 Intonation processing model for lines 2 and 3 of Extract (9.1).

Tone is responsive to hers, in Figure 9.2 we have drawn an arrow connecting his mother's turn to his turn at this level of the model, i.e. Level 1. In line 4, Robin's mother then matches his fall, indicating that her turn aligns with his. There is also an arrow from the right-hand box to show that Robin has drawn on some prior knowledge of the Tone system.

Focus choice and Tonic placement

The next step is to select the topic that will be the Focus of the action that was formulated at the first step. As explained in Chapter 3, it is not always necessary for the speaker to make Focus explicit through intonation. The exchange in (9.1) illustrates some of the factors that determine this. In line 2 of her first turn, Robin's mother repeats THIS from line 1 and also locates the Tonic on it, which serves to pick out THIS as the Focus of her turn, rather than REMEMBER or YOU, for example. Although Robin's turn in line 3 does not contain any words that are readily identifiable to a listener from their phonetic shape, he appears to mark the final syllable as the narrow Focus of his own turn, by making it a Supertonic: it carries a wide rise-fall pitch movement, it is noticeably louder than the preceding syllables and it follows a pause. Thus, it seems that Robin already uses the resources of intonation to convey Focus; and that he uses Focus to indicate the part of his response that is topically most relevant to his mother's prior question. Evidence to support this view is found in his mother's next turn (line 4) where she presents "top" as her repetition of that final word of Robin's. She thus treats his Supertonic word [pɒkx] as being co-referential with her own "this" in lines 1 and 2. On this basis we can conclude that Robin's choice of Focus and of Tonic placement was responsive to his mother's turn. We have therefore drawn an arrow joining the two boxes at Level 2. There is also an arrow from the right-hand box, indicating that Robin has drawn on some prior knowledge of the Supertonic/Tonic system.

Turn construction, syntax and Intonation
Phrase structure and syntax

The next step for the speaker is to construct the turn that will express the action and topic that have been formulated. This involves generating in parallel the syntactic and the intonation structure of the turn. As we saw in Chapter 2, Intonation Phrase structure can function like traffic lights to display whether a turn is still in progress by using the Head as a red light; whether it is about to end by using the Tonic as a yellow light; or whether for all practical purposes the turn is over by using the Tail as a green light. In lines 1–2, Robin's mother produces a turn of two IPs, as shown in (9.1.1):

(9.1.1)

1	M:	L	‖ now 'whats (.) 'whats `this ‖
2	M:	=	‖ cn you re'member what `this is ‖
3	R:	=	ʔə (.) ʔɛdʒœː ʔɪʒ₃ (0.7) ⇑ ˆpɒkx
			F
4	M:	=	‖ `top‖ thats `right‖ `top ‖

The first IP, in line 1, demonstrates the combined role of syntax and intonation in maintaining the progress of the turn. Although they are followed by a pause, the first two words, "now whats", do not project the end of her turn, first, because there is no Tonic pitch movement on either syllable; and, second, because the final consonant of "whats" projects something more in the clause. If both these features had been different, as in ‖ `now what‖, the two words could have been heard as a complete question, expecting a reply from Robin. In the event, following this hitch, Robin's mother completes the IP with a Tonic, simultaneously completing the clause with a subject: "whats `this". Interactionally, line 1 is potentially the first part of a question-answer pair, where an immediate response from Robin would normally be expected. In the event, in line 2, his mother extends her turn with a reformulation of the question that suggests more precisely that her interest is Robin's label for the spinning top piece. Line 2 has a more complex syntax than line 1, as the object of the matrix sentence is an embedded clause, "what this is". It also has a slightly more complex IP structure, with a Tail, as shown in (9.1.1). As it turns out, from an intonational perspective, it is the IP in line 1, ‖whats ˋthis‖, that is reflected most directly in Robin's next turn in line 3, since Robin's IP is structured as a Head + Tonic, with the Tonic on the final syllable, like the reformulated final part of the IP in line 1. On this basis we suggest that Robin's IP structure could reflect that of the first line of his mother's turn. We have therefore drawn an arrow joining the two boxes at Level 3. The arrow from the right-hand box indicates that Robin has also drawn on some prior knowledge of how to construct an IP, since he is not simply echoing his mother's IP structure.

Motor planning and Foot structure

The fourth step involves lexical selection, i.e. choosing the words and phrases that will fill the syntactic slots provided at the third step, turn construction. Part of the stored representation of a word or phrase is its motor program, a set of instructions for the achievement of gestural targets that result in a match for the auditory target that is stored as the word's phonological representation (Stackhouse & Wells, 1997). The stored motor program for a word or formulaic phrase has its own rhythmic structure, determined by the lexical stress pattern that is a part of the phonological representation of that word or phrase. The concatenation of the words and phrases selected gives the Foot structure of the Intonation Phrase, as described in Chapter 1. Once the words have been selected, they are fitted into the IP structure created at the previous processing step. For example, in line 2, the words that Robin's mother actually uses are: "can you remember what this is". This gives the Foot structure ‖ _ _ _ ˈ _ _ _ ˈ _ _‖, where each dash represents a syllable. However, she could in theory have chosen slightly different words, for example: "Can you tell me what this is called". This has one fewer syllables in the first foot of the Head, and one more syllable in the Tail, compared to the 'original', resulting in a different rhythmic pattern within the same overall IP structure of Head + Tonic + Tail: ‖ _ _ˈ_ _ _ ˈ_ _ _‖.

The selection of words and their order may be influenced by the prior speaker's turn. However, this is not evident in Robin's response in line 3 to his mother's turn. We have therefore not drawn an arrow joining the left and centre boxes at Level 4. The arrow from the right-hand box indicates that Robin has drawn on some prior knowledge of words with their motor programs, notably the monosyllabic final word TOP, pronounced by Robin as [pɒkx].

Motor execution

The last step is the physical production of the utterance that results from the realization of the motor plan created at the previous step. If there is an influence of the previous speaker's turn at this level, it will be evident in an audible attempt by the current speaker to match the phonetic detail of the prior turn. An example might be if instead of using her own pronunciation of TOP in line 4, Robin's mother had produced [pɒkx], presenting back to Robin his own pronunciation, perhaps as a stimulus to get him to self-repair in a way favoured by speech and language therapists (cf. Stackhouse & Wells, 2001: 417). This kind of precise phonetic imitation of the prior speaker's turn is an interesting feature of immediate echolalia, as described in the case study of a child on the autistic spectrum by Local and Wootton (1995) (see also Chapter 11 of this volume). There is no evidence in line 3 of Robin attempting to match the phonetic detail of his mother's prior turn. Instead he relies on his own motor plan for the production of his turn. For this reason, there is no arrow at Level 5 that joins the left and centre boxes.

In summary, we can see from Figure 9.2 that the intonation of Robin's turn in line 3 derives in part from his previously acquired and stored, though as yet incomplete, knowledge of Tone selection, Tonic placement, IP structures and lexical motor programs. However, the application of this knowledge is shaped by the demands of the interactional context, which in this instance influences his Tone selection, Tonic placement, use of Supertonic and possibly choice of IP structure.

Summary

In this chapter we have presented two complementary models of children's intonation: a developmental model and a processing model. The developmental phase model summarizes the unfolding trajectory of children's intonation over time, in relation to internal and external factors. The processing model can be used for the microanalysis of specific utterances that the child produces in order to pinpoint the effects of immediate context as it interacts with the child's own knowledge at a particular time point.

In the following chapters, we will see how the information about a child that is summarized on the IIP, described in Chapter 5, can be interpreted with reference to the intonation processing model and the developmental phase model for intonation. This will enable us to understand the trajectories of typical and atypical intonation development as well as the range of profiles that we encounter in children with atypical intonation. One benefit that can be derived from a processing model of this type is that it can enable us to hypothesize different types of 'breakdown' and their impact on children's prosodic output. For example, if a child has mis-specified phonological representations of stored words or phrases, in term of their stress pattern, leading to inaccurate motor programs, then this will impact at the level of motor planning, disrupting the rhythm of the IP, even though IP structure in terms of Head, Tonic and Tail may be accurate. Such cases will be discussed in Chapter 10.

Once we have identified the locus (or loci) of difficulty that child has with prosodic processing, we can suggest rational strategies for intervention and management. Apart from our own studies using this framework, evidence is available from studies that other researchers have carried out, using a variety of theoretical frameworks and methodologies. In order to evaluate these studies in a theoretically consistent way, so that their findings can be compared, we will review them from the perspective of our interactional framework and model.

CHAPTER 10

Speech, language and literacy impairments

In Chapter 9, a model was presented of how the intonation pattern of an utterance is produced, in terms of the speaker's own processing system and also in relation to the prior turn of the other participant in the conversation. This provides a basis for understanding what might be happening in the case of a speaker whose intonation is atypical in some respect, e.g. in terms of its sound, or in terms of its fit with the context. In addition, a developmental phase model was introduced, enabling us to see how the individual child with communication difficulties compares to the typical path of development. This will be explored in more detail in the remaining three chapters. In this chapter we first consider school-aged children who have been diagnosed as having persisting difficulties primarily with their speech development, i.e. at a segmental level. We then turn to children whose difficulties are identified as being primarily at other levels, e.g. with grammar and vocabulary. Finally, we consider children with dyslexia, whose difficulties are primarily with learning to read and spell.

Speech output impairments

One of the most striking manifestations of impairment to speech output is found in children with cerebral palsy whose physical disabilities are so severe that they are unable to coordinate breath flow and movement of the organs of the vocal tract in order to produce intelligible speech. Clarke and Wilkinson (2007) analysed peer dyad interactions of English school-aged children where one of the two children was affected in this way. One child with cerebral palsy, Jamal, had no intellectual impairments and in fact at the age of CA 7;11, when the study as carried out, had a language comprehension level well above that of his chronological age, although he was confined to a wheelchair and had no intelligible speech. In order to communicate, he used an electronic voice output communication aid (VOCA), operated by a head-mounted infrared light. This was capable of producing single words, thus in this respect Jamal, like the typically developing infant up to the age of around 18 months, was at the one-word stage with regard to 'speech' output. Although the production of turns using the VOCA was extremely slow, Jamal was able to participate in conversation with his friend Colin, including sharing jokes. However, Jamal's total reliance on the VOCA meant that the resources of intonation were not available in order to mark the

Children's Intonation: A Framework for Practice and Research, First Edition. Bill Wells and Joy Stackhouse.
© 2016 John Wiley & Sons, Ltd. Published 2016 by John Wiley & Sons, Ltd.
Companion website: www.wiley.com/go/childintonation

end of the turn, in the way that typically developing children are already beginning to do in the second year of life, i.e. in the Paradigmatic phase. Equally, since Jamal's VOCA did not have a pitch-generating facility that he could manipulate, he did not have a resource for conveying interactional alignment by Tone matching or action initiation by using a non-matching Tone, something that children at this phase are already doing. Thus, for Jamal, the severity of his speech output impairment means that he is not only very limited in his ability to produce intelligible utterances that convey lexical and grammatical meanings: in addition, he is unable to make use of intonation to communicate meanings related to Turn-taking, Focus and Actions. By contrast, as we shall see in the remainder of this section, children who have specific speech output difficulties in the absence of severe motor impairments are likely to retain the ability to communicate interactional meanings through intonation.

Specific speech difficulty

When a child is diagnosed as having a *phonological delay, speech delay, phonological impairment, phonological disorder, specific speech difficulty, persisting speech difficulty* or some similar label, this is done primarily on the basis of the child's segmental production, above all of consonants, and its impact on intelligibility (Rvachew & Brosseau-Lapré, 2012). Prosodic difficulties are most often referred to in relation to lexical stress, e.g. if the child omits unstressed syllables. Intonation is not generally considered to be affected. Later in this section, we will investigate further whether that is always the case. Initially, however, we consider a child who has a persisting speech difficulty that is most evident in consonant production.

We first met Mick in Chapter 8, in the context of his interaction with two school friends, Johnny and Fred, all aged 5. Mick attends a mainstream school in a rural area of the English Midlands. His hearing is normal and his school work is reported to be at least average. His understanding and expressive language are not a concern. However, his teachers are worried about his speech production. In class, he has been observed to give up on interactions with teachers, to avoid answering questions and to show frustration during interactions with adults. This has sometimes also been observed with peers, although Mick is reportedly a popular boy and, despite his speech difficulties, Mick is in many respects competent to manage peer interactions at school (Tempest & Wells, 2012).

Mick's consonant production has features that are found in much younger, typically developing children, including context-sensitive voicing, velar fronting, cluster reduction and gliding. In addition, his articulation of emerging final and medial fricatives is atypical. The utterance transcribed in (10.1), taken from the recording of peer interaction that was presented as Extract (8.1), illustrates some of these features. A gloss of the presumed target words is provided beneath the phonetic transcription:

(10.1) [ən nɛʔ wi nid   ən nɛts wi nid   ʌvə   d̥ɪʂ]

     and next we need - and next we need (another of) these

Mick's competence in intonation is evident in Extract (8.1), which is reproduced here, minus nonverbal information, as (10.2). A completed IIP form, profiling Mick's contributions to the interaction transcribed in (10.2), is presented in Appendix 6.

Although Mick's contribution amounts to only eight lines of transcript, the IIP shows that he is competent in using and responding to intonation in relation to the three areas of Turn-taking, Focus and Alignment. Specific examples from this extract of his use of intonation were discussed in Chapter 8. The case of Mick suggests that a relatively mild, albeit persisting speech difficulty, restricted to consonant production, will not seriously impinge on a child's ability to learn and deploy the intonation systems of English in conversation. On the contrary, intonation can function as a resource that enables a child with speech difficulties to participate in peer and other interactions.

(10.2)

```
01   J:   L   'no Mick 'Mick let(.)  'lets make a ⇑ `long 'water pipe
02   M:   ≠   'theres ˇgreen 'ones
03   F:   =   we need  ´-
              (2.05)
05   J:   ∅   yeah and we 'nee[::d]
06   M:   ∅                   [and] we 'need
07   J:   ≠   'oh ^wait
08   M:   ≠   'nother 'one of (.)´them
09   F:   ≠   need a  ` red one Johnny `dont we
10   M:   =   mm red ones `on (.)
11   M:   ≠   and a ´green
12   J:   =   and we 'have ´that 'one::
13   M:   =   'and we need a ´bendy 'one
14   J:   ∅   yeah 'Mick [Mi::ck
15   F:   =   then we 'need a ´ˇyellow 'one
16   J:   ∅   yeah and we 'nee::d
17   M:   =   and we need an ˇorange 'one
18   J:   =   and 'then we need ´this 'one
19   F:   ≠   no(.)[no     no    no      `n o :]
20   J:   =        ['Freddie we 'dont need a `small] one
21   F:   ≠   'yeah we ´do
22   J:       'Freddie
23   F:   ≠   'it- 'its a^long bit
24   J:   =   'Freddie 'that bit isnt `long
25   M:   ≠   and 'next we need and 'next we need 'other one of ´these
26   J:       yeah thats it Mick
```

Childhood apraxia of speech

Where a child's persisting segmental speech output difficulties are severe, there is a potential impact on prosodic aspects of speech production. This will now be explored with reference to the condition variously referred to in the literature as Childhood Apraxia of Speech (CAS), Developmental Apraxia of Speech (DAS) and Developmental Verbal Dyspraxia (DVD). This is a condition for which prosodic features have been invoked as potential diagnostic markers. A key issue that has implications for diagnosis and intervention is whether the atypical prosodic features of the child's speech result from an underlying prosody-specific deficit or whether they are the consequence of the difficulties with segmental (consonant and vowel) production.

Shriberg, Aram and Kwiatkowski (1997) compared the spontaneous spoken output of speech disordered children who met clinical criteria for Developmental Apraxia of Speech (DAS) (n=53), to children diagnosed as having speech delay (n=73). In an attempt to determine whether there was a single diagnostic criterion that would distinguish these children from others with speech delay, a very comprehensive range of segmental and prosodic features were examined in spontaneous speech samples. The only one that appeared to distinguish a sizeable subgroup of the children with suspected DAS from other speech delayed/disordered children was the feature the authors called inappropriate stress. They found that just over half the children in the DAS group had inappropriate stress, compared to 10% of the children with speech delay. It was suggested that the children in the DAS group who had inappropriate stress may represent a specific subtype of severe speech disorder.

This diagnostic feature principally involved inappropriate *phrasal* stress: the system of "stressing and destressing words according to their morphological and syntactic function in a phrase" (Shriberg, Aram, & Kwiatkowski, 1997: 309). The disruption to this system took the form of "excessive/equal/misplaced stress", which is one of the categories used in the perceptual assessment tool employed for the study, the Prosody-Voice Profile (Shriberg, Kwiatkowski, & Rasmussen, 1990). According to the manual for the profile, this coding subsumes a diverse range of prosodic behaviours, including: "monostress" speech characterized by forceful, punctuated stress; misplaced stress on words that would not normally be stressed for purposes of emphasis or affect; sound blocks or prolongations; sing-song intonation which violates English intonation patterns. It may also include the absence of co-articulation at the segmental level (pp. 31–32).

The label "inappropriate phrasal stress" covers various aspects of English intonation. In the terminology of the present book, "phrasal stress" can be understood as equivalent to the Tonic, there being one Tonic per Intonation Phrase (IP) for typical speakers. In Table 10.1, the criteria for "inappropriate phrasal stress" (left column) are mapped onto the English intonation system (middle column), along with the potential interactional impact on the listener (right column).

Shriberg and colleagues argued that the inappropriate stress is likely to result from a deficit in the linguistic representation of stress, rather than in motor planning or execution. They speculated that this may link to deficits in stress comprehension/perception, suggesting that these children's segmental difficulties may arise from the prosodic deficit. However, they did not investigate the children's input processing in their study and, in fact, their hypothesis that there is an underlying deficit with stress perception and representation is not supported by the available evidence from input testing, as will be shown later in this chapter. Further, Shriberg and colleagues argued that the stress deficit they discovered is independent of segmental phonological difficulties, on the grounds that some of the older children with inappropriate stress had only mild segmental difficulties, as measured by PCC. However, the argument that there is a dissociation between segmental difficulties and prosodic difficulties in this group is problematic on two counts. First, it calls into question the 'clinical' criteria that have been used to identify the group in the first place. Second, since it is older children who are reported to have milder segmental speech difficulties, it is quite possible that these children have already undergone therapy that has alleviated their

Table 10.1 Mapping the criteria of Shriberg et al. (1990) for "inappropriate phrasal stress" onto the English intonation system and its interactional functions.

"Inappropriate phrasal stress"	Intonation	Interaction
Sound blocks	May extend or disrupt the Head of the IP (Intonation Phrase)	Affects the signalling of Red traffic light. Listener may be unsure if child will reach end of the IP
Forceful, punctuated stress	Multiple Tonics within a sentence, creating multiple IPs	Yellow light may be signalled early, so listener may start speaking in overlap Multiple points of Focus, so Topic not clear
Sound prolongations	May give effect of extra Tonics, as lengthening is a cue to prominence	Possibly multiple points of Focus, so Topic not clear
Misplaced stress	Tonic placement does not coincide with intended with Focus	The Focus of the turn is not signalled accurately to the listener
Sing-song, non-English intonation	Atypical pitch realization of Tone	Child may not signal clearly if he or she is matching/not matching the Tone of the previous speaker; so may not communicate interactional alignment

segmental problems, while having no effect, or possibly even a negative effect, at the prosodic level (cf. Wells, 1994).

There is an alternative interpretation of the atypical prosodic features manifested in the group identified by Shriberg et al. (1997), namely, that the main underlying difficulty for such children concerns motor planning (see Chapter 9). Difficulty in sequencing syllables and segments is likely to disrupt the rhythm of the Foot and thence the sequence of Feet that make up longer IPs. Rhythmic disruption could account at least for the first four of the five characteristics of 'inappropriate stress' provided by Shriberg et al. (1990) and listed in Table 10.1. In order to explore this possibility in more depth, we consider the case of a young girl, Zoe, who had severe speech difficulties as the segmental level, which had led to a possible diagnosis of CAS, though there were no obvious generalized motor difficulties. Psycholinguistic and phonological aspects of Zoe's speech processing have previously been reported (Stackhouse & Wells, 1993; 1997) as have features of her connected speech (Wells, 1994).

Zoe: a case of severe and persisting speech difficulties

Zoe lived in the West Midlands of England and the speech of her family showed features of the local accent. At the time of recordings discussed here, she was aged 5;11.

There had been no medical problems at Zoe's birth, and her health was good. Her coordination and motor skills have throughout been normal for her age. Hearing and vision were satisfactory when tested. Zoe had had no problems apart from her speech and language. She started speech therapy at CA 2;10. There was no family history of speech and language problems. Educational psychologists' reports suggested that Zoe was a child with academic potential within the average range. She performed significantly better on visual tasks than on verbal tasks when tested at C.A. 5;0. She scored poorly on a test of short-term auditory memory, as assessed by digit span. The scatter of scores suggests that she has a specific expressive verbal difficulty. Her performance on measures of language development revealed relative strengths in comprehension and word-finding, in contrast to poor expressive grammatical development: in the session recorded, the most complex clause structure found was "and he waiting ambulance come".

Extract (10.3) presents a transcript of part of a session in which the speech and language therapist (J) is eliciting a targeted speech sample, using the pictures in Weiner, (1979) and following the elicitation procedure recommended there. The transcription of Zoe's speech does not attempt to capture the segmental detail of her pronunciation other than for the target word PIG (see Stackhouse & Wells, 1997, for further examples). Both Zoe and J talk at a slow rate throughout. Uncle Fred is the cartoon character who appears on each page of the material, getting up to unusual activities that are designed to elicit target words for different consonantal simplifying processes, both in isolation and in connected speech. In this extract, the targeted process is prevocalic voicing, the targeted word being PIG. In the picture, Uncle Fred is riding on a pig.

Zoe's speech output displays several of the behaviours grouped by Shriberg and colleagues as "inappropriate stress" (see Table 10.1). "Forceful, punctuated stress" could be used to describe the loud syllables on "sit" and "the" in line 11. "Misplaced stress on words that would not normally be stressed for purposes of emphasis or affect" could apply to the falling pitch and loudness on the final "it" in line 6; sound prolongations are evident on "ride" in line 6 and "pig" in line 11. "Sing-song intonation which violates English intonation patterns" could be used to describe the effect of line 6 resulting from the slow tempo combined with several pitch movements. "Absence of co-articulation at the segmental level" is evident throughout Zoe's speech, as described in Wells (1994). However, all these features could also be viewed as phonetic means that Zoe employs to communicate meaning in the face of her segmental speech problems.

(10.3)

```
1   J:  L   ‖ 'this is a `pig ‖(1.0)
2   J:      ‖ Uncle`Fred ‖ (.) ‖ its 'not a `horse ‖ 'its a (0.6)



3   Z:  =    p ɪ
                {ff}
4   J:  =   ‖ `pig ‖
5   J:  =   'whats 'uncle 'Fred `doing ‖ (0.8)



6   Z:  =    having ri::de on it
                {{f}lento{f}      }
7   J:      ‖hes 'riding a


```

```
 8   Z:   =    p ɪ:g=
               {ff}
 9   J:   =‖ 'thats ˆright ‖
10   J:   ≠    ‖⇒ whats 'uncle Fred ´doing ‖ (1.0)
```

```
        ⌣   ⌣   —    _    ⟋
```

```
11   Z:   =    sitting on the  p ɪ:
               {f}           {f}  {f}
12   J:   ≠    ‖ 'good `girl‖ (.)
13   J:   =    ‖ `this is a 'funny one 'Zoe ‖
```

Turns and traffic lights

The IIP form is used to analyse Zoe's performance.

Does Zoe project the end of the turn by using the Tonic? (Zoe uses yellow light)

The following phonetic features are characteristic of the ends of Zoe's turns:
• pitch movement on the final word (lines 4, 8, 11), even when the Focus and main pitch movement are earlier in the IP, as in line 6 (see Focus below);
• increase in loudness as in lines 4, 6, 8 and 11;
• lengthening of the vowel, relative to non-final position; as in line 11.

The role of these features in delimiting Zoe's turns is attested by the fact that they regularly occur at the end of her turns, i.e. a change of speaker follows. These features are exaggerated versions of the pitch movement, lengthening and final aspiration used by typical English speakers in turn-final position (Local & Walker, 2012). Thus, although Zoe's use of phonetic features as markers of turn delimitation may appear somewhat idiosyncratic, the phonetic ingredients are not intrinsically 'unEnglish'; rather, they are a more extreme version of what is typically done.

We saw in Chapter 7 that children who have not yet developed adult intonation systems tend to make the ends of their turns particularly phonetically prominent. The prominence is often achieved by locating the major pitch movement on the last word or syllable and also by means of extra loudness and duration. Exaggerated phonetic marking of turn endings may therefore be characteristic of both normal and atypical development.

Does Zoe produce a turn of more than one word by creating an IP with a Head? (Zoe uses red light)

Zoe creates a Head, as in line 11, by avoiding the use of the above turn-final features in non-turn-final position. J does not overlap the Head.

Does Zoe refrain from taking a turn until the current speaker has projected the end of his/her own turn? (Zoe observes red light)

With regard to Zoe's understanding of the role of intonation in turn-taking, she always waits for a Tonic in J's turn before starting her own turn. However, on three out of four occasions in this short extract, there is an intervening silence of at least (0.6) seconds. It is therefore possible that Zoe is unsure whether J has in fact ended her turn. Alternatively, Zoe may need a little time to work out what kind of answer is expected in this rather artificial assessment procedure where J is trying to elicit the word PIG in a phrase. Zoe shows awareness of IP structure in lines 3 and 8, where she completes J's incomplete IP. On each occasion, J produces a Head, inviting Zoe to complete the IP with a Tonic, which she duly does.

Tonic placement and Focus

Does Zoe indicate broad Focus over the whole IP by using final Tonic placement?

Zoe produces turns with broad Focus, in which maximum pitch height occurs on the lexically stressed syllable of the final word and maximum loudness occurs on the final syllable of the IP. An example is line 11.

Does Zoe indicate narrow Focus on a non-final word of the IP by using non-final Supertonic placement?

Zoe's narrow Focus turns contain one new or important word, occurring in non-final position. Maximum pitch height in the turn occurs on the first, normally the stressed, syllable of the focussed word. Loudness peaks are located both on the focussed word and on the final word. An example is the narrow focus on "ride" in line 6, which represents the new, important information that she is contributing to the development of the topic. The old information, "on it", is placed in the Tail. "Ride" has the main pitch movement, although there is also some pitch movement and loudness on the final word, "it". Further examples are presented in Wells (1994). Zoe marks the new information with a peak of pitch and loudness, as in the Tonic of the English intonation system that she is exposed to. The main difference is that in Zoe's narrow Focus turns, there is also some pitch movement and loudness prominence on the final word of the utterance, whereas in the adult variety the post focus stretch, i.e. the Tail, tends to be on a low level pitch and to be relatively quiet (cf. Chapter 3). Thus, Zoe has the ability to manipulate the placement of the main pitch and loudness prominence in accordance with requirements of information Focus, at least when the focussed word is in non-final position. She therefore has a more mature system than some language-impaired children, for example, David, whom we met in Chapters 3 and 5, who routinely have a single peak of pitch and loudness on the final word or syllable of the sentence, irrespective of Focus considerations (see also later in this chapter).

Does Zoe indicate narrow Focus on the final word of the IP by using final Supertonic placement?

Zoe's intonation system for Focus is mostly similar to the system found in the variety of English spoken around her. However, her realization of the system differs some-what from standard varieties of English with reference to broad Focus, in that she often has a step-up in pitch to the final word, and maximum loudness on the final syllable: this is more like a Supertonic (cf. Chapter 3). In the standard variety, a Supertonic on the final word is associated with narrow Focus on the final word of the

IP, i.e. when the final word alone represents new information. In broad Focus IPs in adult standard varieties of British English, the final word is unlikely to start at a higher pitch than the preceding syllables, and is unlikely to be the single loudest part of the sentence. Unfortunately, we do not have examples in the recordings of turns where final narrow Focus would be contextually expected so we are unable to determine whether she in fact distinguished final narrow Focus from broad focus.

Tone matching and alignment

There is evidence that Zoe and J use Tone matching to align with each other, and in J's case, also to initiate a new direction in the talk. In line 1, J uses a falling (L) Tone. In line 2, she produces two further IPs but with a fall-rise, projecting that she has not yet completed her turn. She then starts a fourth IP but does not complete it with a Tonic. As noted above, Zoe duly completes in line 3, matching the Tone of J's original production of PIG in line 1. Zoe thus has managed to skip back to the relevant IP that she needs to match in order to align with the model for labelling action that J produced. In line 4, J's tonal matching serves to acknowledge Zoe's IP in line 3 as an acceptable version of PIG. A non-matching, i.e. rising Tone could have been heard as a request for clarification, i.e. the initiation of a new action. There is no evidence that either J or Zoe treat line 4, with its matching Tone, as such a request.

In line 5, J matches her own Tone from line 4, progressing her agenda, which is to get Zoe to produce PIG in a connected speech sentence. Zoe in line 6 duly produces some connected speech which is topically relevant. Although her main prominence is on "ride", which has a rising pitch, the final pitch movement on "it" is falling, thus matching J's Tone. Had Zoe used a final rise, it might have been heard as requesting confirmation from J that Zoe had provided an appropriate answer. However, J does not treat it as such a request. Instead, in line 7 she recasts part of Zoe's turn in such a way that it forms the Head of an incomplete IP (as she did earlier in line 2) inviting Zoe to complete the IP with a Tonic. Grammatically and lexically, J's turn in line 7 is designed to invite Zoe to complete it with the word PIG, which was missing from line 6. Zoe duly complies in line 8, matching her own falling Tone from line 6, again showing that she is not asking for confirmation. In line 9, J matches Zoe with a fall, then moves rapidly to a further IP with a non-matching, i.e. rising Tone in line 10. J uses this for an IP which exactly repeats the words she had used in line 5, "what's Uncle Fred doing", with the same Tonic placement, on "doing". J's non-matching Tone serves to signal that although the question has been asked before, the answer Zoe provided in line 6 was in some way inadequate, even though the follow-up in lines 7–9 ended in a positive acknowledgement from J, "that's right". Thus, by using a non-matching Tone in line 10, J re-launches her original action as a new action. In line 11, Zoe provides a response with a matching (rising) pitch movement at the end. This meets the dual requirement of J's elicitation agenda: not only has Zoe produced a response that is a connected speech sentence (like line 6) but one that also now contains the target word PIG (from line 8). In line 12, J positively assesses this response, "good girl". She does this with a non-matching Tone, a fall, which is then matched by her next IP in line 13. This moves the agenda on to the next picture, which is of a PUMPKIN. The Tonic is on "this", indicating Focus on the new picture. Thus, by using a non-matching Tone, J disengages the talk from the current topic (PIG) and moves it on to the next one.

In summary, we can see that the system of Tone matching and alignment plays a central role in the management of the exchange between Zoe and J. J exploits it to ensure that her therapist's agenda is addressed by Zoe, and she relies on Zoe's own use of Tone matching to monitor Zoe's understanding of what is required. We suggest that Zoe's competence in the intonation systems of Tone matching, Tonic placement and Turn projection is shared by many children like Zoe who have severe and persisting speech difficulties at the segmental level. Although the child's prosodic production, like Zoe's, may sound unusual as a result of the disruptions to rhythm and timing caused by speech production difficulties, she can still participate in interaction successfully by drawing on these systems. This possibility is enhanced when her interlocutor, like J in this extract, is skilled in her own use of these systems.

Intonation production of children with language impairments

In this section we turn from children whose most evident difficulties are at the level of phonology to children whose primary difficulties are with grammar and semantics, who may or may not have some segmental speech difficulties too.

Tonic placement and Focus

Baltaxe, Simmons and Zee (1984) compared intonation patterns in typically developing children and children with language impairments, using acoustic measures without reference to linguistic or interactional functions. They found that the children with language impairments were impaired on a number of features relating to fundamental frequency (pitch) and intensity (loudness). Baltaxe (1984) then studied the use of 'contrastive stress' (i.e. use of Supertonic for narrow Focus) in the same populations, using a procedure similar to that of Hornby (1971), which was described in Chapter 7. There were seven children in each group, groups being matched for MLU. The age range was 2;5 to 4;0 for the typically developing children and 3;8 to 10;10 for the children with language impairments. The children with language impairments performed significantly worse than the typical group. However, in one respect, the two groups were similar: in both groups, the greatest number of errors involved a shift of Tonic to the right, mostly to the last word of the utterance.

Hargrove and Sheran (1989) looked at the location of the Tonic in relation to sentence position (final versus non-final) and Focus (new or given information) in five 3-year-old children with language impairments, matching them by MLU to the children described by Wieman (1976) (see Chapter 7). Whereas Wieman reported that in her typical development children, Tonic placement had been determined by information Focus, this was true for only one of the five children with language impairments described by Hargrove and Sheran: three showed a clear preference for utterance final Tonic placement, irrespective of Focus considerations. These findings are congruent with case studies of (British) English-learning children who show an overwhelming preference for locating the main or nuclear pitch movement of the utterance on its final word or even its final syllable. We have already drawn extensively on one such case study, that of David, as reported in Wells and Local (1993), to illustrate how the present approach to assessing intonation might be used. Perkins (1985) describes a very similar case of a 4-year-old boy who exhibited an overwhelming preference for the final syllable of the utterance as the location of the main pitch movement. In the same vein, Crystal (1987) presents a transcript of a 6-year-old language-delayed girl, Paula, who invariably located the greatest pitch movement on the final word of the utterance. The subjects of these case studies had obviously atypical prosodic output, along with speech and language impairments at other linguistic levels. In summary, from the evidence available, it seems that some children with a language impairment are less sensitive to requirements of Focus, exhibiting a preference for Tonic placement at the end of the utterance.

A quite different compensatory use of the Tonic system is reported by Camarata & Gandour, (1985) in a case study of a child learning American English. It offers an intriguing example of the use of intonation as a compensatory resource for morphological and phonological deficiencies of the kind found in some children with language impairments. At the age of 3;8, their participant G.G. had at least normal receptive language and nonverbal IQ, but only produced one-word utterances. His phonological system was highly impaired: fricatives, affricates, liquids and clusters were absent, as were all word-final consonants except for target nasal codas, which were all realized as a voiced velar nasal. With regard to inflectional morphology, G.G. was able to distinguish English grammatical morphemes perceptually, and to signal the progressive morpheme -ING consistently in his speech output, with a syllable ending in a velar nasal, e.g. RAINING → [wawaŋ]. The focus of the case study was on his production of singular – plural noun pairs like BOAT – BOATS, SHOE – SHOES, GLASS – GLASSES. For each pair, the authors observed no segmental difference between singular and plural in G.G.'s productions. However, prosodic differences were noticed, which were subsequently confirmed by acoustic measurements. Based on the description provided by the authors, a transcription of the differences between singular and plural forms is presented in Table 10.2.

G.G.'s plural forms were consistently longer in duration and had a larger pitch movement; in most cases the plural was also louder. As we saw in Chapter 3, these features characterize the Supertonic used in English intonation to mark narrow Focus, and so have been notated in Table 10.2 by the supertonic diacritic ⇑. Thus, to signal an important morphological contrast in English, G.G. used prosodic features of the kind found in American and British English to convey narrow Focus in the intonation system. Presumably this was a compensatory strategy for him, the usual realizations of the plural morpheme, which involve the addition of an alveolar fricative as illustrated in the 'Plural Target' column of Table 10.2, being unavailable to him because of his highly restricted system of coda consonants. G.G.'s strategy of adding

Table 10.2 G.G.'s production of singular and plural forms of monosyllabic nouns (adapted from Camarata & Gandour, 1985).

Lexical item	Singular target	Plural target	G.G.: singular	G.G.: plural
BOAT	ˋboʊt	ˋboʊts	ˋbo	⇑ˋbo:
BALL	ˋbɑl	ˋbɑlz	ˋbɑ	⇑ˋbɑ:
SHOE	ˋʃu	ˋʃuz	ˋdu	⇑ˋdu:
GLASS	ˋglæs	ˋglæsɪz	ˋgæ	⇑ˋgæ:

more prosodic ingredients – extra length, loudness and pitch prominence – may reflect that the plural refers to 'more' than the singular. This mirrors regular plural formation in English, where the addition of an extra fricative, as in BOAT/BOATS, or syllable as in GLASS/GLASSES, also reflects the fact that semantically plurals refer to 'more' than singulars. Thus, it appears that G.G. has found an alternative way to signal this morphological contrast that indirectly mirrors the standard system to which he is exposed.

Cases such as G.G.'s, where a child learning English uses prosodic features with a grammatical function, may be quite rare (or at least rarely observed), even among children with impaired phonological and expressive language development, though in Chapter 3 a comparable instance was noted in the speech of Robin, a child with typically developing speech, at the age of 19 months (Extract 3.14). What G.G. has ended up with is something like the kind of system that is found in some Tone languages, where some of the morphology is expressed by Tone rather than by segmental additions and alterations (see Chapter 6). The case of G.G. suggests that a child's path to discovering that English is a non-Tone, intonation-only language may not always be entirely straightforward.

Turns and traffic lights

As we saw in Chapter 2, two prosodic features that have been traditionally associated with utterance final position in English are major pitch movement and lengthening. Snow (1998) undertook a study to see whether children with specific language impairments (SLI) used these features in the same way as typically developing children. Participants were ten children with the phonological-syntactic type of SLI and ten age-matched children with normally developing language between the ages of 4;0 and 4;11, from the USA. They took part in recorded play sessions centred round a baby doll. Specific spontaneous utterances were then measured for mean length of utterance (MLU), duration and fundamental frequency contour. Snow had anticipated that the final prosodic features, i.e. falling Tone and syllable lengthening, might not be found to the same degree in the children with SLI, since their grammatical abilities were less than those of the normally developing children. In the event, both groups showed similar use of these parameters. This suggests that the features studied by Snow are not associated directly with grammar, i.e. they do not serve to mark syntactic boundaries, but rather they serve to mark the end of the speaker's turn. Snow's results thus indicate that children with SLI are not impaired in the ability to use a final Tonic to mark the end of the turn.

Tone matching and alignment

In a later study, (Snow, 2001), Snow wanted to find out whether children with SLI had difficulties with intonation production. Participants were eleven 4-year-olds with SLI and a group of chronological age-matched controls. Snow focused specifically on rising and falling intonation contours, which the children were encouraged to imitate at the end of a play session involving hand puppets. Examples of the stimuli are reproduced as (10.4) and (10.5):

(10.4) ‖ the pig has some `socks ‖

(10.5) ‖ did you take some ´socks ‖

Both groups of children imitated the Tone correctly around 75% of the time. Acoustic measures revealed no significant differences between the two groups in how they produced the rise or the fall. The results for this imitation task imply that in conversation such children would have the phonetic ability to match the Tone of the prior speaker, either rising or falling, in order to signal alignment. However, this was an experimental study and did not look directly at the children's functional use of rises and falls, i.e. whether in conversation they actually use Tone matching for alignment.

The children with SLI all had some degree of phonological difficulty, as evidenced by percentage consonants correct (PCC) calculated on data from the recorded play session. Snow found no correlation between performance on the intonation imitation task and their PCC score for the children with SLI. This suggests that there is no relationship between intonational and segmental phonological deficits, as far as the imitation of Tone is concerned. For some children, then, intonation will be a relative strength, which might be used to compensate for grammatical impairments and poor segmental intelligibility.

Intonation processing and language impairment

Despite the conclusions of Snow's studies, it would be premature to rule out the possibility of an association, at some level, between problems with intonation and difficulties at the grammatical level, given the role of intonation in grammatical segmentation as, for example, in the PEPS-C 'Chunking' tasks (Chapter 8).

Clinical and educational assessments of the comprehension of spoken language necessarily have an intonational component, which frequently goes unacknowledged. Every spoken item in a language comprehension test, like any utterance in spoken language, has a rhythm and intonation structure, as well as a grammatical structure. Failure on a spoken test of grammatical comprehension tends to be attributed to immature or deficient grammatical development or alternatively, to limitations on working memory or on perception of segmental timing cues (Bishop, 1997). However, if a child has problems in processing the prosodic component, it can be hypothesized that this too will result in impaired performance on the test.

Children with speech and language impairment: using the PEPS-C battery

The importance of taking into account the perception and comprehension of intonation as well as its production when assessing children with speech and language difficulties was one of the main motivations for developing the PEPS-C battery, the comprehensive set of tasks for investigating intonation in school-aged children with and without communication difficulties that was described in Chapter 8. Using the original manual version of the PEPS-C battery, Wells and Peppé (2003) carried out a study to determine whether, and to what extent, children with speech and language impairments have difficulties with the comprehension and production of different aspects of intonation. Until then, studies had focused, in the main, either on production or on comprehension, and on one or two specific aspects of prosody. There had not been a comprehensive investigation of the different aspects of intonation comprehension and production, with one group of speech or language impaired children.

Eighteen 8-year-old children were recruited who had previously been identified as having significant language difficulties and were receiving specialist therapy in a language unit or special school. Children selected for the language-impaired (LI) group had a deficit of at least 1.5 standard deviations below the mean on one or both of the TROG (Test for the Reception of Grammar) (Bishop, 1989) or the sentence formulation subtest of CELF-R (Clinical Evaluation of Language Fundamentals – Revised) (Semel et al., 1987). Evidence of an overt intonation production difficulty was not a requirement.

In order to investigate whether these children had specific deficits in intonation, they were compared to two groups of typically developing children, who had participated in the normative study using the PEPS-C described in Chapter 8 (Wells et al., 2004). To create a language age (LA) control group, children were matched on grammatical comprehension, on an individual basis, using TROG (Bishop, 1989). One of the groups in the normative study (n=30), which had a mean age of 8;6, served as a chronological age matched (CA) control group. This basic research design has subsequently been used in studies with children with high functioning autism, Williams syndrome and Down syndrome, using the revised PEPS-C (see Chapter 11).

The most striking finding was that there were significant differences on nine PEPS-C subtests between the LI group and the CA controls, suggesting that difficulties with aspects of intonation processing and production may co-occur with speech or language impairments. However, the children with speech and language impairments were not worse on PEPS-C tasks, as a group, than the (younger) LA controls. This suggests that the intonation deficits that are evident in the children with language impairments when compared to their age peers may still be typical of younger children and not more severe than their other speech or language difficulties.

The fewest differences between the LI and CA groups were found on the Output Function subtests. This suggests that many children in the impaired group are like their unimpaired peers of the same age in being able to make use of intonation to convey a range of meanings; thus intonation could function as a valuable communicative resource for them. However, this has to be viewed in the context of more frequent deficits in input processing, particularly on the Focus and Chunking Input Form tasks. Now complete Activity 10.1, which investigates the processing demands of these Input Form tasks.

In Activity 10.1, we saw that for children with normal hearing, failure on the Chunking Input Form task may be attributable either to deficits in the perception of linguistic prosody or to auditory memory. In the study by Wells and Peppé (2003), the children who struggled with Input Form did so on the Chunking and Focus tasks, both of which use stimuli of around five or six syllables. They did much better on the Affect and Interaction Input Form tests, which used stimuli of one or two syllables. This discrepancy suggests that auditory memory is the more likely explanation for their performance. The results for these two Input Form tasks thus support the idea that intonation processing deficits may be implicated in the short-term memory problems of children with specific language impairments.

Many children in the LI group also had problems with the Output Form tasks, which require the accurate imitation of a prosodic pattern. This was rather surprising, given the results of the imitation study by Snow (2001) described above, where there was no difference between children with language impairments and age-matched controls. Now complete Activity 10.2, which investigates the processing demands of the Output Form tasks.

ACTIVITY 10.1

Aim: To analyse the processing skills demanded by PEPS-C Input Form tasks.

The Input Form task for each PEPS-C communicative area comprises 16 test items, each item consisting of a pair of sound stimuli. Each stimulus pair derives from the functional contrast associated with the particular communicative area, as described in Table 8.1 in Chapter 8. The Chunking pair exemplified there is reproduced here as (10.6) and (10.7):

(10.6) ‖ ˇchocolate cake ‖ and ˋbuns ‖ (two foods)

(10.7) ‖ ˇchocolate ‖ ˇcake ‖ and ˋbuns ‖ (three foods)

However, instead of hearing the intonation contour associated with an intelligible phrase, the child is presented with stimuli in a form where the lexical and grammatical information provided by vowels and consonants is not audible. The result is a buzz, a little like the voice of a speaker in an adjacent room. For each test item, the child has to decide whether the two stimuli in the pair are the same or different.
1 If possible, listen to the recordings of 10.6) and (10.7).
2 Based on the description of the task above and, if you have access to them, the recordings of the test items, identify the speech processing skills that the child needs in order to succeed on the Chunking Input Form task. Why might some children with speech and language difficulties find this task difficult?
Check your answer with the Key at the end of the chapter.

ACTIVITY 10.2

Aim: To analyse the processing skills demanded by PEPS-C Output Form tasks.

The Output Form tasks involve repetition. The instructions are: "You'll hear some words on the recording, and I want you to copy them, saying them in exactly the same way as you heard them said on the recording." Digits were used, since their semantic representations, motor programs and articulatory routines at the segmental level were assumed to be familiar to children. It was assumed that there would therefore be less semantic and segmental phonological interference in the task.
    For the Chunking Output Form task, each item is a string of digits, e.g. FORTY, TWO, ONE; or: FORTY-TWO, ONE. In terms of the prosodic phrasing involved, these correspond to Function task items such as those in (10.6) and (10.7) above.
    Based on the description of the task above, identify the speech processing skills that the child needs in order to succeed on the Chunking Output Form task. Why might some children with speech and/or language difficulties find this task difficult?
    Check your answer with the Key at the end of the chapter.

Wells and Peppé (2003) noticed a pattern whereby the children in the LI group who failed on the Focus and Chunking Input Form tasks were likely also to fail on the equivalent Output Form tasks, which also have long items, this time to store and then repeat. One possibility is therefore that for some of these children, the difficulty is as much to do with recall as with intonation production. The importance of rhythmic and intonational grouping in the serial recall of speech has often been demonstrated in the experimental psycholinguistic literature (Morgan, Edwards, & Wheeldon, 2014).

The pattern of deficits on PEPS-C tasks across the children within the LI group did not present a consistent picture. Even when the LI group was divided into three sub-groups according to the particular nature of the impairment (speech and language, language only, additional pragmatic impairment), there was no clear pattern of deficit within each subgroup. This suggests that the relationship between intonation and other linguistic skills is indirect, a conclusion supported by the lack of correlation in the LI group between PEPS-C performance and measures of receptive and expressive language, segmental speech, and performance IQ. Wells and Peppé concluded that for many children with language impairments, intonation may in fact be a relative strength.

However, Wells and Peppé's study was small-scale in terms of numbers, and the sample of children was not particularly homogeneous in terms of diagnosis. Marshall, Harcourt-Brown, Ramus, and van der Lely (2009) in another study drawing on the PEPS-C battery, used tighter selection criteria to identify children with specific language impairments (SLI). Like Wells and Peppé (2003), they found limited evidence for intonation deficits in children with language impairments. The problems that they did find were largely confined to input processing of specific aspects of intonation, mainly ones which relate to grammar.

The diversity of patterns found by Wells and Peppé (2003) among children in their LI group supports a single case type of investigation, to explore associations and dissociations further. Three children from the LI group are presented here to highlight some of the most important findings. Names are pseudonyms and capital letters refer to the child's identifier in Wells and Peppé (2003). In all cases, where 'deficits' on PEPS-C are mentioned, this is in relation to the chronological age matched control group. Their general and PEPS-C profiles can be found respectively in Tables 1 and 6 of Wells and Peppé (2003). All three children had similar nonverbal IQs, with receptive and expressive language difficulties. The PEPS-C profiles of Robin and Jonathan are also discussed in Wells & Peppé, (2001).

Malcolm (Child K)

Malcolm had the most severe segmental speech difficulties of all the children in the LI group, as measured by percentage consonants correct on a picture-naming task (PCC = 64%). Further testing of his speech processing revealed relatively good (seg-mental) auditory processing skills but, unsurprisingly given his speech difficulties, poor performance on tasks of real and non-word repetition. His PEPS-C profile is presented in Table 10.3. In this table, as in Table 10.4 and Table 10.5 below, 'x' signifies a score of at least 1.5 SDs below the CA group mean; 'xx' signifies at least 2.5 SDs below the mean; ✓ signifies a score between -1.5 and +1.5 SDs, and ✓✓ a score of over + 1.5 SDs.

Table 10.3 Malcolm's PEPS-C profile.

		Input	Output
Chunking	Function	✓	✓✓
	Form	x	x
Affect	Function	✓✓	x
	Form	✓	x
Interaction	Function	xx	✓
	Form	✓	xx
Focus	Function	✓	✓✓
	Form	xx	✓

Table 10.4 Robin's PEPS-C profile.

		Input	Output
Chunking	Function	✓	✓✓
	Form	✓	xx
Affect	Function	x	✓✓
	Form	✓✓	x
Interaction	Function	xx	xx
	Form	✓✓	✓
Focus	Function	x	✓
	Form	✓	xx

Table 10.5 Jonathan's PEPS-C profile.

		Input	Output
Chunking	Function	x	x
	Form	x	xx
Affect	Function	✓	✓✓
	Form	✓	x
Interaction	Function	x	x
	Form	✓	x
Focus	Function	✓	xx
	Form	✓	✓

Relative to the CA group, Malcolm performed within normal limits on most of the Input and Output Function tasks, suggesting he can understand and convey intonational meanings. However, on some tasks, e.g. Chunking and Focus Input Function, performing within the normal limits of the CA group does not entail actually scoring above chance on the task, since as a group the 8-year-old CA children did not score above chance either. Malcolm's performance on Form tasks was weaker: on three of the four Output Form tasks he was significantly below the CA group, also on the Input Form tasks with long items, i.e. Chunking and Focus. Problems with input processing particularly where the stimuli are long may give rise to difficulties in remembering the intonation contour when asked to repeat an utterance, as in the PEPS-C Output Form task investigated in Activity 10.2. His low Output Form scores suggest that there may be a relationship between intonation and segmental production: a severe speech impairment may lead to disruption in the motor planning of the utterance, which gives rise to prosodic disruption. This was proposed in relation to Zoe earlier in this chapter.

Robin (Child V)

At the age of 8;4 Robin was described as having a severe-moderate language disorder, scoring below the tenth centile on the TROG (Bishop, 1989), the BPVS (Dunn, Dunn, Whetton & Pintillie, 1982) and the Formulated Sentences subtest of CELF (Wiig et al.). He had no obvious segmental speech difficulties. His speech and language therapist's main concern at this point was with his social skills: she reported that he found activities such as Turn-taking and requesting very difficult, possibly as a result of his growing awareness of his own language difficulties.

Robin's intonation in spontaneous speech did not cause concern. In a transcribed extract from an oral narrative, Robin routinely used Tonic placement to mark the end of a grammatical sentence, constructing his narrative in coherent chunks He also used Tonic placement to focus on new information, using the Tail for 'given' or old information (Wells & Peppé, 2001).

Robin's PEPS-C profile is presented in Table 10.4, using the conventions introduced in Table 10.3. On the input side, Robin had significant deficits compared to the CA group on Input Function tasks, which involve comprehension of intonational meaning. However, his performance on all the Input Form tasks was within or above the normal range. This suggests a dissociation: a difficulty in understanding intonational meaning contrasts with his ability to perceive differences in pitch patterns.

Robin's success on most of the Output Function tasks, which tap the ability to use intonation to convey meaning, is consistent with his apparently proficient use of intonation in spontaneous speech. More surprisingly, he performed poorly on the Output Form tasks, which require repetition of an intonation pattern. This suggests a dissociation: the weakness in imitating sentences or words with the correct intonation pattern contrasts with the strength in conveying meaning through intonation. Unlike Malcolm, Robin did not have overt segmental phonological problems and on tasks of real and non-word repetition, he performed within normal limits. This suggests a further dissociation: age-appropriate segmental production contrasts with a weakness in prosodic production as assessed by the PEPS-C Output Form tasks. Thus, on the output side, Robin seems to have a rather specific difficulty with the accurate imitation of intonation patterns, even though his intonation in spontaneous speech does not sound atypical. However, it is hard to determine whether poor performance, such as Robin's on the Output Form tasks and Input Function tasks, derives from a genuine deficit in intonation knowledge and processing; or whether they derive from a more 'meta' problem in understanding what is required in the task. This issue will be explored further as we turn to the third case, Jonathan.

Jonathan (Child F)

Jonathan, who lived in London, had been delayed in his early language development, only beginning to use expressive language around the age of 5. However, his speech and language therapist reported that, at 8;11, he was very chatty and communicative, able to talk about past and future, his own experiences, to ask questions, and to interact well with other children. While he had no obvious segmental speech errors, he made grammatical errors, e.g. in past tense formation, pronouns and prepositions. He also had problems with comprehension. Jonathan's intonation was described as having a 'sing-song' character. This was regarded as unusual by his parents, as well as by professionals and others outside the family. They noted that this feature had started when he was 7 and had become increasingly evident. Jonathan's performance on standard assessments is summarized in Table 10.5. The PEPS-C tests and other recordings discussed here were made at CA 8;11, when his score on measures of language development was broadly in line with that of a typically developing 5-year-old, as detailed in Wells & Peppé, (2001). Jonathan's performance on the PEPS-C battery is summarized in Table 10.5, using the conventions introduced in Table 10.3.

The profile shows some differences according to communicative area. His performance is relatively strong on the Affect tasks. The Affect tasks are psycholinguistically simple, since the stimuli and responses are short for all tasks, and there is no requirement to integrate verbal with prosodic information. In the output Affect tasks, the response does not involve any lexical material: the pitch has to be produced on the syllable "mm". The remainder of this section will concentrate on his performance in the other three communicative areas which, as noted in Chapter 8, correspond to the three key areas of intonation highlighted throughout this book.

Jonathan scored within normal limits on Input Form tasks, except for Chunking. The latter may be due to his not immediately understanding what he was required to do for the Input Form tasks: Chunking was the first of these that he was presented with and initially it appeared that he had no idea what to do. After ten items he had tuned in and thereafter he scored within normal limits. It therefore seems unlikely that he has a fundamental difficulty with discriminating between different intonation patterns.

Turning to Output Form, Jonathan fell below 1.5 SDs on Chunking and Interaction, which suggests that he may have lower-level difficulties in controlling prosodic patterns in his speech. Although he was adept at using a full range of Tones on utterances that consisted only of the syllable "mm", in the Affect tasks, he succeeded less well in mapping the Tones on to words (i.e. the digits). Jonathan failed to use lengthening and pausing in the Chunking Output Form task to convey the difference between such number sequences as TWENTY, NINE, TWO and TWENTY-NINE, TWO. In this task he demonstrated a tendency to syllable-timing, which can easily obliterate functional differences in syllable-length. When no use is made of pause between utterances the problem is exacerbated. As Jonathan had no problems with segmental phonology, his atypical intonation production may have other causes than motor planning, which was the explanation we proposed in relation to children with persisting speech difficulties like Malcolm and Zoe earlier in this chapter.

Turning now to the meaningful production of intonation as tested in Output Function, Jonathan scored below 1.5 SD on the Chunking, Focus and Interaction tasks. While the syllable timing that was noted above might contribute to his poor performance on longer items, he also had problems with comprehension, scoring below 1.5 SD on the Chunking and Interaction Input Function tasks. Thus Jonathan's results indicate that an overt intonation production problem may also be accompanied by difficulties with intonation comprehension. This opens up the possibility that problems with intonation production may derive, at least in part, from inaccurate representation of the intonation systems of English. If Jonathan is unaware of the subtleties of intonational meaning, or of how intonational meaning can combine with lexis and grammar, this could give rise to some misunderstandings on his part, and thence a failure to realize how he could be making use of intonation in his own utterances to convey meaning effectively.

Jonathan's spontaneous speech

Jonathan's inability to use intonation appropriately in his own speech output, as measured by the Output Function tasks, is a major source of concern. Using questions from the IIP, we will now analyse extracts from his spontaneous speech, to see how this manifests in everyday interaction. The first extract is a fragment of conversation between Jonathan and the researcher when he was being tested on PEPS-C. Extract (10.8) was recorded when he was being asked to name some vocabulary items that would be used in the test. An audio recording of this and the following three extracts performed by actors is available. The transcript of Extract (10.8) embodies the approach explained in earlier chapters. The words are transcribed orthographically for both speakers. For intonation, a systematic notation is used for the researcher (R), who is a speaker of the standard variety of Southern British English. For Jonathan, the transcription is impressionistic, as his intonation is atypical.

(10.8)

```
1  R:  right
```

```
2  J:  fishca:ke   (1.0)    thats not    nice    to have  a  fishca:ke
       {f}                  {f}   {f}    {f}
       {lento                                                    lento}
```

```
3  R:  ‖ 'sounds ^horrible ‖ ^doesnt it ‖
```

```
4  J:  yea:h
5  R:  ‖ ^mm ‖
```

```
6  J:  if   you eat  it   nobody li:kes  i:t
       {f}      {f}       {f}   {rallentando}
```

Compared to typically developing children of a similar age, as described in Chapter 8, and also to Mick and Robin in this chapter, Jonathan's intonation is atypical in several respects. Where speakers of English normally use on-syllable pitch movements to signal a Tonic at the end of an IP, Jonathan more often has level pitch, as in line 6 "likes it"; or else he moves abruptly from one level to another, as on the final syllable of "fishcake" at the end of the line 2. The latter feature also occurs non-finally in the turn, on "nice", suggesting that this may be a way of signalling Focus. Jonathan's speech rate is slow overall and he lengthens vowels very noticeably in the final syllables of his utterances (lines 2, 4, 6), which may contribute to signalling the end of a turn, i.e. a yellow traffic light. Earlier syllables are similar in duration to one another, giving an effect of syllable timing up to the end of the line. Some syllables that are high in the pitch range are also noticeably loud, particularly earlier in the utterance (lines 2, 6). Taken together, these features may account for the 'sing-song' character of his speech noted by his family and others.

In order to check whether these features are found generally in his speech, we turn to a different kind of context. Extract (10.9) is from an interaction between Jonathan and the researcher, R, when he was being tested on the formulated sentences subtest of CELF, in which the child has to make up a sentence that includes the word provided.

(10.9)

1 R: **L** ‖'can you use the 'word (.) ⇑`after ‖(.)

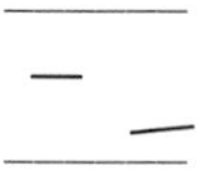

2 J: = after (1.0)
{f}

3 R: ‖'get ⇑`that in 'what you 'say ‖

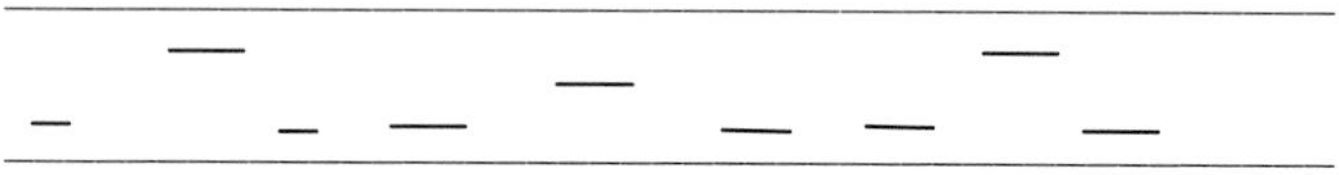

4 J: the people were playing in the summer:(0.5)
{f} {f} {f}

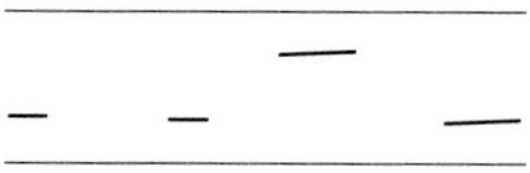

5 and the win:d blew (1.2)

6 R: = ‖ oˇkay ‖ thats very `nice 'Jonathan ‖ well `done

7 ‖(.) `okay ‖ `now(.)the 'last thing
I 'want to cl 'do [is]

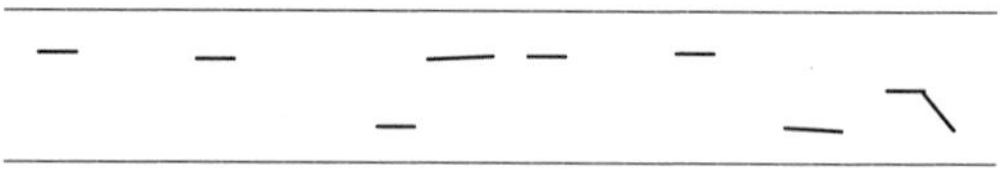

8 J: [what]time will I go back to class:
{f} {f} {f} {dim}

9 R: (1.0) ‖ 'after weve 'played this ´game ‖

Jonathan's pitch patterns in (10.9) are again very different phonetically from R's and those of other standard speakers. However, they are quite similar to his patterns in (10.8).Moreover, in both extracts the patterns seem to bear a systematic relationship to the systems of English intonation. In words of more than one syllable, the lexically stressed syllable is relatively high compared and loud to the unstressed syllable. In (10.9) this is evident in AFTER (line 2), PEOPLE and SUMMER, both in line 4 (PLAYING is produced as a monosyllable). Conversely, function words tend to have low pitch: in line 4, THE, WERE, IN and THE; and in line 8, WILL and TO. Thus, even though Jonathan produces almost all syllables with level rather than moving pitch, and most with roughly equal duration, he systematically distinguishes between stressed and unstressed syllables by means of pitch height and loudness.

In the transcript of (10.9.), we have included phonological notation for Turns, using traffic light highlighting; for Focus, by marking the location of the Tonic and whether it is a Supertonic; and for Alignment, by indicating whether there is Tone matching or not. For R's turns, it is relatively straightforward to notate the traffic lights and the Tonic. The identification of Tone matching depends on being able to identify the Tone of the other participant, i.e. Jonathan, which is more problematic. As for Jonathan, applying any of the phonological notation is quite problematic. This is apparent once we try to answer some of the main questions from the IIP.

Turns
We first consider how Jonathan gains the floor.

Does Jonathan refrain from taking a turn until the current speaker has projected the end of her/his own turn? (Jonathan observes red light)

Does Jonathan routinely start a turn with minimal pause, following the prior speaker's turn? (Jonathan observes yellow and green lights)

In (10.9) we can see that Jonathan takes turns, e.g. in lines 2 and 4, which are appropriately placed following the projection of the end of a turn by R – even if the content of his turn displays a lack of understanding of what R requires. This is also evident in lines 4 and 6 of (10.8). In each case he does this immediately or after only a minimal silence.

We now consider how Jonathan, having gained the floor, holds onto it and then gives it up.

Does Jonathan project the end of the turn by using the Tonic? (Jonathan uses yellow light)

The key question is whether Jonathan signals the Tonic. There is some evidence that he adds lengthening to words with "stress" (as defined above) and before a pause: in (10.9), SUMMER in line 4; WIND in line 5; and in CLASS in line 6, where there is also pitch movement. The same is true of lines 2, 4 and 6 of (10.8), all these having pitch movement. In all cases except line 6 of (10.8), the pitch ends at the base of his pitch range. The ingredients of lengthening, pitch movement and reaching the base of the pitch range, on top of "stress", resemble features that are associated with Tonics in English, as we saw in Chapter 1.

However, it is not altogether clear whether R in fact responds to them as Tonics that project a yellow traffic light, signalling the end of Jonathan's turn. In lines 3, 6 and 9 of (10.9), R takes a turn following his Tonic, though only after a pause of at least a second. After his 'Tonic' in line 4 she does not take a turn, even though he leaves half a second before continuing himself. While this may look as though she is not responsive to these 'Tonics', there are other reasons why she might not answer immediately: in lines 2, 4 and 5, his responses indicate that he probably does not understand the test in progress so R may be waiting for him to correct himself. In line 8 he offers an implicit complaint (that he is getting bored with the test) and she may need time to formulate a suitable response. On balance, we have given Jonathan the benefit of the doubt and attribute to him use of the traffic light system, albeit with somewhat unusual phonetics.

Does Jonathan produce a turn of more than one word by creating an IP with a Head? (Jonathan uses red light)

Jonathan can be seen to do this in lines 4-5 and 8 of Extract (10.9) as well as in lines 2 and 6 of Extract (10.8).

Does Jonathan produce a turn of more than a single IP by creating a non-final IP before the final IP?

Jonathan appears to do this in line 6 of (10.8). He uses a rising pitch movement at the end of the first clause "if you eat it", then a step down to the base of his pitch range, accompanied by lengthening, on the final two syllables of the second clause: "nobody likes it".

The next extract, (10.10), provides further evidence of Jonathan's ability to create extended IPs. It is taken from an interaction between Jonathan and a family member (M) about the film *Rainman*, Jonathan has the floor to himself from line 6 until the end of the extract, following M's invitation to him in line 5. As a result, he does not have to make a specific effort to hold on to the floor or to signal that he has finished a turn. In this respect, it resembles the fragment of 'solo' talk presented in Chapter 7 as Extract (7.4). This was produced by Robin at the age of 19 months, when playing with his mother. Jonathan, like Robin, makes of his interactional freedom to deploy a wider range of intonation patterns than has been evident elsewhere in his talk. This underlines the importance of sampling in different contexts.

(10.10)

1   M: what have you been   doing with Rainman
                                           {f}

2   J: Huh

3   M: have you been doing it   good

4   J: yes (1.2)

5   M: tell tell tell   me   what   happened   (.) with Rainman

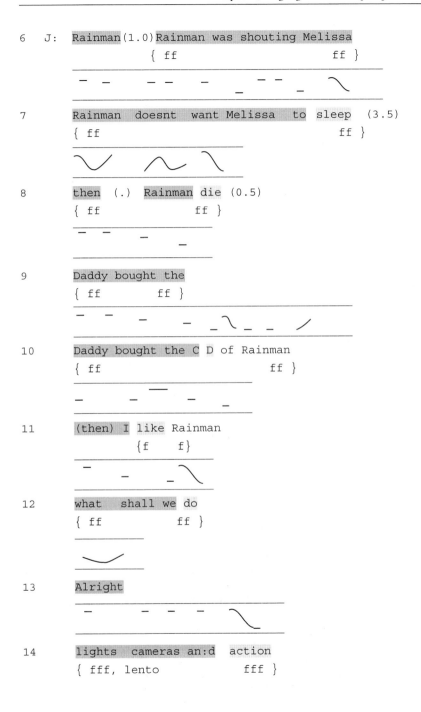

As in (10.8) and (10.9), Jonathan seems to signal word stress by raised pitch, with unstressed syllables having lower pitch. In lines 6 and 7, the first syllable of MELISSA is low. In line 6 WAS is low, while in line 7 TO is low. However, the pattern is slightly different from the one we saw in (10.8) and (10.9): in (10.10) the unstressed syllable that follows a stressed syllable remains high. One result is that the majority of syllables are now high in Jonathan's pitch range. In addition, there is uniformly loud volume but no lengthening, which makes it difficult to identify a Head–Tonic–Tail structure.

From line 8 onwards, there is much more variety of pitch, with dynamic pitch on single syllables, more like English Tones that could readily serve as Tonics to signal a yellow traffic light, e.g. at the end of lines 8, 10 , 12 and 14. Although turn-exchange is not at issue, Jonathan uses pitch devices to chunk his 'narrative' into internally coherent parts. For instance, in lines 6 and 7, reproduced as (10.10.1), he produces two grammatically separate clauses but has not provided BECAUSE between the two clauses to make explicit the causal relationship between the two propositions:

(10.10.1)   `6: Rainman was shouting Melissa`

        `7: Rainman doesnt want Melissa to slee`

Intonationally, however, he produces the two clauses as a single chunk: there is no pause between them and there is a wide fall in pitch to the base of his pitch range on "sleep" in line 7 but no such delimitation at the end of line 6 on "Melissa". Thus, intonation provides the cohesion which is lacking grammatically.

At the same time, line 6 illustrates some limitations in Jonathan's ability to use intonation to chunk the turn into meaningful parts. It is not clear whether line 6 and 7 are to be interpreted as (10.10.2) or (10.10.3):

(10.10.2)   Rainman is shouting, "Melissa!" (because) Rainman doesn't want Melissa to sleep

(10.10.3)   Rainman is shouting (to) Melissa (because) Rainman doesn't want Melissa to sleep

The first version would require the speaker to mark out MELISSA as a separate IP with its own Tonic, which Jonathan does not do. The second version would require a preposition before MELISSA, which Jonathan does not supply either.

The next intonational chunk that Jonathan produces is in line 8, again ending with a wide fall. The preceding two words are produced with wide fall-rises, projecting the continuing turn; this line displays a capacity to use complex dynamic pitch movements in line with the English intonation system, in a way that was not at all evident in (10.8) and (10.9). The following chunk consists of lines 9, 10 and 11. In line 9, Jonathan breaks off at a syntactically and intonationally incomplete point, then in line 10 re-does line 9 with exactly the same pitch pattern, demonstrating his control over pitch production. In the final section, lines 11–13, Jonathan appears to animate the role of a film director making a film (possibly the film of *Rainman*). He produces one side of a conversation. While it is not clear whether this is addressed to M or to an imaginary interlocutor on the film set, he is able to animate his director persona by marking the end of each line in this exchange with a dynamic pitch movement.

The final extract, (10.11), is taken from a session where R is administering the PEPS-C Focus Output Function test to Jonathan. It takes the form of a lotto (bingo) game, in which the child is offered a picture which does not match the ones he has; the child asks for a different picture, emphasizing what differentiates the picture the child wants from the one that had been offered. The variables are the object, which is a form of transport (e.g. car, bus) and its colour (e.g. red, blue).

Here, Jonathan again marks stress systematically but, curiously, his pattern is the opposite of what was seen in the previous extracts: the stressed syllables are low in the pitch range, for example WANT - and BLACK in line 3 or WANT - and BLUE in line 9. Conversely the unstressed syllables are high: I, -ED and A in both lines.

(10.11)

1 R: ‖ sup ˇposing I ˈsay ‖

2 L ‖ˈhow about a ⇑`black ˈcar ‖

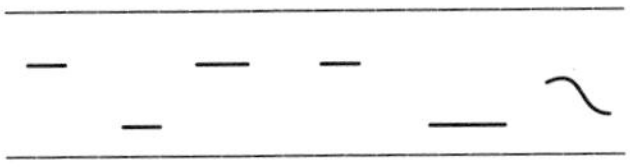

3 J: I wanted a black car

4 R: ‖ ´did ˈyou ‖

5 J: No

6 R: ‖ ˈwhat ˈcolour is your [`car] ‖

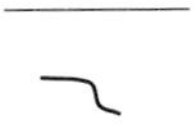

7 J: [blue]

8 R: ‖ ˈso you ˈsay (.) `oh ‖ [I]

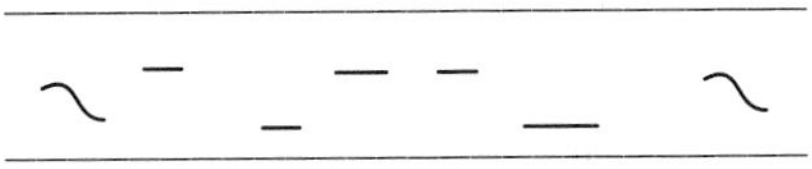

9 J: [oh] I wanted a blue: car:

10 R: ‖ I ˈwant a ⇑ `blue car ‖

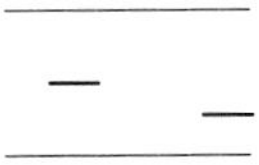

11 J: blue: car:
{f}

12 R: ‖ there you ´go ‖ (2.0) ‖ ˈnow youve got ˈall your ´pictures ‖

13 R: ‖ ˈso you ˈsay (0.3) `bingo ‖

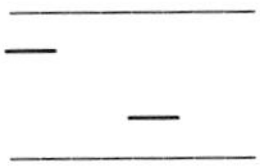

14 J: bingo:
{f}{ff}

15 R: ‖`right ‖

Does Jonathan produce an appropriately designed non-competitive turn in overlap, while the current speaker is still talking?

With regard to turn-taking, in lines 3, 5 and 11 of (10.11), Jonathan comes in immediately following R's projection of a TRP. In line 7, he anticipates this slightly, overlapping the final, Tonic word of R's turn in line 6. His answer is the expected one: it seems that, making use of the context, Jonathan is able to anticipate the answer that R wants, on the basis of "what colour is your..." without actually waiting for the word CAR.

Does Jonathan produce an appropriately designed competitive turn in overlap, in a bid to capture the floor while the current speaker is still talking?

In line 9 of (10.11) Jonathan anticipates the continuation of R's turn in line 8. Again, he anticipates correctly in terms of the required lexical content, though by taking the floor from R he loses the chance to hear the rest of R's turn which would have included correct model of Tonic placement that R would have produced (see next section).

In Extract (10.9), there was another instance of competitive overlap, reproduced here as (10.9.1). When Jonathan starts his turn before R has projected a TRP, there is evidence that he is doing this deliberately to compete for the floor.

(10.9.1)

```
7        ‖(.) `okay ‖ `now (.) the 'last thing
         I 'want to cl 'do [is ]
```

```
8   J:                    [what] time will I go back to class:
                           {f}   {f}    {f}                {dim}
```

First, his turn is designed in the way that is usual for interruptive turns, in that it starts with high pitch and is loud; once he has the floor, the volume reduces. Second, the content of his turn indicates that is getting tired of the test activity and is looking to get back to his usual routine.

In sum, although his pitch patterns can be unusual compared to standard varieties of English, particularly with regard to the realization for stressed and unstressed syllables, Jonathan appears to use prosodic features to manage turn-exchange in the extracts we have presented. This includes the use of competitive and non-competitive overlaps.

Focus and Tonic placement

Does Jonathan indicate narrow Focus on a non-final word of the IP by using non-final Supertonic placement?

As we saw in Chapters 1 and 3, in English there is a relationship between the system of lexical stress and the system of Tonic placement to mark Focus. The Tonic is placed on the lexically stressed syllable of the word that is the new or most important item in the IP.

One of the complications in analysing Jonathan's competence in the Tonic/Focus system results from the difficulty in identifying how he marks lexical stress. For most speakers of English, the stressed syllable of a word of more than one syllable will form the first syllable of a Foot, and will stand out in relation to unstressed syllables by virtue of a combination of pitch prominence (normally raised pitch compared to neighbouring unstressed syllables), relative loudness and relative length. With regard to pitch, we have already noted that the stressed syllable is higher than the unstressed syllables in (10.8) and (10.9), while in (10.10) it is higher than the preceding but not the following unstressed syllable. In (10.11), by contrast, stressed syllables are lower than adjacent unstressed syllables. His use of loudness is quite variable and sometimes unusual, particularly evident in the latter part of the *Rainman* passage in (10.10) where he speaks at very high volume throughout most of his narrative; this has the effect of masking relative loudness as a cue to stress. As for length, Jonathan generally speaks with a syllable timed rhythm, so that syllables are of roughly equal duration except at the end of the IP; this means that he is not using length as a cue to stress.

In line 9 of Extract (10.11), Jonathan's turn is treated by R as containing an error of Tonic placement, which is the subject of a repair operation in the next three lines. We noted above that in this extract, the stressed syllable is made prominent by a step *down*, to the first syllable of "wanted", and "blue" in line 9, as shown in (10.11.1):

(10.11.1)

```
9    J:   [oh]  I  wanted   a   blue:  car:
```

It is hard to tell where Jonathan's Focus is intended to be, on account of the combination of abrupt pitch jumps, low level pitch on the anticipated Focus word BLUE, moving (dynamic) pitch on a different word CAR, and lengthening on CAR as well as BLUE. In most varieties of English, a narrow Focus word will be prominent by virtue of a Supertonic, i.e. being longer, louder and having dynamic pitch that is higher than the surrounding syllables. In the event, R responds by 'correcting' Jonathan's Tonic placement, using a Supertonic on the word in Focus, shown in (10.11.2):

(10.11.2)

```
10    R:   ‖ I 'want a ⇑ `blue car ‖
```

Does Jonathan recognize the current speaker's broad and narrow Focus by attending to Tonic and Supertonic placement? Does Jonathan design the next turn accordingly?

In line 11, Jonathan adjusts his production so that the word BLUE is now higher in pitch, louder and longer than what surrounds it, i.e. closer to the standard system. This meets with R's approval (line 12). Within his own system, however, it is possible that Jonathan was already marking the word "blue" as the Focus in line 9, by the drop in pitch combined with extra lengthening.

Does Jonathan background non-Focus material, by placing it in the Tail after a non-final Tonic?

In extract (10.10) Jonathan produces the name RAINMAN six times following its introduction by his mother in line 1 and line 5 as the topic of the talk. It is notable that he avoids giving the word RAINMAN the most prominence in its IP on any of these occasions. In line 10 and in line 11, reproduced here as (10.10.4), RAINMAN is in the Tail, since an earlier word is more prominent: "CD" and then "like", these being new items and thus the Focus.

(10.10.4)

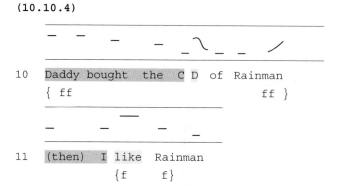

```
10   Daddy bought  the   C D  of  Rainman
     { ff                          ff }

11   (then)   I like   Rainman
              {f        f}
```

Thus, although Jonathan appeared to have some difficulty using narrow focus in the PEPS-C test situation, in his more spontaneous talk he appears to be able to use the Tonic-Focus system quite effectively.

Actions and Tone matching

Does Jonathan align with the action of the co-participant's prior turn by using Tone matching?

We have noted already that in the extracts with the researcher, who speaks Standard Southern British English, Jonathan's use of pitch is strikingly different: he uses more abrupt jumps and level pitches, sometimes with a narrow fall on the final word , whereas R has dynamic falls and rises on the Tonics, whatever their position. Nevertheless, there is evidence that Jonathan can use matching to display alignment. In Extract (10.11), even though there is a mismatch between the speakers regarding the location of the Tonic, Jonathan throughout matches R's falling Tone with a pitch pattern that steps down and a final narrow fall, as in (10.11.3).

(10.11.3)

```
2   R:  ‖'how about a ⇑`black 'car‖

3   J:  I  wanted a  black  car
4   R:  ‖ ´did 'you‖

5   J:  No
```

Does Jonathan recognize that the prior speaker has initiated a new action by use of Tone non-matching, and respond accordingly?

Immediately following the lines just discussed, in line 4 of Extract (10.11.3), R uses a rise to contest Jonathan's statement in line 3. Jonathan recognizes that this is not merely a request for confirmation, which R would have done with a matching fall. Instead he recognizes her non-matching rise as a new action requiring him to repair line 3, which he subsequently attempts to do. Thus, it seems that Jonathan is able to make some use of the system of Tone matching and non-matching for alignment and non-alignment of actions.

In summary, although J's use of pitch, loudness and duration sound is atypical in some important respects, we have seen that he shows awareness of the three key systems of intonation and, at least some of the time, uses them effectively. However, we also noted that some of his atypical prosodic features are nevertheless systematic.

Some of these behaviours may be attributable to a fact about Jonathan's linguistic environment that we have not disclosed until now. His family is of West African origin and their speech had some prosodic characteristics of West African English. Extract (10.12) presents talk that immediately precedes Jonathan's monologue about RAINMAN in (10.11). M, a member of his family, introduces the topic of RAINMAN.

(10.12)

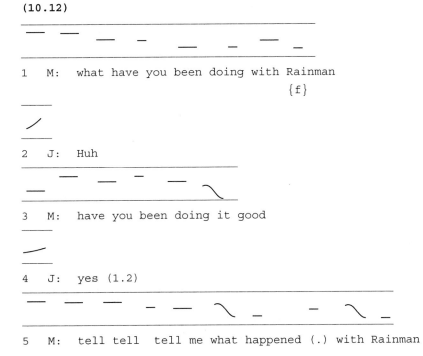

Features of the accent, as described by Gut (2004), that are evident in M's speech include the preponderance of level pitch on syllables other than the IP-final syllable; a tendency to have "stress" pitch movement on the final syllable even when it does not contain new or important information, i.e.as a marker of turn-finality; more equal length of stressed and unstressed syllables compared to British English. These are features that we have already noted in Jonathan's speech, along with high pitch on the stressed syllable and following syllables within the word, with low pitch on grammatical words. It is very likely that this accent background has been a key factor in determining the prosodic patterns that Jonathan uses. From the brief exchange in (10.12) there is some evidence that he is tuned into it; he uses non-matching Tone in line 2 to initiate a new course of action in the talk. Following the fall at the end of M's turn in line 1, Jonathan uses a rising pitch on "huh". This is treated as a request for clarification, as M then recasts her question in line 3. With regard to turn-taking, Jonathan comes in in lines 2, 4 and 6 directly following M's TRP. Her lines 1, 3, 5 all have a similar prosodic pattern, with fall on final word. The final fall serves to delimit the turn, and is followed by a turn from Jonathan, so he is orienting to M's utterances as complete turns. Whether M is always able to identify the end of Jonathan's turns is less clear. In line 3, she immediately comes in following his rising pitch on "huh", so she appears to treat him as having projected a TRP. However, there is a substantial silence between lines 4 and 5; this suggests that M is waiting for Jonathan to add more to his "yes" response which , although adequate in terms of its content, was produced with a mid-level pitch and so does not project a TRP.

It would be misleading to attribute Jonathan's prosodic patterns uniquely to the West African accent. Many children growing up in London are exposed to varieties of West African English, yet these children do not have all the features that characterize Jonathan's speech. Indeed, it was Jonathan's parents who were initially concerned about his unusual intonation, which include his apparently erratic use of high volume evident in (10.11). However, it does seem that Jonathan's difficulties may be compounded by the fact that he is exposed to standard British English as well as West African English, two varieties that have very different intonation characteristics. The consequences of this in real time can be shown by using the Intonation processing model from Chapter 9 to unpick the factors leading to Jonathan's production of one of the turns he produces when interacting with R. The exchange is reproduced here as (10.11.4):

```
(10.11.4)

2   R:   ‖how about a ⇑`black 'car‖

             —    —  —
                 —         —   ╲

3   J:   I  wanted a black car
```

As we have already seen, he does not produce this turn with an intonation pattern that would be expected for a standard variety of English, which instead might be as in (10.11.5), with a Supertonic on the new element, "wanted", to convey narrow Focus:

```
(10.11.5)  ‖ 'I ⇑`wanted a 'black 'car ‖
```

The processing of Jonathan's turn is illustrated in Figure 10.1. at Level 1, that of Action selection, Jonathan potentially conforms to the requirements of R's action: in compliance with the rules of the bingo game they are playing, she has proposed a black car as a selection for Jonathan. Jonathan goes along with this suggestion (albeit, as it turns out, mistakenly since he already has a black car). He uses a falling pitch movement,

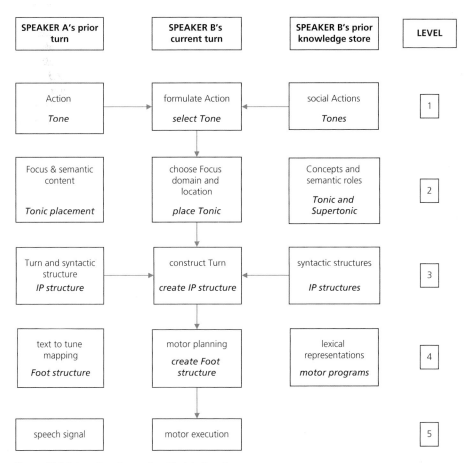

Figure 10.1 Intonation Processing Model: Jonathan.

which thus matches the fall Tone used by R. There is thus an arrow at this level from Speaker A's current turn to Speaker B's prior turn, to show that Jonathan is responsive to R's Tone choice. There is also an arrow from Speaker B's knowledge store, since falling Tones are already part of Jonathan's stored repertoire.

At Level 2, Jonathan does not display understanding of the requirements that Focus exerts on Tonic placement, which would have resulted in (10.11.5). It appears that he is not drawing on knowledge of the English system. We have therefore not shown any arrows here.

At Level 3, Turn construction, Jonathan starts his turn immediately following the end of R's turn, showing his awareness of the traffic light system. In his own turn, he uses a dynamic pitch on the last syllable, which serves as a yellow traffic light to mark the end of his turn, being immediately followed by a new turn from R. We have included arrows at this level since he appears to be using a system of traffic lights effectively, albeit one which probably derives from West African rather than British English, since the pitch movement is on the final word (Gut, 2004).

At Level 4, motor planning, there is no evidence that Jonathan's plan is responsive to R's turn. Moreover, by associating lexically stressed syllables with low pitch rather than high pitch, he does not conform to the West African English system either in this extract. We have therefore not used any arrows. This indicates that his speech production at the level of motor planning seems to be quite idiosyncratic on this occasion. Finally, there is no evidence of Jonathan attempting to imitate aspects of R's phonetic production, so there is no arrow at Level 5, motor execution.

In summary, the processing model in Figure 10.1 shows that when Jonathan produces the intonation for his turn, he makes only limited connections both with relevant stored knowledge and with the intonation of R's immediately prior turn. This suggests that the atypical patterns remarked on by his family and by professionals may derive from incomplete learning of English intonation systems, compounded by the fact that he is regularly exposed to two intonation systems, West African English and Standard Southern British English, that differ in important respects. On the other hand, his results on some of the PEPS-C tests suggest that he has the basic skills needed to acquire an intonation system, in terms of pitch perception and ability to produce a range of different pitch patterns. For Jonathan, a child with delayed language development, the difficulties with intonation seem to arise from having to reconcile conflicting intonation systems and map them onto an insecure grammatical basis.

Literacy impairments and dyslexia

The question of whether prosodic skills are important for reading development has increasingly attracted the attention of researchers. Whalley and Hansen (2006) showed that word identification in reading is easier for typically developing children who have good input prosodic skills. To test such skills, they used the PEPS-C Chunking Input Function task, which taps the ability to identify compound nouns as in (10.6) from lists of separate nouns as in (10.7), the two differing in their rhythm and intonation structure:

(10.6) ‖ ˇcream buns ‖ and ˋchocolate ‖ (two foods)

(10.7) ‖ ˇcream ‖ ˇbuns ‖ and ˋchocolate ‖ (three foods)

Dickie, Ota, and Clark (2012) have argued that adults with developmental dyslexia may not be worse than typical controls on distinguishing such minimal pairs. However, research focussing on stress and rhythm indicates that adults with dyslexia have an underlying difficulty with auditory rhythm perception that persists even if they have compensated for their reading problems (Thomson, Fryer, Maltby, & Goswami, 2006). While it is well known that phonological awareness and phonological processing of relatively small units of speech, such as the onset, rhyme, nucleus and coda of the syllable, can be challenging for many children with dyslexia, it seems that the processing of lexical stress can also be an issue.

In order to investigate prosodic deficits, Marshall et al. (2009) administered three sections of the revised PEPS-C (Chunking, Focus, Long item) to a group of children with dyslexia aged between 10 and 15 years, as well as to children with SLI and to a group with both SLI and dyslexia. The dyslexia-only group performed worse than CA controls on the long item imitation task. This is equivalent to the Chunking and Focus

Output Form tasks of the original PEPS-C, discussed earlier in this chapter in relation to Activity 10.2. The quantitative results suggest that some children with dyslexia may have difficulties in reproducing intonation contours in their own speech, though there is no qualitative analysis of what form their difficulties took. The dyslexia-only group also performed below language-age controls on the Chunking and Focus Input Function tasks, leading the authors to suggest that for children with dyslexia, interactions between prosody and syntax and prosody and pragmatics may be linked to subtle language difficulties. This view was reinforced by the finding that the group of children with both SLI and dyslexia performed the worst on all tasks.

In summary, there is evidence that some children with dyslexia have deficits in stored knowledge relating to lexical stress, IP phrasing and Tonic placement for Focus. It seems that this deficit may involve processing prosodic aspects of the signal and also integrating prosodic form with linguistic function. The question then arises as to how the presence of a deficit might affect the reading aloud of children with dyslexia. Unfortunately this is not a topic that researchers have yet addressed, to our knowledge. In Chapter 8, we described some of the ways in which typically developing children's use of intonation in reading aloud changes as they become more accomplished readers. It was suggested that in some respects they recapitulate steps that as much younger children they passed through when learning to use intonation when talking. Research on the impact of text complexity when reading aloud points to a developmental interaction between reading ability and the complexity of the text being read, in influencing the intonation patterns used. Benjamin and Schwanenflugel (2010) showed that 8-year-old American children's use of prosodic features when reading aloud is affected by the difficulty of the text. They were more dysfluent when reading aloud a text that was difficult in terms of its syntax and vocabulary, compared to an easier text. According to the authors, the ability to use intonation expressively is related to reading comprehension ability. It might therefore be predicted that the intonation of children with dyslexia will be affected on a number of levels when reading aloud: difficulties in comprehension will lead to inaccurate use of intonation phrasing and Tonic placement for Focus; imprecise representations of lexical stress will lead to unclear signalling of Foot boundaries within the Intonation Phrase (IP); and difficulties with orthographic decoding are likely to result in dysfluent reading aloud, of the kind noted for beginning readers in Chapter 8, leading to multiple short IPs for each sentence.

Summary

The studies reviewed and the cases presented in this chapter have highlighted the following key points about intonation in children with speech, language or literacy impairments:

- Children with relatively mild speech difficulties are unlikely to manifest unusual intonation (Mick).
- Children with severe and persisting speech difficulties may manifest unusual intonation in their speech; these are primarily a result of disruptions caused by their segmental speech difficulties (Zoe; Malcolm).
- Some children with language difficulties who do not manifest unusual intonation in their speech may nevertheless have intonation comprehension problems related to a receptive language difficulty (Robin).

- Some children with language difficulties may manifest unusual intonation in their speech as result of inaccurate learning of intonation; this may result from mixed input from different dialects or languages (Jonathan).
- Some children with dyslexia may have deficits in intonation comprehension and production related to language difficulties; it is likely that they will have unusual intonation when reading aloud.
- Analysis of spontaneous speech using the IIP and of test performance on PEPS-C offer complementary approaches to assessing the intonation abilities and performance of a child with speech or language difficulties.
- Interpretation of IIP and PEPS-C analyses using the Developmental Phase model and the Intonation processing model offer complementary perspectives on the child's strengths and limitations.

Key to Activity 10.1

The task addresses hearing ability, insofar as children with severe hearing difficulties may be unable to hear the differences in pitch and loudness between the two stimuli in the 'different' pair. This point will be pursued further in Chapter 12. If a child who has normal hearing nevertheless fails on this task, there must be another reason.

The stimuli, though non-linguistic in the sense of having no lexical or grammatical content, are linguistic in that they incorporate prosodic patterns that are found in languages and which may in fact be specific to the English language. A child who fails to tell apart the two stimuli in the 'different' pair, may have a deficit in perception of these linguistic prosodic features, just as some children have deficits in perception of segmental features such as the voiced–voiceless contrast.

Alternatively, the difficulty may be with auditory memory. The child has to hold in working memory two strings, each of five 'syllables', but with no words or meaning attached to them. The child then has to compare these two strings and make a judgement. Thus, children whose language impairment is accompanied by difficulties in short-term auditory memory may end up guessing on this task.

Key to Activity 10.2

As with Input Form tasks, the child needs to be able to hear the stimuli and perceive the relevant differences. The child then needs to be able to access motor programs for the digits, assemble them in the correct order and produce them as a turn with the appropriate IP phrasing. Difficulties may arise with prosodic discrimination or auditory memory, as for the Input Form task. Furthermore, the child may have difficulty with assembling a turn consisting of multiple IPs and choosing the appropriate Tone for the non-final and final IPs.

CHAPTER 11

Autism spectrum disorders and learning difficulties

In Chapter 10, it was suggested the atypical patterns of intonation in some children with speech and language impairments arise either as a consequence of articulatory difficulties or else as a compensation for linguistic problems that affect intelligibility. In this chapter we will explore the hypothesis that for other children, atypical intonation can be the product of underlying cognitive (including socio-cognitive) deficits. We will again refer to the developmental phase model and the intonation processing model, highlighting the important role of intonation in Turn-taking, Focus and Actions – basic interactional functions that are important for all children, whatever their cognitive limitations. One such group of children is those who are diagnosed as having a disorder on the autism spectrum. In this chapter, we concentrate principally on this group. We then consider the intonation abilities of children with Williams syndrome and of children with Down syndrome.

Intonation and the autism spectrum

Introducing a study of acoustic aspects of intonation, Diehl and Paul summarize a current view of prosody in the autism spectrum disorders (ASD):

> Atypicalities in prosody production, including rhythm, rate, and intonation patterns, are some of the most commonly reported social–communicative features of the disorder … and also some of the earliest characteristics to appear … The perceived difference in prosodic patterns is considered to be one of the most stigmatizing aspects of the disorder.
>
> *(2013: 136)*

In this chapter, we first consider speech behaviours traditionally described as delayed and immediate echolalia. Although these are not particularly transparent descriptions of the phenomena, here we will retain the traditional terminology. We address the intonational aspects of echolalia primarily through a case study of Kevin, an 11-year-old boy with severe autism, who has been described in some detail in publications by Tony Wootton and John Local. As in Chapter 10, we draw on questions from the IIP to structure our analysis. We then turn to children diagnosed as having High

---

Functioning Autism (HFA), focussing mainly on results that have been reported from group studies using the PEPS-C battery (Peppé & McCann, 2003), which was introduced in Chapter 8.

Kevin

Kevin had a diagnosis of severe autism. His expressive language at CA 11;04 was approximately the equivalent of that of a 2-year-old typically developing child. Detailed analyses of audio and video recordings with members of his family and with his teachers are presented by Local & Wootton, (1995) and by Wootton, (1999; 2002). The proportion of different vocal behaviours produced by Kevin in the recordings was (very approximately) as follows. Around half were non-communicative delayed echoes, which made up almost all his spontaneous talk, "that is, talk which is not a direct response to something like a question from another person" (Wootton, 2002: 146). Labelling responses to questions made up around 30% and immediate echoes, which were produced only in response to questions, around 15%. Initiations, which were always requests, made up 5%. Instances of these categories will be discussed from the point of view of Kevin's use of intonation.

Extract (11.1), which is an adapted transcription of Fragment 11 from Local and Wootton (1995), was earlier presented in Chapter 4. Kevin and his mother are playing a game that involves throwing dice. In line 1, Kevin's mother asks him whose turn it is to throw the dice:

(11.1)

```
1  M:   ‖ˈwhose ˋturn is it‖
        (1.5)
2  M:   ‖ˈwhose ˋturn is it‖
        (1.5)
3  M:   ‖ˈwhose ˋturn is it‖
        {      lento       }
        (.)
```

```
4  K:      turn is it
        { lento   }

5  M:   ‖ˈwhose ˋturn is it‖
```

```
6  K:   Kevins  turn
        {f}
7  M:   ‖ˇhonest‖
        (sound of shaking dice)
8  M:   ‖ˈwhatve you ˋgot Kevin‖
```

Kevin's mother produces the same question four times. On the first two occasions (lines 1 and 2) Kevin does not respond. Her third production (line 3) is slightly slower. It is followed by an instance of immediate echolalia: Kevin produces the final three words of his mother's turn, i.e. the Tonic + Tail; the pitch, loudness and tempo features are echoed with great precision. This shows that Kevin is able to produce a well-formed intonation contour of English. Nevertheless, his mother does not treat his utterance in line 4 as a fitted response: instead, she reiterates her question a fourth time (line 5).

Focus and Tonic placement

Our observations about Kevin's functional use of intonation are formulated as answers to questions from the Intonation in Interaction Profile (IIP), which was described in Chapter 5.

Does C indicate narrow Focus on a non-final word of the IP by using non-final Supertonic placement?

Does C background non-Focus material, by placing it in the Tail after a non-final Tonic?

In line 6 of Extract (11.1), Kevin produces the same prosodic contour as in his line 4 and his mother's line 5, but with different words. Slotting KEVIN into turn-initial position means that, with this Tonic + Tail pattern, KEVIN carries Tonic prominence and is thus presented as narrow Focus. This fits the context since the other word, TURN, is already well established as a topic. Unlike line 4, line 6 is treated as a fitted response by Kevin's mother. In line 8, she no longer pursues the same question as hitherto. Instead, with "honest?" she teasingly queries whether Kevin is telling the truth, that it really is his turn in the game. Thus in line 6 ,Kevin has produced a turn that is both lexically and intonationally fitted to the context.

However, we cannot automatically infer from this that Kevin intended to use the Tonic in order to signal narrow Focus. It may be that the appropriate Tonic placement is an accidental by-product of a prosodic routine that has just been established. In line 6, Kevin uses the same pattern as that of his mother's "(whose) turn is it," (lines 1–3, 5) and his own "turn is it" (line 4). Moreover, his 'correct' Tonic follows (and ends) a repair sequence that had been initiated and pursued by his mother. The ability to deploy Tonic placement for the purposes of Focus may not be fully productive for Kevin but instead may be parasitic on the immediate context. This example illustrates how consideration of the wider context can affect our interpretation of a child's intonation ability as demonstrated in a particular utterance.

Turns and IP structure

Does C project the end of the turn by using the Tonic? (C uses yellow light)

To investigate further how far a child with autism is able to use intonation productively, it is important to consider his topic initiations, since by definition a topic initiation will not be parasitic on the preceding context. In line 1 of Extract (11.2), which is adapted from Fragment 1 in Local and Wootton (1995), Kevin initiates talk following a lapse in the conversation:

(11.2)

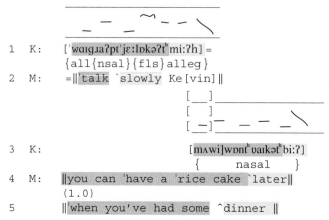

```
1   K:    ['wɑɪɡɹaʔpt'jɛ:lɒkəʔtʰmi:ʔh] =
          {all{nsal}{fls}alleg}
2   M:    =‖'talk `slowly Ke[vin]‖
                                 [__]_____
                                 [  ]
                                 [_-]¯ _ _ ¯ _____
3   K:                          [mʌwi]wɒntʰʋaɪkətʰbi:ʔ]
                                {    nasal    }
4   M:    ‖you can 'have a 'rice cake `later‖
          (1.0)
5         ‖'when you've had some ^dinner ‖
```

The phonetic delivery of Kevin's turn in line 1 is quite unusual, with very wide fluctuations in pitch, including a long falsetto vowel, pervasive nasality, and rapid speech rate. The segmental content is not readily interpretable. Despite its speed and unintelligibility, his turn is immediately followed by a turn from Kevin's mother, suggesting that she knows that Kevin has reached the end of his turn. It is likely that the pitch fall to the base of Kevin's pitch range on the final syllable, in combination with lengthening of the final vowel and the strongly aspirated release of the final consonant, contribute to his mother's identification of the end of his turn. Similar features are found at the end of Kevin's utterance in line 3, which, like line 1, is followed immediately by a turn from his mother. This suggests that despite some strikingly atypical phonetic features in his initiations, Kevin can nevertheless deploy intonation resources to indicate the completion of his turn, displaying a yellow traffic light.

Does C refrain from taking a turn until the current speaker has projected the end of his or her own turn? (C observes red light)

Does C routinely start a turn with minimal pause, following the prior speaker's turn?(C observes yellow and green lights)

Line 3 demonstrates that Kevin is able to modify prosodic features of his talk: following his mother's request in line 2, Kevin's turn in line 3 is both a little quieter and lower in pitch, though not in fact slower. It also provides some evidence of his orientation to intonation features of his mother's talk: the start of his turn in line 3 overlaps the Tail of his mother's turn in line 2. As we have seen, the Tail is vulnerable to terminal overlaps in English conversation, so Kevin's incoming here is not atypical. In general, his incomings are placed following the end of the prior speaker's IP. However, he does not take a turn after line 4 of Extract (11.2), even though his mother has displayed a yellow light. After a second's pause, she is obliged to continue. Similarly, in Extract (11.1) we saw that initially Kevin did not take a turn at all, even when asked a question.

However, when he did take a turn, he did so straight away without undue pause, as in lines 4 and 6. Thus, there is evidence that despite his severe autism, Kevin shows orientation to some basic interactional practices, including the intonation features that English speakers use to manage turn-taking (see Local & Wootton, 1995 and Wootton, 1999, for further discussion).

Does C produce a turn of more than one word by creating an IP with a Head? (C uses red light)

Kevin's two turns in Extract (11.2), in lines 1 and 3, each consist of six syllables. In each case the turn-demarcative fall in pitch occurs on the last syllable, there being no major pitch movement earlier in the turn. Thus, even though his words are unintelligible (at least to an outsider), for each turn, Kevin has created a Head + Tonic IP structure, displaying a red light followed by a yellow light.

In summary, Extracts (11.1) and (11.2) show that Kevin is able to produce well-formed IP structures. To some extent, Kevin demonstrates the ability to use intonation functionally, for the projection of turn endings vs continuations. He appears able to respond to his co-participant's use of intonation to project turn endings. He himself routinely uses a pitch fall to signal turn-completion.

Actions and Tone matching

Does C align with the action of the co-participant's prior turn by using Tone matching?

If so, what actions does C align with? For example, Assessments; Repairs; Requests; Offers

Sometimes Kevin produces standard Tone matching, using the same pitch direction as the previous speaker, as in Extract (11.3), which is adapted from Fragment 3 of (Local & Wootton, 1995):

(11.3)

```
1  M:   ‖'what ´is it‖
         (1.9)
2  M:   ‖'its a w::‖
         (0.7)
3  M:   ‖'wa-
         (1.1)
```

```
4  K:    pex   zi  koh
         {   ppp       }
```

```
5  M:   ‖'no its a ⇑`wateringcan‖
```

```
6  K:   `wateringcan
```

```
8  M:   ‖'what dyou `do with a 'watering'can ‖
```

In line 6, Kevin repeats a correct label provided by the co-participant, using Tone matching, as happens in the labelling sequences involving very young typically developing children described by Tarplee (1996) and discussed in Chapter 7. He seems to do this for the purposes of interactional alignment (cf. Chapter 4). His mother treats it as an appropriate move, as is evident by her progressing the topic in line 8. There was a similar case of Tone matching in line 8 of Extract (11.1). In both cases, he aligns with a request from his mother.

However, in addition, Kevin produces 'unusual' pure echoes, like the "turn is it" example in (11.1). Here, the pitch is very precisely matched, as are the duration and the segmental articulation; but the rhythm of his echo turn is disjoined from the rhythm of the prior speaker's turn. Local and Wootton point out that Kevin only produces these unusual pure echoes as his first response to adult questions (which otherwise he tends to make no reply to). So we can regard this as an atypical use of Tone matching, to fill a rather specific interactional function, namely to acknowledge that a response is required but without committing to any semantic content in that response: he merely repeats his mother's word. Nor does he commit to any interactional or pragmatic content, e.g. to indicate a problem with hearing or understanding by requesting a repeat or clarification – which would be conveyed by using a non-matching Tone. These unusual repeats or echoes do not have a counterpart in normal development, according to Local and Wootton (1995). Kevin overextends the Tone matching resource that exists in English intonation: he uses Tone matching not only to align with an ongoing action, but also, as one of a cluster of imitative features in his speech, to provide a response that is semantically and pragmatically empty. It thus appears that Kevin uses both the kinds of "prosodic repetition" described by Couper-Kuhlen, (1996). First he uses repetition of the prior speaker's Tone but adapted to his own pitch register. In addition, however, he uses repetition of the Tone with "absolute" register matching. Couper-Kuhlen shows how in adult interactions this latter type of mimicry is used by speakers to tease or annoy the prior speaker. This may be one reason why the unusual echolalia produced by some speakers on the autism spectrum can be quite irritating for the interlocutor. It may also be unsettling for the observer, who perceives a mismatch between the precision with which the child with autism replicates the speech of the typical speaker, which contrasts dramatically with other highly atypical behaviours that the person with ASD may display.

Does C initiate a new action, different from the action underway in C's preceding IP in his own current turn, by using Tone non-matching?

The fact that Kevin hardly ever initiates a topic or action (other than a request) makes it seem unlikely that he will use non-matching of Tone functionally, as this is typically used in a situation where the speaker wants to initiate a new course of action in the interaction, e.g. to initiate a repair sequence. Kevin, like other children on the autism spectrum, rarely does this. Returning to the sequence transcribed in Extract (11.1), it is possible that if Kevin had used a non-matching Tone in line 4, such as a rise, his mother would have explicitly acknowledged his turn in line 4 as a fitted response, e.g. as a clarification request, as in the hypothetical sequence in (11.1.1). This is based on (11.1) but lines 4 and 5 are invented:

(11.1.1)

```
3  M:  ||'whose `turn is it||
       {       lento        }
       (.)
4  K:  'turn is it
5  M:  'yeah
```

Such instances of Tone non-matching to initiate a new action are not produced by Kevin.

On the other hand, Kevin, like other children with autism, frequently produces a "delayed echo" which, by virtue of having a fixed and invariant intonation contour, may result in Tone non-matching with the prior speaker's turn. "Delayed echo" is a term that is used in the autism literature to refer to a linguistic form that the child has heard and remembered, originating, for example, from an adult speaker such as a parent or teacher, from a film or a TV programme. The child then reproduces this form verbatim in subsequent interactions, where the original phrase is likely to make no sense. For these reasons, delayed echoes are unlikely to be sequentially fitted in terms of interactional moves; and because they have a set intonation pattern, they are often liable to be heard as non-matching and therefore disaligning with the prior speaker's agenda.

Extract (11.4) illustrates some of the important intonational and interactional features of Kevin's delayed echoes. Kevin is with his sister (S) and his mother (M). He has done a piece of drawing or writing (it is unclear which from the recording). The words of the delayed echo are "that's a naughty boy" – a formulation that occurs some 30 times in the course of the 4.5 hours of recording examined by Wootton (1999).

(11.4)

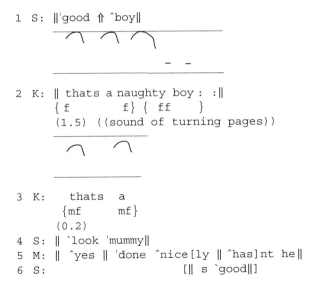

```
1  S:  ||'good ⇑ ^boy||




2  K:  || thats a naughty boy :  :||
       { f          f} { ff    }
       (1.5) ((sound of turning pages))




3  K:     thats   a
          {mf       mf}
          (0.2)
4  S:  || `look 'mummy||
5  M:  || ^yes || 'done ^nice[ly || ^has]nt he||
6  S:                   [|| s `good||]
```

In line 1, Kevin's sister praises him, apparently for his drawing/writing. Kevin immediately produces an utterance that is recognizable from many other places in the recorded data as one of his delayed echoes. This is followed by a gap where only the sound of papers can be heard. Then in line 3, Kevin produces an utterance that repeats the first two syllables of line 2, with virtually identical intonation. After a short gap, in line 4, his sister addresses the mother only ("look Mummy"), apparently showing her Kevin's work. In line 5, the mother responds, praising Kevin's work, but addressing her comment to the sister only, as is evident from the use of the tag "hasn't he", rather than "haven't you". Throughout the recordings, as here, Kevin's interlocutors routinely do not respond to his delayed echoes: for the purpose of progressing the interaction, these delayed echoes are ignored. This is particularly striking in the fragment under consideration here, since if we were not aware of the status of "that's a naughty boy" as one of Kevin's delayed echoes, we might interpret his use of BOY as topically related to his sister's mention of "boy" in line 1, and that by modifying "boy" with "naughty", and giving it Tonic prominence, he might therefore be formulating a disagreement with his sister's assessment. However, as we have seen, there is no orientation by Kevin's sister or his mother to the possibility that Kevin's turn in line 2 might have any bearing on their positive assessment of his drawing, since they seem to disregard it and him in their subsequent talk. Nor does Kevin make any further move to display the relevance of line 2 to line 1. On the contrary, by precisely redoing the first part of line 2 at line 3 but then breaking it off without apparent reason, he reinforces the status of his phrase in line 2 as a delayed echo.

Line 2 illustrates the salient prosodic characteristics of Kevin's delayed echoes as described by Wootton (1999):

- dynamic pitch change: there are three rise falls on the first three syllables;
- very high and or very low pitch : the three first syllables of line 2 have a peak of above 730 Hz while the final syllable is around 250 Hz, a drop of around 20 semitones from the first syllable of "naughty" to "boy";
- marked stress patterns: the first three syllables are loud or very loud;
- prolongations: the final syllable, "boy" is sustained on a level pitch for c. 400 ms.

These prosodic features are important for characterizing and identifying instances of delayed echoes (Wootton, 1999: 364–365).

In his analysis of Kevin's delayed echoes, Wootton (1999) presents further observations that are relevant to our understanding of their intonation. First, delayed echoes can be four or five words long, as in "that's a naughty boy", whereas Kevin's immediate echoes are usually just one or two words. Second, the lexical items found in delayed echoes are not confined to the delayed echo. Wootton provides the example of the word SMACK. Sometimes Kevin uses this word in a sequence which is treated as interactionally relevant by his interlocutors. In such cases his pitch pattern matches the Tone of the interlocutor in the conventional way to indicate alignment. In Extract (11.5), Kevin and his parents are playing a game that they often play together, in which Kevin is presented with various pairs of alternatives and has to choose the one he wants. Here Kevin chooses the second alternative, "smack", and produces it with a falling pitch, matching the falling Tone just used by both his mother (line 1) and father (line 2). Following Kevin's turn, the game continues, with the mother presenting the next pair of alternatives, suggesting that they treat Kevin's turn in line 3 as a fitting move in this interactional game.

(11.5)

```
1   M:   dyou want [ 'kiss::::::::::::::::]:  or:: a `smack   (.)
                    [                      ]              {f}
2   D:              [‖ 'cuddle or a `smack ‖]
```

```
3   K:   smack
         {f}
```

On many other occasions, Kevin produces the word SMACK as part of a delayed echo. On these occasions, it is always produced with falling pitch from very high in Kevin's pitch range towards the base of his range, and the vowel is lengthened. Thus, as a delayed echo, SMACK has its own distinctive contour. However, variations are possible, in that the echo phrase may be extended or interrupted. Wootton (1999: 371) presents the examples in (11.6), from within one 10-minute interaction where Kevin and his father are drawing pictures:

(11.6)

```
(i)    S:ma:::ck to: dora::n re-
(ii)   S:ma::ck todododo
(iii)  Ta: y: s:ma:::ck
(iv)   To: s:ma::::ck nu
(v)    Sma:::ck yor sma:::ck yor sma:::ck( ) sma:::ck
(vi)   To: sma- ma: ma: ma: ma: ma: sma:ck
```

As is evident, the word SMACK may be preceded and/or followed by other material. However, it always has the pitch fall and vowel sustention described above. Where there is a word or syllable preceding the word "smack" , as in (iii), (iv) and (vi), that word is low in the pitch rage, so there is a big step-up in pitch to the start of "smack". Syllables following "smack", present in all the examples except (iii), are low in the pitch range, until there is another production of "smack" as in (v) (Wootton, 1999: 372).

The potential for extension suggests that delayed echo phrases may not be entirely fossilized forms; they may also be broken off, as in line 3 of the "that's a naughty boy" extract (11.4). In spite of this structural flexibility, they are nevertheless characterized by fixed pitch patterns. The resilience of these echoes through an interaction, as described by Wootton (1999), suggests the "inflexibility" that Muskett, Perkins, Clegg, and Body (2010) show to be characteristic behaviour of children on the autism spectrum, used as a way of controlling the interaction.

Delayed echoes from developmental and interactional perspectives

The association of a relatively fixed Tone with a stored linguistic form, in this case, a delayed echo such as Kevin's SMACK in (11.6), parallels the phenomenon of lexical Tone in a Tone language (cf. Chapter 6), where a word stored in the lexicon has a fixed Tone associated with it. An interesting manifestation of such Tone language-like behaviour in a child learning English, is the case of Kenneth, aged 3;09, described by Tarplee & Barrow, (1999). Kenneth had been diagnosed as having an autistic spectrum disorder. His developmental level for language and other behaviours was around two years or below. Interactions with his mother were characterized by delayed echolalia. Specifically, he used words and phrases from a favourite cartoon film to initiate talk with his mother:

> For instance, a vocalization produced three times by one character in the cartoon takes the form *yap yap yap*. On each of these occasions this utterance is produced with roughly equal prominence on all syllables, with level pitch on each syllable, and with an overall pitch contour of either one or two upward steps. In the data, a version of this utterance is produced 17 times by Kenneth and 11 times by his mother. Each time, although tempo and pitch height vary, those prosodic characteristics outlined above are retained.
>
> *(Tarplee & Barrow, 1999: 454)*

The following extract (11.7), adapted from Fragment 1 in Tarplee and Barrow (1999), gives a flavour of how delayed echoes are used by Kenneth (K) and his mother (M).

(11.7)

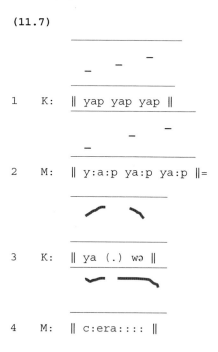

Another favourite for Kenneth was the cartoon character name CERA, which he consistently produced with a narrow rise-fall high in his pitch range, as in line 3. While these phrases were not necessarily accurate or consistent in terms of their consonantal and vocalic segments, Kevin consistently produced them with the same pitch pattern, which was the pattern used in the original cartoon film. One benefit of this Tone consistency may be in helping his mother to identify the word that Kenneth had produced, so that she can repeat it back. She routinely did so, as in line 4 of (11.7). In this respect, the distinct Tone patterns of Kenneth's delayed echoes are comparable to the use of lexical Tone in a Tone language such as Mandarin: as there are many potential homophones in the language, the segmental content of a Mandarin syllable is often insufficient to uniquely identify to the listener the word that the speaker intends, so the additional information provided by Tone is necessary. In terms of the developmental phase model, Kenneth's delayed echoes may thus indicate that he does not yet appreciate that English is a non-Tone language. This can be interpreted as arrested development at the Paradigmatic phase, which lasts until around the age of 18 months in typically developing children (cf. Chapter 6).

While both Kenneth and Kevin frequently produced delayed echoes, there is an important difference between them in how these delayed echoes were treated by their interlocutors, which Tarplee and Barrow (1999) discuss. Kenneth's mother would often repeat his delayed echo, as a way of engaging in a Turn-taking interaction with him. Sometimes she would even be the first to produce the delayed echo phrase, attempting to draw Kenneth into conversation by encouraging him to repeat after her. Both these strategies would incidentally result in Tone matching between Kenneth and his mother and thus an intonational display of interactional alignment, as in Extract (11.7).

By contrast, as we saw in (11.4), Kevin's interlocutors typically did not respond to his delayed echoes. They would only acknowledge and build on utterances by Kevin that were recognizably not echoes, either delayed or immediate. Wootton (1999) makes an interesting connection between Kevin's delayed echolalia and so-called crib talk of typically developing young children, i.e. the kind of solo-play talk that we observed from Robin at the age of 19 months (see Chapter 7). Just as Robin's solo play talk is not designed to be interactive, and is not treated as such by his mother, so Kevin's delayed echoes are used in a non-interactive way and are not treated by his co-participants as contributions to the talk.

However, it does not follow that Kevin lacks awareness of interactional issues. He can use a delayed echo to mark a disengagement from ongoing talk, while continuing to interact nonverbally, e.g. continuing to play a board game with his parent while producing delayed echoes. Thus, the nonverbal actions that accompany his delayed echoes may actually be addressing the interaction in hand. Moreover, Wootton (1999) points out that Kevin times his delayed echoes in such a way as to avoid overlap. This displays Kevin's orientation to Turn-taking mechanisms even when his talk (i.e. the delayed echo) is not addressing the co-participant.

Thus, it appears that for Kevin both immediate and delayed echoes display awareness of some of the requirements of talk-in-interaction and awareness that intonation is part of the display. He produces immediate echoes where a response from him is expected. As part of a package of vocal imitative features, the immediate echo includes Tone matching, thus potentially indicating interactional alignment. However, this is at odds with the verbal content of the echo which, by being a mere repeat of the prior speaker, fails to satisfy the requirements of a response. Delayed echoes, on the other hand, are placed by Kevin in a much wider range of sequential positions. For instance, "that's a naughty boy" in (11.4) follows a positive assessment from his sister, "good boy". Whether or not there will be Tone matching is unpredictable: because the delayed echo has a fixed pitch pattern, it is a matter of chance whether or not it will match the Tone of the prior turn. Even though his sister in line 1 had used a rise-fall Tone with a wide pitch movement, Kevin's turn in line 2 uses such an extreme pitch range, with repeated dynamic rise-fall pitches on the first three syllables, that it does not lend itself to being interpreted as a match to her Tone and thus an alignment with her positive assessment. This Tonal non-matching highlights the function of Kevin's delayed echo to disengage from the talk in progress.

From a psycholinguistic perspective, immediate echoes and delayed echoes reflect different prosodic processing abilities. Figure 11.1 illustrates the processing of an immediate echo found in Extract (11.1.2). To produce an immediate echo with the precision that Kevin demonstrates, the speaker needs to have excellent phonetic perception,

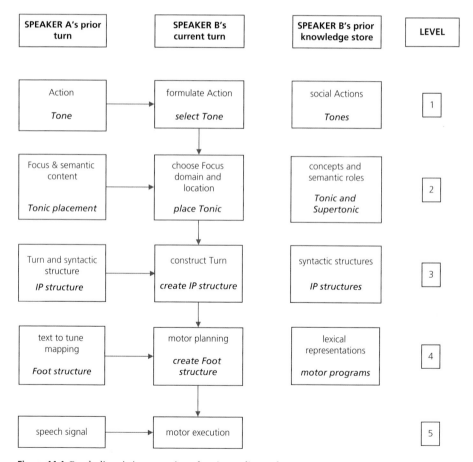

Figure 11.1 Psycholinguistic processing of an immediate echo.

some capacity for short-term storage of verbal material, the ability to map from short-term stored representation to a motor plan and, finally, a high degree of articulatory control. The production of the immediate echo derives entirely from the prior speaker's turn. At each level there is an arrow that points from the box in the left-hand column, representing the mother's line 3, to the parallel box representing Kevin's line 4. This illustrates that each processing step underlying Kevin's turn in line 4 is parasitic on the corresponding step taken by his mother in line 3. Conversely, the immediate echo does not depend on the current speaker's stored knowledge at all, hence the lack of any arrows from the boxes on the right to the corresponding boxes in the middle.

(11.1.2)

```
3   M:    ‖'whose `turn is it‖
          {        lento        }
          (.)
4   K:    `turn is it
          { lento  }
5   M:    ‖'whose `turn is it‖
```

To produce delayed echoes, the speaker needs some capacities that are not required for immediate echoes: to be able to store a representation of a phrase in all its phonetic, including prosodic, detail, with an invariant motor program and motor plan. The speaker needs to be able to retrieve the phrase from this store and then, as with immediate echoes, have excellent motor execution. Figure 11.2 illustrates the processing of the delayed echo in line 2 of Extract (11.4.1):

(11.4.1)

```
1   S:    ‖'good ⇑^boy ‖


2   K:    ‖ thats  a naughty boy::‖
          { f           f} { ff  }
          (1.5) ((sound of turning pages))


3   K:       thats   a
          {mf        mf}
          (0.2)
4   S:    ‖ `look 'mummy‖
5   M:    ‖^yes ‖ 'done^nice[ly ‖^has]nt he‖
6   S:                  [‖s `good‖]
```

There is just one arrow from 'stored knowledge' on the right. This is at Level 4, the lexical motor program, indicating that Kevin accesses the formula "that's a naughty boy"

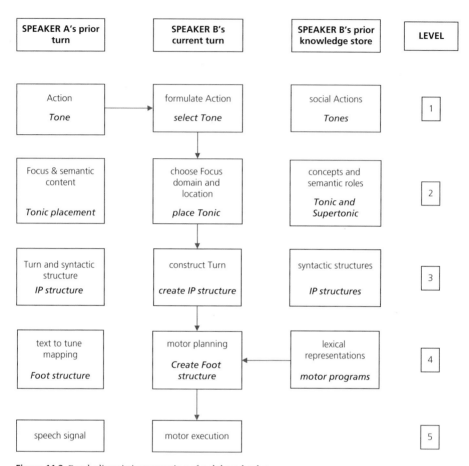

Figure 11.2 Psycholinguistic processing of a delayed echo.

as a gestalt, as if it were a single word with its associated articulatory and prosodic plan. The only arrow from his sister's first turn to Kevin's turn is at Level 1, Action formulation. This is to indicate that the action of producing a delayed echo, as a way of disengaging from the interaction, is interactionally responsive to his sister's attempt in line 1 to engage him in interaction by addressing directly to him a positive assessment of his work. At the other levels, there is no influence of his sister's turn on Kevin's turn. Although the lexical item BOY is common to both turns, it was argued earlier that this is not treated as relevant to the interaction by any of the three participants.

While the immediate echoes and delayed echoes used by Kevin are different in their processing demands, they share an important feature: neither demonstrates, in their intonation or any other level, a generative ability to build up more extended or complex prosodic structures out of simple elements. Moreover, neither immediate nor delayed echoes, as used by Kevin, demonstrate the ability to use intonation contrastively to signal different kinds of meaning, i.e. to combine the same word or string of words with different Tones, in the way that, as we saw in Chapters 6 and 7, typically developing children are able to do by the age of 2. Although he is eight years older than Kenneth (Tarplee & Barrow, 1999), judging from his echoes, Kevin too seems to be arrested at the Paradigmatic phase of intonation development (see Appendix 4). On the other hand, in Extract (11.2) Kevin produced longer, albeit unintelligible, turns when initiating a request. These are reproduced here in (11.2.1):

(11.2.1)

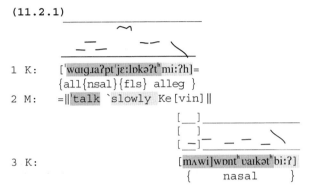

```
1 K:   ['wɑɪɡɹaʔptˈjɛːlɒkəʔtʰmiːʔh]=
       {all{nsal}{fls} alleg }
2 M:   =‖ˈtalk `slowly Ke[vin]‖
3 K:                    [mʌwi]wɒntʰʋaɪkətʰbiːʔ]
                        {    nasal    }
```

This suggests that Kevin may be beginning to move into the Syntagmatic phase, described in Chapter 7. In that respect he would be like Robin, the typically developing child aged around 19 months described in earlier chapters. Like Robin, Kevin is still unable to integrate accurate and intelligible motor programs into the longer and more complex IP structures that he is now attempting.

Our discussion of intonation in relation to echolalia has focussed mainly on Kevin, a child with severe autism. However, it is evident that children on the autism spectrum may use echolalia to a greater or lesser extent and in different ways, both interaction-ally and intonationally. It also seems to be the case that with time many children with autism grow out of echolalia– an observation which supports the value of considering the intonation of children with autism from the perspective of a developmental model. One of the ways in which the rigid intonation associated with echolalia may be miti-gated is described by Sterponi & Shankey, (2014) in a case study of echolalia produced by a 5-year-old American boy, Aaron. Like Kevin, Aaron produced delayed echoes that seem to originate in controlling or reprimanding phrases that he has heard in the past from parents and others. However, unlike Kevin, he showed the ability to vary the intonation of the echoed phrase. Moreover, he deploys them at places where they are interactionally relevant. From the perspective of the developmental phase model, this suggests that Aaron is further on in the Syntagmatic phase, than Kevin, who still has at least one foot in the Paradigmatic phase.

The following activity provides an opportunity to analyse an interaction involving a child on the autism spectrum who demonstrates a great deal more expressive language ability than Kevin or Kenneth. Interactions with this child have been analysed by Muskett & Body, (2013). Jacob (J) is an 8-year-old boy with a diagnosis of autism spectrum disorder and associated learning difficulties. Sally (S) is a 19-year-old female student. In Extract (11.8), Jacob and Sally are sitting at a table and playing with a set of *Thomas the Tank Engine* toys that both parties are removing from a bag. *Thomas the Tank Engine* is a popular series of books and TV programmes, in which the principal characters are steam locomotives that have names. Thomas, Mavis and Toad are three such characters. An audio recording of this interaction performed by actors is available.

(11.8)

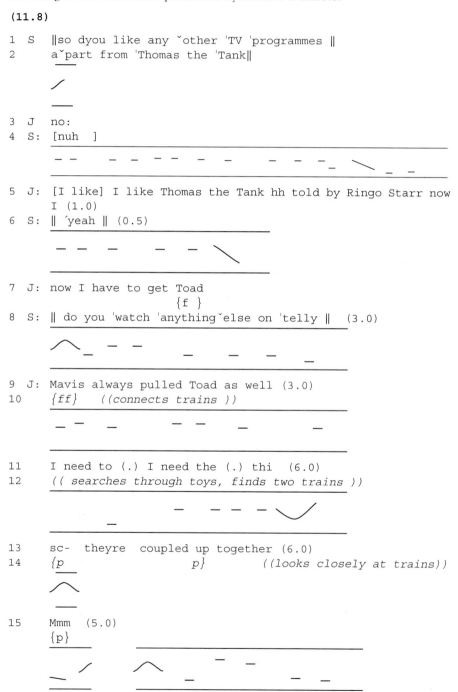

```
1   S    ‖so dyou like any ˇother 'TV 'programmes ‖
2        aˇpart from 'Thomas the 'Tank‖


3   J:   no:
4   S:   [nuh  ]


5   J:   [I like] I like Thomas the Tank hh told by Ringo Starr now
         I (1.0)
6   S:   ‖ ´yeah ‖ (0.5)


7   J:   now I have to get Toad
                        {f }
8   S:   ‖ do you 'watch 'anything ˇelse on 'telly ‖  (3.0)


9   J:   Mavis always pulled Toad as well (3.0)
10       {ff}    ((connects trains ))


11       I need to (.) I need the (.) thi  (6.0)
12       (( searches through toys, finds two trains ))


13       sc-  theyre  coupled up together (6.0)
14       {p                    p}        ((looks closely at trains))


15       Mmm  (5.0)
         {p}
```

```
16    scoruh (.)M:avis a far far (company)
17                          ((stands up and looks in bag))
```

```
18    now I'm going to be (now)   (1.0)
      {ff}
```

```
19    (in a)while I'm going to get(1.0) the twins
20 S: ‖ ˇJacob ‖ 'why dya `like 'Thomas the 'Tank ‖
21    (( J drops toys ))
```

ACTIVITY 11.1

Aim: To complete the questions on the IIP for a child with a diagnosis of moderate-severe autism.

For this activity you will need to refer to the phonological transcription of (11.8), presented as (11.8.1). You will need a blank IIP form (Appendix 3).

(11.8.1)

```
 1   S        ‖so dyou 'like any ⇑ˇother 'TV 'programmes ‖⇒
 2        H   a⇑ˇpart from 'Thomas the 'Tank ‖
 3   J    =   ‖ˊno ‖
 4   S:   Ø   [ nuh ]
 5   J:   ≠   ‖[I like]I like 'Thomas the'Tank 'told by'Ringo `Starr now I ‖
              (1.0)
 6   S:   ≠   ‖ˊyeah ‖ (0.5)
 7   J:   ≠   ‖now I have to 'get `Toad ‖ (0.5)
 8   S:   ≠   ‖do you 'watch 'anything ⇑ˇelse on 'telly ‖   (3.0)
 9   J:   ≠   ‖⇑ˊMavis always pulled Toad as well ‖(3.0)
10            ((connects trains ))
11        Ø   I need to (.) I need the (.) thi  (6.0)
12            (( searches through toys, finds two trains ))
13        ≠   ‖s c-  they   coupled up toˊgether ‖ (6.0)
14            ((looks closely at trains))
15        ≠   ‖ˊmm ‖ (5.0)
16        =   ‖ˇscoruh(.)⇑M:avis‖⇒ the far far `company ‖
17            ((stands up and looks in bag))
18        =   ‖⇑ˊnow Im going to be (next)‖   (1.0)
19        =   ‖in a 'while Im 'going to 'get(1.0) the `twins ‖
20   S:   ≠   ‖ˇJacob ‖ 'why dya `like 'Thomas the 'Tank ‖
21            (( J drops toys ))
```

Turns

1 The phonological transcription in (11.8.1), uses the traffic light notation. Referring to this, complete the 'Gaining the floor' section on the IIP. Attempt to answer each question by referring to the phonological transcript (11.8.1), also referring as necessary to the phonetic transcript (11.8)

and the recording. If your answer to a question is *Yes* or *No*, then fill in the line number(s) that provide evidence for your answer. Use the comment box for any further observations relating to the question. Check your answer with the Key to Activity 11.1 at the end of the chapter.

2 Repeat this procedure for the four questions relating to 'Holding the floor'.

3 Repeat this procedure for the four questions relating to 'Giving up the floor'.

Focus

1 In each line of the phonological transcript in (11.8.1), underline words/phrases/clauses that represent new information, i.e. topics which have not previously been mentioned.

2 Complete the 'Focus' section on the IIP. Answer each question by referring to the phonological transcript, as you did for 'Turns'.

Actions

1 For each IP the phonological transcript in Extract (11.8.1) indicates if the Tone matches (=) or does not match (≠) the Tone of the preceding IP. Complete the 'Aligning' section on the IIP. Answer each question by referring to the phonological transcript, as for 'Turns'.

2 Repeat this procedure for the four questions relating to 'Initiating'.
A Key to Activity 11.1, with a completed IIP can be found in Appendix 7.

The completed IIP captures the inconsistency with which Jacob uses the intonation systems of English. At some points he produces turns that seem to display a command of intonation for Turn-taking, Focus and Actions, yet on other occasions he produces turns that do not conform to these systems. With regard to Turn-taking, Sally comes in immediately when Jacob has produced a Tonic at the end of an IP and only then; she does this even when her own turn is not closely topically related to J's prior talk. This suggests that she is orienting to Jacob's final Tonic as a yellow traffic light. However, sometimes Jacob's turn is confusing in this respect. For instance, in line 5, he produces an IP in which the Head and Tonic contain material that addresses the question that Sally has just asked. However, he then adds a Tail consisting of two words quite unrelated to what precedes: "now I". This seems to project more talk, so Sally does not take a turn immediately; but a full second passes without further talk from Jacob. This is an example of the kind of mismatch between grammar and IP structure that children would typically have sorted out before the end of the Syntagmatic phase, i.e. in the preschool years (Chapter 7). Similarly, with regard to Focus, there are IPs in which final Tonic placement marks broad Focus appropriately; however, there are examples in line 9 (MAVIS) and line 18 (NOW) of Supertonic placement on the very first word of the IP, indicating non-final narrow Focus, but there is no strong contextual reason for Focus to be on that word. Again, sorting out appropriate placement of the Tonic in relation to Focus is a feature of the Syntagmatic phase, as we saw in Chapter 7. With regard to Tone matching for Action alignment, Jacob again seems to be inconsistent. He apparently displays his orientation to this system, e.g. at the very beginning in line 3 when he answers her question about other TV programmes. However, when he responds to Sally's second question, in lines 8–9, he prefaces his response with a long pause, then uses a non-matching Tone, while the content of his turn does not acknowledge Sally's question at all. Instead he reverts to his own prior agenda of playing with the toys on his own. The non-matching Tone underlines that his actions are not aligned with Sally at this point. In summary, these different facets of Jacob's inconsistent use of intonation conspire together to create a dysfunctional interaction in which Jacob secures the floor for extended periods and controls the agenda despite Sally's repeated efforts to get him to answer questions.

High-functioning autism

Current clinical diagnostic practice, as expressed, for instance, in DSM-V, takes the position that there is a spectrum of autism-related conditions. So far, we have considered the intonation of children diagnosed as having severe or moderate-to-severe autism. At the other end of the spectrum is the condition referred to in the literature as High Functioning Autism (HFA), although this diagnostic label is not used in a consistent way:

> The use of the term *high functioning* is generally used to refer to individuals with autism who are in the average to above average range of cognitive functioning, although some studies have used general language measures to make this distinction. As such, there is no accepted or recognized definition of "high functioning."
>
> *(Diehl & Paul, 2013: 158)*

The PEPS-C battery (Wells & Peppé, 2001), which has already been discussed in Chapter 8 and Chapter 10, has been used in its revised, computerized version (Peppé & McCann, 2003) to investigate the prosodic processing characteristics of children at the higher end of the autism spectrum, many of whom have received the diagnosis of HFA. Peppé, McCann, Gibbon, O'Hare, and Rutherford (2007) administered the PEPS-C battery to a group of 31 children with HFA, aged 6–13 years and a larger control group of typically developing children, matched on receptive vocabulary using the British Picture Vocabulary Scales (Dunn, Whetton, & Burley, 1997). The study was carried out in Scotland. It was a selection criterion for the HFA group that the child had had language delay before school entry. The children with HFA performed significantly lower than controls on seven of the 12 PEPS-C subtests: the four Form tasks (Input and Output); the two Affect (Function) tasks; and the Focus Expression task, which was formerly known as the Focus Output Function task.

On the Form Input tasks, the child hears pairs of intonation patterns derived from low-pass filtered real speech utterances, so that the words are not intelligible, as illustrated in Chapter 10. Unexpectedly, the main error among the HFA group was to interpret pairs of identical stimuli as different, rather than vice versa. This result suggests that their problem may have been less one of pitch perception and more one of making sense of the task. On the Output Form tasks the requirement is to imitate the pattern that they hear. Given the phenomenon of immediate echolalia discussed earlier in this chapter, one might expect children on the autism spectrum to find this relatively easy. Again, a possible explanation for the result is that the children with HFA had a problem with understanding what the task is about, namely that not simply the words but also the intonation pattern of the stimulus has to be imitated.

Turning to the Affect results, again, there is an indication that the children with HFA failed to understand the task requirements. On the Input task, the child has to decide whether the speaker of the stimulus likes the item of food in question. The children tended to respond according to their personal preferences about the food, rather than to respond to the emotion expressed by the voice on the computer. This could be due to the lack of theory of mind that is often attributed to people with ASD (Peppé et al., 2007: 1023).

The result that reflected prosodic disability most purely was on the Focus Expression task. The children with HFA showed an inappropriate preference for placing the Tonic in a non-final position, when the expected response was a final Tonic. The tendency to use an early (non-final) Tonic location was observed in the child with moderate-severe ASD (Jacob) who was the subject of Activity 11.1. We found that this related to his non-interactional and inflexible handling of the topic of the interaction. It may be that this tendency is one that is reflected more widely among the HFA population. Interestingly, it runs contrary to the pattern of typical development outlined in Chapters 7 and 8, where children tend to put the Tonic on the final word as a default, even when the context implies non-final narrow Focus.

Some more general findings from the study support the view that PEPS-C tasks principally tap into the child's meta-intonational awareness, as outlined in Chapter 8 and in Chapter 10. Peppé et al. (2007) found that in their control group of 72 typically developing children, aged 4–11 years, performance on PEPS-C broadly correlated with age, suggesting that in typical development children perform better on intonation tasks as their general level of understanding and experience improves with age. This is comparable to the findings of Wells et al. (2004) using an earlier version of PEPS-C, which was reported in Chapter 8. It is further underlined by the results for a group of adults that Peppé et al. (2007) tested, who scored close to ceiling on all subtests, suggesting that in the typical population the ability to do this kind of task continues to improve with age. In the HFA group, by contrast, performance did not correlate with age, even though for each subtest there were some children scoring at ceiling. This suggests that there is a good deal of non-age-related variability, pointing to substantial individual differences among children given the diagnosis of HFA.

In a subsequent study, Peppé, Cleland, Gibbon, O'Hare, and Castilla (2011) compared the HFA group just described to a group of children with Asperger's syndrome (AS) aged from 5–13 years, defined for the study as children with the same features as HFA, including normal nonverbal IQ, except that there was no evidence of preschool language delay. The study focussed on performance on the six expressive subtests of the PEPS-C, the HFA and AS groups being compared to each other and to control groups of typically developing children matched on either language level or chronological age. The HFA group performed significantly worse than the AS group on all but one of the subtests, the Chunking Output Function task. For the AS group, scores on five of the PEPS-C subtests correlated with expressive language scores, whereas for the HFA group this was found for just two of the PEPS-C subtests. As the AS group was differentiated at the outset from the HFA group by the absence of a preschool language delay, these results suggest that better language skills and better prosodic skills may go hand in hand. Although the AS group performed better than the HFA group, they still performed more poorly than age-matched controls on three of the six PEPS-C tasks: the Chunking Output Function task and the two imitation (Output Form) tasks. The relatively poorer performance on the imitation tasks rather than function tasks suggests that while children with AS are generally able to convey meaning through intonation, they may still sound unusual.

This idea has been further explored in a study of 24 American children with HFA, aged 8–16 years by Diehl and Paul (2013). Their particular interest was the children's performance on expressive (output) tasks, since they wanted to explore in depth the commonly reported view that children on the autism spectrum have unusual prosody. With this in mind, they used acoustic measures to investigate the children's responses on the PEPS-C expressive tasks, and compared these to the responses of a control group of typically developing (TD) children, as well as a rather heterogeneous group of children with learning difficulties. As in other PEPS-C studies, there was a lot of variation in the results for each group, including, on each subtest, a substantial minority who scored full marks. There was no significant difference between the ASD group and the TD group on any of the expressive subtests in terms of the ability to convey the required meaning to a listener using intonation, as measured by accuracy of responses.

On the acoustic measures, there were rather few differences between the ASD group and the TD group. On the Affect task and the 'Turn-end' task (formerly the 'Interaction Output Function' task) the children with ASD tended to produce utterances of longer duration than the TD children, while on the Focus task the group with ASD had significantly greater ranges and standard deviations for fundamental frequency (pitch). The differences were found for responses that were judged to be correct, as well as some of the incorrect responses. This indicates that the children with ASD on some occasions successfully signalled the correct meaning to the listener but did so in a way that was somewhat different from the TD children.

To summarize, the results of group studies of children with HFA offer little support for the commonly held view that problematic prosody and intonation are a pervasive characteristic of ASD. The most important finding is the amount of variability within this population. Children with HFA may demonstrate one or more of the following:

1 problems with understanding functional aspects of intonation;
2 problems signalling the correct or expected meaning for some of the functions of intonation;
3 the problem of being able to signal the correct meaning but doing so in an atypical way;
4 problems at a meta-intonational level, as demonstrated by poor performance on imitation tasks;
5 no difficulties with intonation.

From a developmental perspective, it seems that children with HFA manifesting these difficulties are still sorting out aspects of intonation that typically resolve in the Syntagmatic phase and so have not yet moved into the Meta-intonation phase that characterizes the school years (Chapter 8). Since the reports of group studies do not routinely present profiles of performance for the individual children in the group, it is not easy to ascertain how much overlap there is between the children listed in (1)–(4) above. However, for the purposes of intervention for prosodic difficulties, information at an individual level is crucial. With this in mind, some of these practical implications are now explored with reference to an interaction-based case study of a boy with HFA.

Sammy: a child with High Functioning Autism

Kelly and Beeke (2011) present the case of Sammy, aged 7;11 and from the Midlands of England, who had a diagnosis of HFA. He also had notable language impairments, scoring at the 13th percentile (age equivalent 3;11) on the receptive part of the CELF-3, and at the 19th percentile on the expressive part. Unusual prosodic features characterized his speech at this stage. These included a sing-song effect brought about by pervasive level pitch with sustained vowels; monotone; frequent pauses and extended vowels; creaky and hypernasal phonation. The analysis by Kelly and Beeke (2011) was based on a video recording of Sammy and his mother playing a board game. Their study focussed on Turn-taking, and specifically on Sammy's ability to use prosodic features to project the end of his turn.

Analysis of a range of turn exchanges from the recording led the authors to a number of observations. Sammy sometimes used typical prosodic resources, in conjunction with syntactic completion, to mark the end of his turn, and this was responded to appropriately by his mother. He sometimes successfully signalled the end of his turn, even when conventional turn-ending features such as notable pitch movement, creaky phonation and final lengthening were preceded by atypical features of creak and vowel lengthening earlier in the turn. These atypical prosodic features did not necessarily impede Sammy's ability to mark the end of his turns effectively. However, his word-finding difficulties frequently gave rise to long pauses within his turn. In the stretch of talk before the pause he did not always manage to signal that his turn was not yet finished, so the other participant might start talking before he had finished.

By contrast, on other occasions Sammy appeared to project the end of his turn and yet continued to talk. In line 1 of Extract (11.9), adapted from Extract 3 of Kelly and Beeke (2011), he produces the word "drawing" with a falling Tone to the base of his pitch range and a lengthened vowel. These are features that potentially signal the end of the turn. His mother therefore starts to talk (line 2) , but immediately breaks off having found herself in overlap, as Sammy immediately produces "again", once more with falling Tone and lengthened vowel (end of line 1). In line 3, his mother repeats his phrase from line 2, thereby displaying that she had heard what he said even though she had been talking in overlap with him.

(11.9)

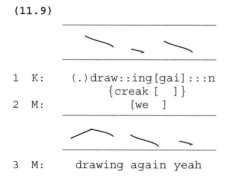

```
1  K:     (.)draw::ing[gai]:::n
                {creak [   ]}
2  M:              [we  ]
```

```
3  M:     drawing again yeah
```

This is reminiscent of an interaction involving Robin at the age of 21 months and his mother, discussed in Chapter 2. Robin produced the words SMOKE and FUNNEL in succession, each with a falling Tone. His mother started to speak after SMOKE and so found herself overlapping his FUNNEL. As with Robin, the production of two successive Tones raises the question of whether Sammy understands the dual interactional implications of producing a Tonic: while highlighting the Focus of the turn, it also projects the end of that turn.

The analysis of Turn-taking provided the basis for speech and language therapy intervention which focussed on issues to do with trouble in conversation. This involved playing extracts of the video recording to Sammy and his mother, in order to raise awareness about how Turn-taking works and how prosodic features are involved. The intervention was reported to have broad and positive effects on Sammy's communicative competence. The study thus illustrates how individualized analysis of interaction can lead to targeted intervention relating to intonation and its functions.

In this chapter we have explored the functional use of intonation by children at lower functioning and higher functioning points on the autism spectrum, in naturalistic interactional and in formal testing contexts. It has traditionally been claimed that such children have atypical intonation and that this is indexical of ASD, with an implication that this characteristic is in some sense a reflex of the underlying condition of autism. Taking a functional rather than an indexical approach to the analysis of intonation, we have seen that intonation is a resource that can be drawn on in social interaction by children with ASD, even those at the lower end of the spectrum. At the phonetic level, i.e. the level of 'form', there is evidence that some, possibly many, children with ASD present with unusual speech characteristics, including voice quality, which may be reacted to either consciously or unconsciously by the co-participants in the interaction (Bone et al., 2014). In the case of Kevin (Local & Wootton, 1995), we saw that such phonetic idiosyncrasies may be sensitive to the particular kind of action the child is performing, in his case, initiations as opposed to responses. In the PEPS-C studies of children with HFA, we saw that children with HFA, including Asperger's syndrome, performed relatively poorly on the PEPS-C Output Form tasks, yet this did not generally stop them signalling the meanings that intonation communicates. Since a good deal of variability in the ability to use intonation for the different interactional functions has been reported, the lesson we can draw from single case studies is that it is important to consider each child as an individual on his or her own terms, to try to understand intonation as part of that individual's bank of communicative resources.

In the remainder of the chapter, we turn to children with two other types of learning difficulty: Williams syndrome and Down syndrome.

Williams syndrome

Williams syndrome (WS) is a rare genetic disorder which results from a gene deletion on chromosome 7. It has attracted significant research interest because of proposals that individuals with WS present with a dissociation between relatively strong linguistic (i.e. grammatical and semantic) abilities, and low general cognitive functioning and abilities in the nonverbal domain. Subsequent research has questioned this (Stojanovik, Perkins, & Howard, 2004). Stojanovik and colleagues have extended the scope of the research to include prosody, using the PEPS-C battery.

In the first such study, Catterall, Howard, Stojanovik, Szczerbinski, and Wells (2006) presented case studies of two boys with WS, child B aged 12 and child C aged 13 and compared their performance on the original version of PEPS-C to data from typically developing children matched on chronological age and on language comprehension, taken from Wells, Peppé and Goulandris (2004). Child C presented with deficits particularly on Input Function and Output Form tasks, but was able to convey intonational meaning appropriately on the Output Function tasks. Child B, conversely, was weak across all four Output Function tasks, and also had a particular problem with all four Focus tasks. Thus, although both children had difficulties with PEPS-C tasks, the patterns of difficulty were not at all alike, suggesting that there is no simple relationship between the cognitive and linguistic deficits characteristics of WS and the difficulties they experience with intonation.

Using the computerized and revised PEPS-C, Stojanovik, Setter, and van Ewijk (2007) carried out a group study of 14 children with WS aged between 6;4 and 13;11, comparing results to a group of age-matched children as well as a group of children matched on language comprehension, who had a mean age of 5 years. As a group, the PEPS-C results of the children with WS were similar to those of the (younger) group matched for language comprehension, however, they were significantly lower than the scores of the chronological age-matched group. Overall, this indicates that the children with WS had intonation skills in line with their linguistic level, although correlational analysis showed there was not a strong relationship between language scores and PEPS-C scores. According to Stojanovik (2010), the results of the PEPS-C studies indicate that children with WS follow an atypical path in their intonation development compared to chronological age controls. Specifically, the ability to signal Focus is delayed in the onset of its development, while the other intonation skills have a slow rate of development. However, intonation development is in line with the children's mental age, leading Stojanovik to conclude that there may be a relationship between non-verbal cognitive ability and intonation ability as measured on the PEPS-C battery. From a developmental perspective, the WS children seem to have not yet entered the Meta-intonation phase, presumably due to their low cognitive level.

Down syndrome

The genetic condition of Down syndrome (DS) is one of the most common causes of learning disability, usually having a major impact on speech and language development. The understanding and use of intonation by people with Down syndrome have been little studied. In this section we present a brief overview of available research.

As part of a study of interactions involving children with severe learning difficulties, Edwards (1990) analysed the intonation of Toby, a boy with DS who was CA 4;7 at the start of the project. Edwards made video recordings of Toby separately with his mother and with his teacher, for a total of approximately eight hours. Edwards reported that Toby had poor control over the muscles of the vocal tract, noting: "The reduced muscle tone, a characteristic of DS children, reduces the child's control over fine muscular adjustments, including the vocal tract and hence phonation" (Edwards, 1990: 215).

Despite this limitation, she found that 72% of his utterances could be categorized in terms of their nuclear Tone. Of these, 50–60% were falls, the remaining Tones being distributed across other Tone types fairly evenly. However, she noted that the proportion of rises was low compared to adult English.

Although Edwards' own analysis of Toby's intonation takes a different starting point from the one used in this book, her examples suggest that Toby may be capable of using Tone both to show the end of his turn and for the purpose of interactional alignment. He does not produce many IPs of more than a single word and Edwards does not mention whether he is able to use Tonic placement for narrow Focus. In Extract (11.10), adapted from Edwards (1990: 228), Toby (T) and his teacher (A) are playing a picture matching game. In the labelling sequence, Toby's Tone in line 2 matches the Tone of his teacher in line 1.

(11.10)

```
      (Toby takes a picture card)
1  A  ‖ `oh ‖ what have you `got ‖
2  T  ‖ `dʌk ‖
3  A  ‖ whos got the `dog ‖ `I have ‖
```

This is like the labelling sequences analysed by Tarplee (1996), involving typically developing young children around the age of 2, which were considered in Chapter 7. Toby aligns with the request to label that the teacher has initiated in line 1 by matching her falling Tone. The teacher treats this as a fitted reply in line 3, moving directly to the next picture.

There is also some evidence that Toby can using a non-matching Tone to initiate a new course of action. In Extract (11.11), from (Edwards, 1990: 230), his mother asks him a closed question about what happened to his toy car. In line 2, Toby does not answer the question directly with YES or NO. Instead he points to the camera operator (Sue), using a falling pitch, which does not match the rise on his mother's final IP in line 1. This suggests that Toby may be using non-matching pitch to initiate a new direction in the talk.

(11.11)

```
      ((Toby is playing with small cars))
1  M  ‖ went under ^there ‖ ´did it ‖
2  T  ^da `nu: (points to camera operator)
1  M  ‖ Sue got it for you ‖
2  T  ‖ ´yeh ‖
3  T  ‖ wasnt that kind ‖
```

Edwards (1990: 233–237) provides a series of transcribed fragments where Toby repeatedly demonstrates a pattern of using a rising pitch on items he is enumerating, ending the sequence with a fall. This occurs in play routines where there is a series of toys in a set. An example is given in (11.12), where Toby is with his teacher:

(11.12)

```
1  A  ‖ ´how many `people are there ‖
2  T  ‖ ´wʌ ‖    ((touches own plate))
3  T  ‖ ´nə ‖    ((touches next plate))
```

According to Edwards: "The rising tones used here give the utterances the appearance of enumerating, a response which would be appropriate to the question" (1990: 233). This use of successive non-low tones in counting sequences is indeed typical, as mentioned in Chapter 7 with reference to research on classroom interaction (Arrowsmith, 2005).

In sum, Toby appears to have the ability to use intonation in conventional ways, as might be expected of a younger typically developing child, like Robin at the age of around 21 months who was described in Chapter 7. The picture of delay in mastering intonation systems, connected to the overall profile of delayed language development in Down syndrome, is also found in a small-scale group study using PEPS-C. Vesna Stojanovik (2011) tested nine children with DS, aged 8;3 to 12;5, matched to two groups of typically developing children, one on chronological age and the other on non-verbal mental age, the latter having a mean age of 5;05. The children with DS scored significantly lower than the CA matched group on all tasks; they were significantly lower than the mental age-matched group on two of the Function output tasks: Affect and Focus. Moreover, there were no results for the Chunking tasks as the majority of children with DS were unable to cope with these tasks. On the Form tasks, the scores of the children with DS were significantly lower than those of both the other groups. Stojanovik also found some evidence to support the view that with regard to intonation functions, the children with DS were slightly better at understanding than at expressing the functions measured on PEPS-C.

Although small in scale, this is a valuable study in that it opens up research into how much children with DS may be able to understand and use intonation to communicate meaning. Stojanovik and Setter (2011) compared groups of nine children, each with Williams syndrome and Down syndrome, matched for mental age. They found that the children with WS did significantly better than the children with DS on many of the PEPS-C tasks. The fact that the children with WS had slightly higher language comprehension skills, as measured on TROG, may be one reason. However, it seems likely that there are other factors leading to the poorer performance on PEPS-C tasks by children with DS, such as the incidence of hearing loss in this population as well as the physical issue of muscle tone, mentioned above in relation to Toby, which may affect the child's ability to produce more complex pitch patterns. Respiration is also commonly affected in Down syndrome. In a detailed case study of the speech output of Ken, an adult in his thirties with DS, Heselwood, Bray, and Crookston (1995) suggest that respiratory difficulties may the reason why Ken's speech is partially unintelligible in the Head of his IPs: he rushes through to the Tonic word, which is more intelligible and which typically, as one would expect, is also the Focus of his turn. Moreover the late and distinct occurrence of the Tonic is valuable interactionally in marking the end of his turn.

While children with Down syndrome, Williams syndrome or even low-functioning autism may be expected to develop language comprehension and production to a certain level, the situation is different for children with profound intellectual disabilities who have no language at all. One approach to intervention with this population, Intensive Interaction, is explicitly based on the idea that the teacher interacts with the child using behaviours found in carer–child interaction with typical preverbal infants (see Chapter 6). Important components include Turn-taking and following the child's lead with regard to topic. The teacher is also encouraged to imitate the child's behaviours, including the child's vocalizations (Firth, 2006). This vocal echoing can be described, in terms of the framework used in this book, as the teacher using Tone matching to align with the child's action in their prior turn. Although to our knowledge there are no research studies that explicitly analyse the intonation component, the reports of interventions using Intensive Interaction (Kellett, 2000) suggest that Tone matching of this kind can help promote the child's own use of contingent vocalizations, as well as having wider benefits.

Summary

The cases presented in this chapter, along with group studies that have been reviewed, highlight the following key points about intonation in children with autism spectrum disorders (ASD) and other learning difficulties:

- *Low functioning ASD.* Prevalence of delayed and immediate echoes indicates arrested development at the Paradigmatic phase of intonation development. The child is unable to mediate or combine external information from the prior speaker with internal information (stored knowledge about intonation and other linguistic systems) in real time to produce a fitting turn.
- *Moderate-severe ASD.* Children show evidence of some ability to integrate grammar and lexis with the three systems of intonation but this is inconsistent and thus leads to dysfunctional interactions, lack of interpersonal alignment, difficulty in establishing and maintaining shared topic, along with inconsistent use of and response to traffic light cues to Turn-taking. This suggests arrested intonation development in the earlier part of the Syntagmatic phase.
- *High functioning ASD.* Children's lack of meta-awareness about intonation, apparent in relatively poor performance on Form tasks in PEPS-C, may be indicative of lack of awareness that as speakers they may sound atypical. More age-appropriate performance on Function tasks suggests an understanding of the relation between intonation and interactional functions. This indicates intonation development is approaching the end of the Syntagmatic phase but has not yet progressed to the Meta-intonation phase.
- *Williams syndrome.* Children seem to have not yet entered the Meta-intonation phase, presumably due to their low cognitive level.
- *Down syndrome.* Evidence suggests that they have passed through the Paradigmatic phase, as they are able to use Tone matching for alignment. While there is some evidence of having entered the Syntagmatic phase, they do not yet integrate longer grammatical strings with Turn-taking and Focus requirements. Cognitive and physical difficulties (muscle tone, respiration, hearing) impact on comprehension and production of intonation systems.

CHAPTER 12

Hearing impairment and cochlear implants

The extremely poor speech discrimination that results from a profound congenital or early acquired hearing loss gives rise to well-documented challenges for speech and language development (Marschark, Rhoten, & Fabich, 2007; Sarant, Holt, Dowell, Rickards, & Blamey, 2009). Management for the hearing loss may be through digital hearing aids or through cochlear implantation, both of which usually mitigate the speech perception problems, albeit in different ways. Nevertheless, children with hearing loss are more likely to experience difficulties in social communication than their typically developing peers and generally may not achieve as well academically (Stacey, Fortnum, Barton, & Summerfield, 2006). Moreover, the hearing loss may co-exist with other speech and language difficulties, compounding the challenges faced by the child, the family and the professionals involved with care in establishing effective modes of communication within the family and in the school setting.

Given the varying individual profiles of hearing, speech and language difficulties that children with profound or severe hearing impairments (HI) may thus display, it is important to adopt an approach to the assessment of the child's speech, language and communication needs that can take account of individual differences between children with HI in their profile of strengths and weaknesses. The importance of an individualized approach is illustrated in a case study (Ebbels, 2000) of TG, a 10-year-old girl with a bilateral sensori-neural hearing loss, for which she had used bilateral hearing aids since early childhood; and in a similar study (Pascoe, Randall-Pieterse, & Geiger, 2013) of NG, a 6-year-old girl with a severe/profound bilateral hearing loss who had received a cochlear implant at the age of 3. Using the psycholinguistic framework of Stackhouse and Wells (1997) to investigate input and output processing of single words, the authors of both studies were able to pinpoint the difficulties that each child had with specific levels of speech processing, with sound contrasts and with particular kinds of words (in both cases, mainly multisyllabic words). Although some of these difficulties could be predicted from the hearing loss, this was by no means always the case.

Studies of speech processing and discrimination abilities in English-speaking children with hearing impairments, like the two just mentioned, have almost always been confined to the level of the word and of segmental speech perception, i.e. discrimination of consonants, vowels and sometimes lexical stress. However, as we have seen in earlier chapters, the aspects of the speech signal that convey meaning above the level of the word, notably the features of pitch, loudness and duration that are implicated in

---

Children's Intonation: A Framework for Practice and Research, First Edition. Bill Wells and Joy Stackhouse.
© 2016 John Wiley & Sons, Ltd. Published 2016 by John Wiley & Sons, Ltd.
Companion website: www.wiley.com/go/childintonation

ACTIVITY 12.1

Aim: To investigate what aspects of intonation are available to the child with a severe or profound hearing impairment.

Materials: Simulations of speech as perceived by a child with hearing impairment using conventional hearing aids, e.g.in a classroom setting: http://www.ndcs.org.uk/family_support/audiology/hearing_loss_simulation/two_minute_walk.html. Listen to the simulations of hearing with a high frequency loss using conventional hearing aids. The speaker is a female teacher in a classroom. You will find that the words of the speaker are mainly unintelligible to you.

1 Decide if you can identify changes in terms of:
  a pitch;
  b loudness;
  c timing and duration.
2 Consider what intonational information the listener might be able to access that is relevant to
  a Turns;
  b Focus;
  c Actions.
3 Refer to the questions on the IIP (Appendix 3) as required.
Compare your answers to the Key to Activity 12.1 at the end of this chapter.

intonation systems, are also centrally important to communication. Consequently, the presence of a hearing impairment provides an opportunity to look at the effects of input processing limitations on children's intonation. In this chapter we explore the role of intonation in the communication of children with HI, with reference to Turn-taking, Focus and Actions. On this basis, it may be possible to suggest ways in which speech and language therapists, teachers and other professionals can integrate work on intonation to promote the development of mutual understanding between the child with HI and others in talk-in-interaction.

If changes in pitch and loudness are involved in managing Turn exchange, Focus and the alignment of social Actions, then it suggests that children who have difficulties in processing these phonetic parameters may have difficulty in recognizing and pro-jecting a turn-ending. Input difficulties such as those found in congenitally profoundly deaf children mean that there will be problems with the perception and the signalling of communicatively important phonetic features, including pitch and loudness (Parker, 1999). It has been reported that such children often fail to perceive and produce the meaning differences conveyed through the subtle pitch and volume changes involved in intonation and stress (Northern & Downs, 2002), giving rise to difficulty with social interaction. However, as will be shown in the remainder of this chapter, we need to be wary of jumping to over-simplistic conclusions about the impact of a hearing impair-ment on intonation systems.

Intonation in interactions with deaf children

In the body of research that has investigated spoken interactions involving deaf chil-dren, both in the home setting and in the school, intonation rarely gets a mention. One exception is a study of conversations with young deaf children in families where Sylheti (the language of the Bangladeshi community in East London) is the first language and English is an additional language (Mahon, 2003). It has been reported that in 2013, 12% of deaf children in UK education had English as an additional language (Consortium for Research into Deaf Education, 2014). The issue of how to advise families on language and communication issues is an important one for professionals working in this field.

Mahon (2003) presents the case of Khalid, CA 6;10, who has a pre-lingual moderate-severe bilateral hearing loss. At home, his father speaks to him in English, whereas his mother, who does not know English, uses Sylheti. Extract (12.1), adapted from Mahon's transcription, shows that Khalid and his father use Tone matching to establish that they have a shared agenda and shared understanding of the conversation. They are in the living room at home, looking at pictures together.

(12.1)
```
1   F          what else there (1.0) what this
2   Kh         this
3   F     L    ‖ `mm ‖ (.)
4   Kh:        ‖ `flowers ‖
5   F:         ‖ `flower ‖ (.)
6   F:         what colour is (.) look
7   Kh:        ‖ 'red `green ‖ (1.3)
8   F:         ‖ 're:d and `gree:n ‖
```

In lines 1–5 and in lines 6–8 there are two short sequences of the kind described by Tarplee (1993; 1996) that we considered in Chapter 7. Each begins with a question from the father. Following the first question, Khalid responds with a clarification request in line 2. In line 3, his father produces a confirmation with a falling Tone. As Mahon (2003: 45) explains, Khalid's answer in line 4 is evidence that the clarification sequence has been successful. In line 5, his father then acknowledges Khalid's answer. The use of the matched falling Tone in lines 3, 4 and 5 reinforces the interactional alignment between Khalid and his father. The same Tone matching can be observed in lines 7 and 8. Both participants are on the same topic and each demonstrates that he understands the other's contribution.

This contrasts with Extract (12.2), from an interaction between Khalid and his mother, who speaks to him in Sylheti (translated and transcribed in italics in line 1) while he responds in English (Mahon, 2003: 46).

(12.2)
```
1   M          Say what the man is doing
               ((both Kh and M look down at Kh's school reading book))
2   Kh:        ‖ oh playing with the `boxing ‖
                                       ⎯

               ⎯⎯⎯

3   M:         ‖ mm ‖
4   Kh:        ‖ `boxing ‖ (2.9)
```

Having initiated a sequence in line 1, which is responded to by Khalid in line 2, his mother takes a further turn in line 3, the third turn of the sequence. By using "mm" rather than a word that has more semantic content, she fails to make it clear whether or not she has understood Khalid's turn in line 2. Moreover, her level pitch does not match his fall on "boxing" in line 2. This potentially signals disalignment, further suggesting that she is not taking on board the content of Khalid's turn. In line 4, Khalid treats his mother's potentially disaligning turn in line 3 as request for further clarification: he repeats "boxing", matching his own falling Tone from line 2. This is followed by a long silence, implying that there is still no shared understanding.

The breakdown in communication in (12.2) is attributable to the lack of a shared language. Nevertheless, in the course of it, Khalid displays orientation to the system of Tone non-matching to signal disalignment, just as in (12.1) he displayed Tone matching to signal alignment. It appears that, despite his hearing loss, Khalid has managed to attain competence in this interactionally important aspect of intonation. In addition, he seems to have some awareness of and control over the use of the Tonic to mark the end of a speaking turn. For instance, in line 2 of (12.2), he produces a noticeable fall in pitch to the base of his range on "boxing", the final word of his turn, though such pitch movement is absent on earlier words.

The ability to use intonation to construct turns of varying length is evident in the children studied by Mahon, including children growing up in monolingual English-speaking families (Mahon, 1997). The following extracts are taken from a recording of a 7-year-old boy, W, and his father, who are from London. W has a severe-profound hearing loss which had been diagnosed at 11 months following meningitis. He uses conventional hearing aids. In lines 1 and 2 of Extract (12.3), W's father asks him how they travelled to Austria for their holiday.

(12.3)

```
1   F:    ‖ how did we `get there ‖ (.)
2         ‖ did we `fly ‖ in an ˇaeroplane ‖
3   W:    ‖ ´no ‖ we 'went in the ˇcar ‖
4         ‖ and 'then n the 'boat and 'then in the `car ‖
5   F:    ‖ 'in the car (.) to the ˇboat ‖ (.)
6         ‖ then in the 'boat (.) thats ˆright ‖ we `did ‖ (1.0)
```

W provides an extended answer in a single turn (lines 3 and 4). This can be segmented into three IPs, each of which ends with a notable pitch movement: rise, fall-rise and fall respectively. His first IP, "no", directly answers his father's second question: " Did we fly in an aeroplane?". W's second and third IPs provide a response to his father's first question from line 1. W lists the three stages of the journey. The IP ‖ we 'went in theˇcar ‖, which describes the first stage, ends with a fall-rise Tone, which projects that his turn is not yet completed, as is evident both by father not coming in at this point and by W himself continuing to talk. W's account of the second stage in the journey, "and 'then n the 'boat" is incorporated into the Head of the final IP. He does this by avoiding putting a Tonic on "boat". Thus, W uses the two main ways of securing an extended turn through intonation, described earlier in Chapter 2 and Chapter 7.

In Extract (12.4), W shows that he is able to use the system of Tonic placement to convey Focus. It occurs while W and his father are ˆlooking at photos from the family holiday in Austria. His father wants W to talk about what is in the holiday photos, invoking the pretext that he (the father) cannot remember what they did on holiday. In line 6, W queries his father's claim, pointing out that seeing the photo should enable his father to remember what they did. His father concedes this in line 7.

(12.4)
```
1  F:  L  ||  'Daddy 'just wants you for a `minute ||
2  F:  =  ||  cos I 'want you to 'tell me about `this || in `Austria ||
3  F:  =  ||  'cos its im`portant ||
4  F:  =  ||  cos 'I cant re`member || (.)
5  F:  =  ||  'I cant re`mem[ber ||
6  W:  =               ||  [you can ⇑`see and remember ||
7  F:  =  ||  I `know but ||
```

In line 6, W uses a Supertonic on the word "see": there is a big step-up in pitch from "you can", to a point high in his pitch range, then a wide falling pitch that starts on "see" and continues through the Tail ,"and remember", to the base of his range. The word "see" is also by far the loudest syllable in the turn. In this way W highlights the word "see" as the key new information, to point out that seeing the photo will enable his father to remember what they did on holiday.

W's accomplished use of the Tonic placement system for Focus is in striking contrast to his segmental production of this turn: [jukan⇑`θianɹɪmːɛmɑ]. Aspects of W's consonantal and vocalic production that potentially reduce the intelligibility of this turn include the dental articulation of the fricative at the onset of the word "see"; the lengthening of the onset of the second syllable of "remember"; the absence of a voiced bilabial plosive at the onset of the last syllable of "remember"; and the vocalic nucleus of that final syllable, which is not the expected schwa but a more open back unrounded vowel. In addition, there is no perceptible prominence on the second syllable of "remember", which normally would carry lexical stress and thus start a new Foot (cf. Chapter 1). As a result, W's turn is potentially hard for a listener to decode and therefore to interpret. The fact that his father apparently has no difficulty in making sense of it may be attributable not simply to his familiarity with W's segmental speech patterns but also to W's ability to highlight the key word "see" with a Supertonic and background the words that follow. Because backgrounded words are often ones that have just been used by a prior speaker (cf. Chapter 3), the listener is able to make the inference that the last three syllables of W's turn represent the word "remember", re-used from lines 4 and 5 of his father's turn.

In summary, both W and Khalid demonstrate the ability to use interactionally important intonation systems of English in the course of conversation with family members. This contributes to the maintenance of shared understanding and the progression of their conversation. Moreover, it may compensate in some ways for the potential loss of intelligibility that results from the impact of the hearing loss on consonant and vowel systems.

Phonological analysis of intonation in deaf children's speech

The effects of deafness on a child's development of contrastive phonological systems, including intonation systems, have been described by Parker & Rose (1992). They point out that in addition to analysing a spontaneous conversational interaction, it is often important to elicit intonation patterns in a more structured way, since opportunities such as led to W's turn in line 6 of the above extract may not arise. An elicitation procedure is presented as part of the PETAL assessment (Parker, 1999), using short dialogues in which the Focus required of the response is manipulated by altering the context sentence. This type of elicitation has been exemplified in Chapter 3 (Activity 3.1) and in the PEPS-C Focus-Output Function task that was described in Chapter 8. Parker and Rose (1992) illustrate the variety of patterns that may be produced by different deaf children with reference to this system of Tonic placement to mark narrow Focus. We have reproduced some of these in Extracts (12.5) to (12.8), retaining the identifying letters for the children that were used by Parker and Rose (1992).

In Extract (12.5), Child A demonstrates a typical realization of Tonic for Focus through pitch obtrusion and movement, as well as loudness. We saw that W was able to do this when talking with his father in Extract (12.4).

(12.5)
```
T:  ‖ is it a `blue car ‖
```

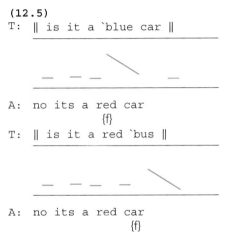

```
A:  no its a red car
                {f}
T:  ‖ is it a red `bus ‖
```

```
A:  no its a red car
                {f}
```

In Extract (12.6), Child D uses length contrasts with high pitch and increased loudness to mark narrow focus. This is similar to the pattern we observed in Jonathan in Chapter 10, a child with language difficulties but no known hearing problems.

(12.6)
```
T:  ‖ is it a `blue car ‖
```

```
D:  No::its a re::d car
    {ff}           {ff}
T:  ‖ is it a red `bus ‖
```

```
D:  No::its a red car::
    {ff}              {ff}
```

Child C in Extract (12.7) uses falling pitch on the final word, irrespective of Focus considerations. This pattern of invariant final placement of the main pitch movement, signalling the end of the turn, is one we observed in young typically developing children in Chapter 7 and in David in Chapter 5, though David used a rise rather than a fall.

(12.7)

T: ‖ is it a `blue car ‖

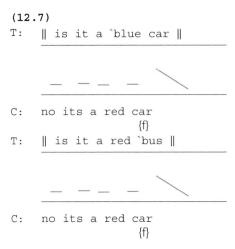

C: no its a red car
                {f}
T: ‖ is it a red `bus ‖

C: no its a red car
                {f}

Child E, whose responses are shown in Extract (12.8), was described as follows: "Severe system reduction and high variability. Much phonetic variation of pitch which is not related to linguistic context. Higher pitch used for certain vowels, which confuses the picture further" (Parker & Rose, 1992: 103).

(12.8)

T: ‖ is it a `blue car ‖

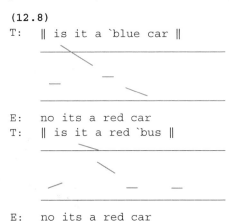

E: no its a red car
T: ‖ is it a red `bus ‖

E: no its a red car

While we noted that the patterns described for Child D and Child C have counterparts in the speech of some children who do not have a hearing impairment, Child E is different: the amount of apparently unconstrained pitch variability and the use of high pitch as an exponent of particular vowels are features that seem to be specific to some deaf children. It is likely that the wide use of early cochlear implantation will reduce the number of children with such extremely unusual intonation patterns, since the implanted children will have better access to the patterns produced by typical speakers. This issue is followed up in the next section.

To summarize, some deaf children can use the Tonic placement system to communicate Focus, either accurately (Child A) or with unconventional phonetic realizations (Child D). Still other children may present a mixed picture, like another child (Child F) described by Parker and Rose (1992: 102) who is able to mark non-final narrow Focus but in the same turn also uses pitch movement on the final word to mark the ending. Other children, like Child C and Child E, are apparently not able to use the system of Tonic placement to mark narrow Focus at all. It seems likely the variability across children reported by Parker and Rose (1992) and illustrated here bears some relation to the nature and severity of the child's hearing impairment, in which case, one would anticipate a relationship between a child's performance on this kind of output task and on a matching input task, such as the PEPS-C Focus Input Function task. This issue is taken up in the following section.

Cochlear implantation

Conventional digital hearing aids, such as those used by Khalid and W, aim to fully exploit the child's residual hearing by amplifying the speech signal. Cochlear implantation (CI), which is now a frequently adopted treatment for profound deafness, takes a different approach. By copying the function of an unimpaired cochlea, it makes a link between external sounds and the CI user's auditory nerve fibres. In a surgical operation, an electrode array is inserted into the cochlea. The user wears a removable headset comprising a speech processor and microphone. The microphone picks up sounds and inputs them to the speech processor, where various computational algorithms, referred to as a speech processing strategy, translate the sound signal into a series of frequency bands. These are then transmitted as electrical impulses via the electrode array in the ear, to the auditory nerve fibres (Barry et al., 2002). Now complete Activity 12.2.

In this section we explore the potential impact of cochlear implantation for the child's understanding and use of intonation.

ACTIVITY 12.2

Aim: To investigate what aspects of intonation are available to children using a cochlear implant

Materials: Simulations of speech as perceived by a child with hearing impairment using a cochlear implant: http://www.ndcs.org.uk/family_support/audiology/hearing_loss_simulation/cochlear_implant.html. Listen to the simulations of hearing using a cochlear implant. The speaker is a female teacher in a classroom.
1 Decide if you can identify changes in terms of:
  a pitch;
  b loudness;
  c timing and duration.
2 Consider what intonational information the listener might be able to access that is relevant to
  a Turns;
  b Focus;
  c Actions.
3 Refer to the questions on the IIP (Appendix 3) as required.
Compare your answers to the Key to Activity 12.2 at the end of this chapter.

Hearing via a cochlear implant differs from normal hearing in a number of important ways, one of which is particularly relevant to intonation: representation of fundamental frequency (F0) is poor. As we saw in Chapter 1, F0 is the main acoustic correlate of perceived pitch for unimpaired listeners. However, most CI listeners report changes in F0 as timbre, rather than pitch per se. Most and Peled (2007), in a study of Hebrew-speaking children, found that a cochlear implant did not improve the child's ability to perceive prosodic features such as pitch to the same extent as for segmental features. In their study, children with a CI were significantly less able than children with conventional hearing aids to recognize intonation and stress differences.

Thus, even after cochlear implantation, it seems that listeners will have considerable difficulty with the perception of intonation. This is most likely due to the emphasis in CI design on signal processing strategies that help with the identification of spectral (consonant and vowel) features, which has led to the relative neglect of the prosodic features involved in stress, intonation and in many languages, lexical or grammatical Tone (Barry et al., 2002). This may be compounded by the finding that child-directed speech to children with a CI does not differ, in terms of its pitch, from child-directed speech to normal-hearing children with the same amount of hearing experience (Bergeson, Miller, & McCune, 2006), suggesting that the child with CI may not be getting any extra help from the environment in identifying intonation features.

For children growing up as CI users, this may result in delay and difficulty with understanding and producing the tone and/or intonation systems of the language being acquired. This is likely to be an obstacle to active participation in conversations, where, as we have seen, the management of turn-taking, topic and social actions requires the production and comprehension of systematically used prosodic and temporal features. One behavioural consequence can be that the CI user withdraws from conversation, particularly where multiple speakers are participating and overlap is prevalent. There may be other consequences too. Thus, Tye-Murray and Witt (1996) reported that in dialogues between adult CI users and unfamiliar hearing conversational partners, the CI users made significantly more interruptions than their partners. Furthermore, some of the CI users were seen to dominate their conversation with the hearing partner because they used a lot of overlapping talk.

The above account presents a rather discouraging picture for the child with a CI wanting to engage in social interaction. However, recent research suggests a more complex situation and perhaps a more encouraging outlook. It appears that over time the pitch contours produced by children with a CI progressively approximate more closely to those of the ambient speech community, at least in terms of their range, i.e. the span of the falling or rising intonation contour that the child produces. This was found in an analysis of recordings collected at 6, 9 and 12 months post-implantation, from 18 American children from English-speaking families who were aged between 8 and 35 months at the time of implantation. It also appears that the implanted children generally followed the same developmental path as normal-hearing children in acquiring adult-like pitch range (Snow & Ertmer, 2009; 2012). However, these researchers do not report on whether the children use the intonation patterns functionally in the same way as young typically hearing children.

In addition to pitch, cues of amplitude (perceived as relative loudness) and duration are important for the perception of functional intonation contrasts in English, and these may be more easily accessible to implanted children. This possibility was investigated by O'Halpin (2010), who conducted three experiments with 17 English-speaking children with CIs, aged 5;7 to 16;11, in Ireland. In the first experiment, the children listened to a disyllabic nonsense word BABA in a range of different patterns of F0 (pitch), duration and amplitude across the two syllables. To detect a pitch change in a 'male' voice (i.e. low in the pitch range), all but one of the children needed a pitch change of at least half an octave, and for half of the group a change of over 0.8 of an octave was needed. With a 'female' voice, higher in the pitch range, some of the children fared better, eight children being able to detect differences of less than half an octave. Most of the CI children were better at detecting differences in duration and amplitude than differences in pitch.

In the second experiment, the children with CI and a matched group of hearing controls listened to natural speech stimuli, using a minimal pair paradigm. There were three subtests. The Phrase test targeted the contrast between compound nouns and adjective-noun phrases, as Atkinson-King (1973) had done with typically developing children (cf. Chapter 8). The two-element Focus test and the three-element Focus test use stimuli similar to the task described by Parker (1999) in the PETAL assessment. Examples of the stimuli are given in Table 12.1.

In the Phrase test pairs of corresponding pictures (e.g. BLUEBELL and BLUE BELL) appeared for each spoken stimulus and the child was required to click on the appropriate picture. In the Focus 2-element test two pictures (e.g. BLUE and BOOK) appeared for each stimulus, and in the focus 3-element test three pictures (e.g. BOY, PAINTING, BOAT) appeared with each stimulus. Children were asked to decide which word in the stimulus sounded the most important and then click on the appropriate picture. The two-element Focus task is similar to the Focus Input Function task from the PEPS-C battery described in Chapter 8, while the Phrase task, using compound nouns, resembles the PEPS-C Chunking Input Function task.

In both the CI group and the matched hearing control group, older children tended to do better than younger children on these tasks. Although on all three subtests, the children with CI performed worse as a group than the normal-hearing group, some nevertheless performed above chance level: 6/16 on the Phrase task and on the Focus 2-element task; 12/16 on the Focus 3-element task. For most of the children with CI, performance on the Focus subtests correlated with their F0 discrimination performance on Experiment 1, as might be expected since pitch is such an important cue to the Tonic. However, some children who had very poor F0 perception on Experiment 1 nevertheless managed to perform above chance on Focus tasks, presumably by

Table 12.1 Examples of experimental stimuli used by O'Halpin (adapted from O'Halpin, 2010, Table 3.1).

PHRASE TEST: Compound noun vs. Adjective + Noun		
give me the bluebell give me the blackboard	give me the blue bell give me the black board	
FOCUS TEST: two elements		
it's a BLUE book it's a GREEN door	it's a blue BOOK it's a green DOOR	
FOCUS TEST: three elements		
the BOY is painting a boat the GIRL is baking a cake	the boy is PAINTING a boat the girl is BAKING a cake	the boy is painting a BOAT the girl is baking a CAKE

drawing on other cues such as duration and loudness. In fact, it was duration perception performance in Experiment 1, rather than pitch perception, that correlated most consistently with the CI children's performance on the Focus 2-element task. With regard to perception of amplitude (loudness), the results suggested that this too may be used by a few of the CI users to help identify the Focus element.

To summarize the results of these perception experiments, a range of acoustic cues are available to CI listeners to identify the Tonic, and therefore the item that is in Focus. Although CI users may vary in their ability to respond to the different cues of pitch, loudness and duration, they may be able to exploit their individual strengths when responding to actual language examples, for instance, by focussing on duration if their pitch perception is poor, or vice versa.

In a third experiment, O'Halpin investigated the spoken production of the children with CI. This was tested under different Focus conditions, using one of the three-element Focus stimuli used in the perception experiment just described: THE BOY IS PAINTING THE BOAT. The child has to produce this sentence having heard a prior turn spoken which is identical apart from one element. The task thus resembles other tasks already mentioned in this book, including the one in Activity 3.1 of Chapter 3; the Focus-Output Function task from the PEPS-C battery (Chapter 8) and the elicitation procedure used in PETAL (Parker, 1999). The dialogues are presented in (12.9), where T represents the tester and C the child being tested:

(12.9)
Focus position 1:
T: Is the GIRL painting the boat?
C: No, the BOY is painting the boat.

Focus position 2:
T: Is the boy WASHing the boat?
C: No, the boy is PAINTing the boat

Focus position 3:
T: Is the boy painting the CAR?
C: No, the boy is painting the BOAT

Each condition was elicited five times. O'Halpin judged whether the speaker conveyed Focus appropriately, and also carried out acoustic measurements of F0, duration and amplitude for each word under each Focus condition. She reported that 4/16 of her CI users were consistently able to communicate Focus to the listener. One speaker achieved this by a combination of F0 and amplitude, the other three by a combination of duration and amplitude. A further six CI users conveyed Focus most of the time, i.e. on at least 11/15 occasions. While three of these used all three features (F0, duration, amplitude), the remaining three did not use F0 at all. These results suggest that it is not essential for a CI user to produce an appropriate pitch pattern in order to mark Focus appropriately: duration and amplitude can be sufficient. This exploitation of duration and loudness is similar to what Parker and Rose (1992) described for child D, illustrated in Extract (12.6).

Finally, O'Halpin explored the possibility of a relationship, at an individual level, between ability to perceive these features, as tested in Experiments 1 and 2, and the ability to produce them, as in Experiment 3. Only two of the four children with CI who consistently signalled Focus in their own speech had shown good F0 perception in Experiment 1. Furthermore, six CI users who had demonstrated good F0 perception did not use pitch in their own speech to mark Focus. O'Halpin concluded that for CI users there is not a straightforward link between production and perception. CI users may make use of a set of cues in the perception of Focus that are different from the features they use to convey the Tonic, and therefore Focus, in their own speech. This led O'Halpin to the following broad conclusion:

> The results support the view that F_0 is not a necessary cue to focus ... and indicate that CI children should be able to acquire abstract phonological representations of prosodic contrasts such as Tonicity and focus using whatever acoustic cues are available to them through the implant.
>
> *(O'Halpin, 2010: 289)*

Thus, the three-part study by O'Halpin, like much of the research reported in this and earlier chapters, emphasizes that the task for the child is to gain access to the phonological systems of intonation that are used and shared by other speakers of English. The child can then interpret the meaning of other speakers and use these systems as a basis for communicating meaning in their own speech. Different children may gain access to these systems in different ways depending on the child's individual profile of speech processing strengths and difficulties.

Auditory neuropathy/dys-synchrony spectrum disorder

In the second part of this chapter we present a case study of Ricky, a boy who was fitted with a cochlear implant following a diagnosis of auditory neuropathy. He also has specific speech and language learning difficulties, despite normal non-verbal IQ (Anstey & Wells, 2013). Our main aim here is to investigate the positive role that intonation may play in the interactions of a child with a very complex set of difficulties, including hearing impairment, which have resulted in extremely limited verbal resources.

The condition known as auditory neuropathy (AN) or auditory dys-synchrony, first described in the mid-1990s, is estimated to include approximately 8% of newly diagnosed cases of hearing loss in children each year (Roush, Frymark, Venediktov, & Wang, 2011).

> One main characteristic of AN is the disrupted auditory nerve activity with concurrently normal or nearly normal cochlear amplification function ... The other main characteristic of AN is a significantly impaired capacity for temporal processing and difficulty in speech understanding, particularly in noise, that is disproportionate to the degree of hearing loss measured by pure-Tone thresholds.
>
> *(Zeng & Liu, 2006: 367)*

According to Roush et al. (2011), the characteristics of this condition include difficulties with speech perception that exceed what would be expected from the child's hearing threshold, as well as difficulty with hearing in noise. The hearing loss can range from normal to profound. Opinions are divided as to whether cochlear implants are to be preferred to conventional hearing aids as treatment for AN. As mentioned earlier, for individuals with profound sensori-neural hearing loss, implantation generally improves access to (segmental) speech-relevant auditory information, thus enhancing access to spoken language and facilitating accelerated language development (Most & Peled, 2007). However, these advantages are less evident for individuals with auditory neuropathy. Zeng and Liu (2006) showed that under experimental conditions, implanted individuals with auditory neuropathy had greater difficulty in understanding spoken sentences, not only compared to normally hearing controls but also compared to implanted individuals without AN. The difficulties of the individuals with AN were exacerbated by the presence of noise and also when the speech stimuli were presented in 'conversational' style rather than in 'clear' style, the latter being slower and with more amplitude modulation. Low frequency perception is thought to be particularly affected for people with AN (Zeng & Liu, 2006). This implies that implanted children with AN will be unable to fully perceive the relevant pitch contrasts when learning the ambient language, whether it is a language that uses pitch for intonation only, like English, or a Tone language like Thai or Cantonese. As a result, children with AN are unlikely to make optimal use of these features in their own speech. An idea of how speech may sound to an individual with AN can be gained by listening to computer simulations such as the ones at: http://hesp.ent.uci.edu/drupal/simulations

Case study: Ricky

Ricky was aged 9 years 11 months at the time of this study. He has an older brother who has similar, albeit milder, difficulties with hearing and language development. Ricky initially attended a school using British Sign Language as the mode of communication but did not progress beyond using some largely inaccurate two-sign combinations. This may be in part attributable to an apraxia that gives rise to motor planning problems in signing as well as in speech. Ricky and his brother now attend a non-maintained school for the deaf using oral communication, in the north of England. Ricky has a younger sister whose development in all areas has been age-appropriate. Ricky's parents are university-educated with high socio-economic status, speaking with a South Eastern British English accent.

At the age of 9 months, Ricky was diagnosed with auditory neuropathy (AN). He received a cochlear implant at the age of 2, which he uses consistently. The present account of Ricky's speech, language and communication skills is based on standardized and non-standardized assessments, informal tasks and class-based observation carried out around the time that the video recordings referred to in this chapter were made. Details of test results are presented in Anstey and Wells (2013).

Ricky follows simple context-based instructions in class, e.g. 'Get your maths book!' He can respond to speech without looking at the speaker. He uses gesture that is sometimes recognizable. It is thought that he can read up to three-word sentences if he is familiar with the words. In conversation, he uses mostly single words though in an assessment situation he is able to produce three-word sentence structures. His expressive phonology, grammar and vocabulary correspond approximately to those of a typically developing 2-year-old, his comprehension to that of a 4-year-old. It has been proposed that he has oral and possibly verbal dyspraxia.

He has used a Dynavox voca communication aid with a touch screen, though only in teaching sessions. Using it, he could create a sentence up to his level (i.e. three words). In terms of pragmatics, while able to name and respond, he rarely makes requests or initiates talk. He has some repetitive routines and does not like change of routine. His use of eye contact is inconsistent and he is generally unresponsive.

In summary, despite a supportive family, normal physical development, good health, age-appropriate nonverbal intelligence, access to sound through cochlear implantation and prolonged, intensive intervention, Ricky has very limited speech and language skills.

Inevitably there are severe constraints on Ricky's ability to engage in social interaction. It is reported that in school, he only interacts with familiar people and where there is a shared context, e.g. he plays the same game with the same person. He is reported to be predominantly passive, although cooperative and pleasant, not displaying the level of frustration that might be expected from a child with such severe communication difficulties. However, at home, Ricky's interactions with his mother provide evidence of shared attention and joint action, routinely giving rise to the achievement of mutual understanding.

Our aim here is to identify some of the intonation resources that are deployed by Ricky and his conversation partner, in this case, his mother, and to demonstrate how they promote mutual understanding, thereby sustaining the progression of their talk, despite Ricky's very limited linguistic abilities. The analysis is based on video data of interactions that occur between Ricky and his mother. An episode of shared reading of *Eugene the Plane Spotter* (Lodge, 2001) was recorded, lasting almost 8 minutes. Like the use of shared pictures, when working with an unintelligible child, shared book reading brings the advantage of focussing on a limited set of possible referents. For Ricky's family, it appears to be one of the richest linguistic contexts available, given his profound communication difficulties.

Even though the book was already very familiar to Ricky and his mother, Ricky himself did not attempt to read aloud from it, unless prompted. In the course of the activity, either Ricky or his mother would turn the page, then at some stage, his mother would read the text aloud. Ricky or his mother would point to features of the pictures on the page, this often being accompanied by spontaneous talk. An extended transcription from the recording is presented as Extract (12.10) in Appendix 8. During this extract Ricky produces 24 spoken turns. The limitations of his expressive speech and language are evident in the extract, which include some of the linguistically most complex turns for which we have evidence. Glosses are derived principally from his mother's real-time interpretation of Ricky's turn in the interaction. A phonological transcription of the same extract, using the traffic light notation, is presented in Appendix 8, as Extract (12.10.1). This has been used as the basis for the completed IIP for this extract, also included in Appendix 8. Appendix 8 thus provides a worked IIP analysis for readers who may be interested in carrying out a full intonation analysis of a child using this approach.

Carrying out an IIP analysis of Extract (12.10) presents a number of challenges. To a large extent this is because of Ricky's unintelligible speech and the paucity of standard features of English intonation evident in his turns. In the final part of this chapter, we consider the role of intonation in the interaction in some depth, by focussing on three portions of the recording and transcript. In this way, we aim to show how, despite his limitations, there are ways in which Ricky and his mother are able to use intonation as an important resource for establishing a shared understanding of what is going on. They accomplish this not just by the choice of Tone and placement of the Tonic, but also by precisely timing where they start to talk in relation to the other speaker's ongoing turn.

The first portion to be analysed is presented in phonological transcription as (12.10.2):

```
(12.10.2)
1   M:   L      ‖he 'looked out of the ˋwindow‖ (.)
2   M:   ∅      ‖'everything seemed 'so:‖
3   R:   =      ‖'mo:[ jɛ ]‖
4   M:   ≠           ‖'[whats] that ˇword‖
5   R:   ≠      ‖ˋmo:‖
6   M:   =      ‖ˋsma:ll ‖thats ˋright‖(.)
7              ‖'after the 'plane had ˇlanded‖(.)
               ‖the 'first thing 'Eugene ˇspotted‖(.)
```

In line 2, his mother produces mid-pitch and prolongation of "so": she thereby constructs the Head of an IP but does not produce the Tonic that would complete it. This exemplifies a common feature of his mother's interaction with Ricky, whereby she actively offers him the opportunity to speak: in line 2 she invites Ricky to join in. Such offers, which happen frequently during storybook reading, have particular phonetic features. These include prolongations of vowels and sometimes of consonants; pausing at word boundaries and sometimes within words at syllable boundaries; and level or slightly rising intonation. It is a device that we observed in the carer–child interactions of Robin at the age of around 18 months, with his mother, in Chapters 2 and 7. In line 3, Ricky responds by completing the IP with a single syllable that has falling pitch to the base of his pitch range, which can therefore be heard as a Tonic.

His mother responds to Ricky's Tonic in line 3 as projecting the end of his turn, by starting her own turn (line 4). Ricky then produces what appears to be a version of YES, presumably agreeing with the proposition they had jointly constructed in lines 1–3, namely that everything seemed small. However, his mother, who apparently has not understood his first version of SMALL in line 3, initiates a repair (line 4), in overlap with Ricky. Her incoming in overlap in line 4 halts the progress of the reading activity in order to start a pedagogical sequence. Here his mother's incoming is triggered by Ricky's [mo:] as projecting the end of his turn since it is a sufficient response to her turn in line 2 and has a fall to the base of his pitch range. In line 4, she herself uses a rise, so her Tone does not match the fall used by Ricky in line 3. The non-matching Tone functions to mark her turn as a new action, i.e. a repair initiation. In response to this, Ricky then produces a further version of SMALL. He does not match his mother's rise but instead redoes the fall that he had used himself in line 3. This may indicate that he is not able to fully use the matching /alignment system. When his mother acknowledges his repaired version in line 6, thereby closing the repair sequence, she uses a fall, matching Ricky in line 5. She then resumes the reading activity (line 7). Thus, Ricky's mother makes full use of the system of Tone matching and non-matching to manage this interaction, even though Ricky himself may not be fully in command of the system. On the other hand, both Ricky and his mother seem to show awareness of the role of intonation in signalling the end of a turn.

The next portion we will consider, presented as Extract (12.10.3), starts at line 13 and is a sequence that is quite characteristic of this recording: Ricky turns the page in the book, then his mother reads the text (line 13). They are looking at the picture on the page depicting the place where Eugene has now arrived on his round-the-world plane trip, which he has won as a prize.

(12.10.3)

```
13       L  hhh(.)||'everywhere he 'went Eugene ['spotted] `planes||
14  R:  ≠                                         ||[  ´nɪʔ  ]||
15  M:  =   ||'whats ´this||
16  R:  ∅   ||nəuŋ||
17  M:      ||'Eiffel ˇTower|| (.)
18      ≠   ||'where `is it ||(0.3)
19  R:  =   ||`k̹ɛ::əm||
20  M:  =   ||`fra:nce|| (1.0)
21  R:  ≠   || ˇɑ̰ː[:    ]||
22  M:  ≠       ['Ricky](.)`fra:nce||=
23  R:  =   ||frɑ̰ː||
24  M:  =   ||'thats r oh[well [`done]Ricky ||⇒['good(.)with your `ef]||
25  R:  ≠                [ʔe::        ]        [e:      ɪ:       ]
26  M:      ||['whats he g]'whats he 'doing `here||(.)=||`ski[ing = ||`y]eh||
27  R:        [ɑ::           ]              = i::    = [bɹɑː  ]
28  M:  ≠   ||dyou 'like ´skiing||
```

At line 14, Ricky starts to talk in the middle of his mother's turn, i.e. before she has signalled the end of her turn either through the grammar and the sense or by a Tonic. Ricky's incoming consists of a single, relatively loud syllable with mid-rising pitch. At the same time he points to a picture on the page. His starting to talk in overlap here might be an indication that he is not responsive to the intonation and semantic content of his mother's turn, i.e. he is not aware that she has not finished. This interpretation finds some support from his mother's behaviour: she does not orient to the overlap immediately, e.g. by dropping out to let Ricky continue. Nor does she obviously compete with him to hold the floor by raising her own pitch and volume. She just finishes reading the sentence of text, without obviously attending to Ricky's incoming in overlap.

However, she then shifts to the topic that had been offered by Ricky with his incoming and pointing. She does this by requesting clarification (line 15). Given that she can see what Ricky is pointing at, "what's this" is apparently designed to elicit a spoken label from Ricky, rather than to elicit from Ricky a confirmation of what the object actually is. Moreover, she produces her turn with a rise Tone, which matches Ricky's overlapping turn in line 14, indicating her alignment with the new direction for the talk that he has initiated. He next produces a monosyllabic turn in line 16, which she does indeed treat as a label for THIS, presumably a very truncated version of EIFFEL TOWER. Thus we can see that she eventually treats Ricky's overlapping incoming in line 4 as relevant to the interaction and even as a trigger for talk that develops the topic. His competitive overlap is not ignored; rather, it is built upon. It is not clear whether Ricky deliberately interrupted his mother in order to introduce a new topic; or whether the overlap happened because he does not fully understand the turn-taking system. What is clear is that his mother responds to whatever he produces vocally, using her intonation along with other means to lend interactional sense to his turns.

She then pursues the topic that Ricky has initiated in line 14, by asking Ricky to name the location of the Eiffel Tower. He duly produces a turn, consisting of a single syllable accompanied by a point (line 19). The pitch has a fall, matching his mother's question, which may explain why, even though phonetically [ˋḵɛ::əm] bears very little resemblance to FRANCE, she seems to treat it as an attempt at answering her question rather than another new topic. In line 20, she does not produce a confirming phrase such as "that's right"; she merely supplies the correct label FRANCE, in isolation, with relatively loud volume, a prolonged vowel and matching his pitch. In his next turn (line 21), Ricky apparently treats her turn in line 20 as a prompt to repair his own previous attempt (in line 19) to say the name of place. The vowel in his new version [ɑː] is quite different to that of his original version [ḵɛ::əm] in line 19: in line 21, he mimics his mother's vowel in FRANCE, thereby indicating that he is aware of the need to repair his pronunciation. This is not wholly successful, however: his mother had used a prolonged vowel to draw Ricky's attention to the need to repair and in line 21 Ricky imitates just the prolonged vowel, not the whole word.

His pitch in line 21 has a fall-rise shape, which does not match his mother's fall in line 20. This is potentially confusing, since to align with the ongoing repair sequence and thereby present his turn as a new attempt to answer the question from line 18, he would need to use a matching fall. There is evidence that his mother is indeed confused; she does not obviously treat line 21 as another attempt by Ricky to say FRANCE. In line 22, she comes in, in overlap, using his name. This suggests that she feels the need to regain his attention and keep him on the topic of pronouncing FRANCE correctly. By starting with Ricky's name, she gains the floor, thereby preventing him from digressing to a new topic or activity. She has now to initiate a further repair in order to achieve the desired response. She produces a further version of FRANCE (line 22) that is delivered once Ricky has stopped speaking. Ricky complies with her initiation of repair, by producing a third label attempt, in line 23: [frɑː]. This suggests that he is interpreting his mother's prolongations and increase in volume as a cue to repeat and repair. Although his pitch pattern in line 23 does not accurately match his mother's fall in line 22, the divergence is not as great as on the previous occasion in line 21. Moreover, he matches the duration of her syllable as well as the articulation of onset and nucleus of the syllable FRANCE. In line 24, his mother produces a typical third position evaluation – a positive assessment of Ricky's production of the sound [f] - which serves to close the repair sequence.

Ricky has apparently latched on quickly to the fact that the repair issue is now over, as he comes in, in overlap. His turn in line 25, consisting of prolonged close front vowels, is evidently not a fourth attempt at naming FRANCE. It is treated in line 26 by his mother as the introduction of a new topic, skiing. Nevertheless it seems that, at the start of line 27, Ricky may be temporarily reverting to the FRANCE repair issue by producing an open back vowel again. Here he is possibly responding to his mother's extended positive evaluation in line 24, thereby demonstrating that he was attentive to talk that took place in overlap.

Ricky's line 25 has very similar consequences to line 15, discussed above. In each case, Ricky's incoming overlaps his mother's turn in progress; she persists to the end of her turn, thereby closing the reading aloud sequence; she then responds to Ricky's overlapping incoming as introducing a new topic, which she subsequently develops.

Thus, we can see that Ricky's apparently competitive overlaps do not significantly disrupt the progress of the talk; instead they initiate a new stage in its shared development. In each case, Ricky's competitive incoming in overlap is relatively high in pitch and loud in volume – the conventional phonetic design of a turn competitive incoming.

These examples of overlap by Ricky can be contrasted with his mother's overlap of Ricky in line 22, described above. There, her turn-competitive overlap served to temporarily halt the progression of the book reading activity so that the pronunciation issue could be worked on. In that case, Ricky appeared to orient to the placement of his mother's incoming in overlap; and also to the prosodic design of her productions of FRANCE, as marking them as models for repair.

So far, we have shown that both Ricky and his mother are able to deploy an IP that overlaps the other speaker, for interactional ends. In the case of Ricky, this can be to introduce a new topic and thereby progress the action of picture book reading. In the case of his mother, it can be to temporarily arrest the progress of the reading activity in order to work on an aspect of Ricky's phonetic or linguistic production. However, things do not always proceed in such an orderly way. In the passage starting at line 56, presented here as Extract (12.10.4), the features of overlap already mentioned can be observed but here they interweave in a complex way as Ricky and his mother negotiate two slightly different but related topical agendas, both of which relate to the page of the book that they are looking at.

(12.10.4)

```
56   M:   =    ‖ an dyou 'know 'where ´this is ‖ (0.5)
57   R:   ≠    `bæʔ (.) [ ts e ɪ :      `j e ɪ:   ]
58   M:   =          ‖ [dyou know where `this is] ‖
                        (2.0)
59        ≠    ‖ ´there [he is] ‖
60   R:   ≠             [jɛ: ] `jei:
61   M:   =    ‖ the 'train the 'fa:st [`train ‖`yes] ‖
62   R:   =                          [ fɑ: deɪ ]
63   M:   =    ‖ ['where] is 'this dyou 'know where this `is ‖ (0.5)
64   R:   ≠    [ ʔm ]
65   M:   ≠    ‖ its 'Ja`pan ‖
66   R:   =    `ɹeeee
67   M:   =    ‖ `yes‖nononono`no ≠ ‖ this`coun:try =‖⇒ ˇnot where
               erm Eu'gene is ‖
69        =    ‖ 'this`country‖(.)is Ja^pan ‖(.) where they have
               the 'fast `trains ‖(.)
```

In line 56, his mother poses a question that minimally requires a one-word answer, the answer being JAPAN (see line 65). In line 57, Ricky first produces a single syllable [bæʔ], which may be an attempt by Ricky to produce the second syllable of JAPAN. However, it has a falling pitch pattern, which does not match the rising contour of his mother's question. Perhaps as a consequence of this non-matching Tone, his mother does not treat Ricky's turn as an aligning response, as is shown by her repeat (line 58) of her question from line 56. This is further evidence that Ricky does not use the Tone matching system for interactional alignment. Simultaneously with his mother's turn, Ricky produces a second element to his own turn in line 57; this is marked by a step-up in pitch and increased loudness, with a fall in pitch on the second (last) syllable to the base of his pitch range, thereby matching the pitch of the first IP. This suggests that this second IP is an expansion or elaboration of the first one. As in the extracts discussed above, his mother continues to the end of her own turn (in line 58), then after a pause displays in line 59 an orientation to Ricky's new topic: Eugene, who is in the train, rather than to her original topic, i.e. Japan, the location of the picture. At this point, she does not pursue a response to her own question from lines 56 and 58. Ricky, in line 60, in overlap with his mother, re-presents his new topic, repeating the second part of his turn from line 57, matching its falling pitch contour. At this point, possibly as a result of her own orientation to the picture simultaneously with Ricky's repeat of his disyllabic utterance, his mother in line 61 identifies that disyllabic utterance as Ricky's version of TRAIN. Indeed, it is possible that here Ricky contrives the timing of his turn to coincide with his mother's deictic gesture and utterance, with a view to helping her recognize the meaning of his utterance. In the second part of her turn in line 61, his mother expands "the train" to "the fast train", matching Ricky's fall from line 60, her final word being overlapped by Ricky's own production of "fast train" (line 62). Ricky's "fast train" is thus lexically a completion of his mother's turn. His simultaneous nod provides further evidence that at this point they are absolutely on the same agenda.

In Figure 12.1 we represent one of Ricky's turns from the sequence, presented in phonetic transcription as (12.10.5), in terms of the psycholinguistic processing model for intonation.

(12.10.5)

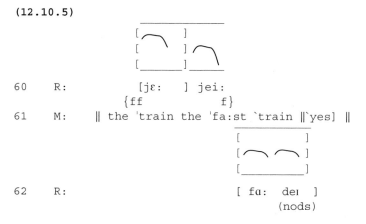

Ricky's turn consists of two words that are apparently his version of two words that his mother used in her prior turn. However, this is not case of immediate echolalia of the kind observed in Kevin, the child with severe autism discussed in Chapter 11. Ricky starts his turn in overlap with his mother. At the point when he starts to talk, he can only have heard "the train the fast" from his mother's turn. In his own turn, he reorders the words into a grammatically accurate order: adjective followed by noun. We can thus credit Ricky with a generative capacity that was not evident in Kevin's immediate echoes, although Kevin was much more accurate at the articulatory level. In terms of intonation, Ricky may be borrowing the level pitch from his mother's productions of TRAIN and FAST, which in his mother's turn are part of the Head. For this reason, there is an arrow from the left box to the centre box at Level 1. The fact that Ricky does not produce a final fall (Tonic) on TRAIN lends credence to this view. On the

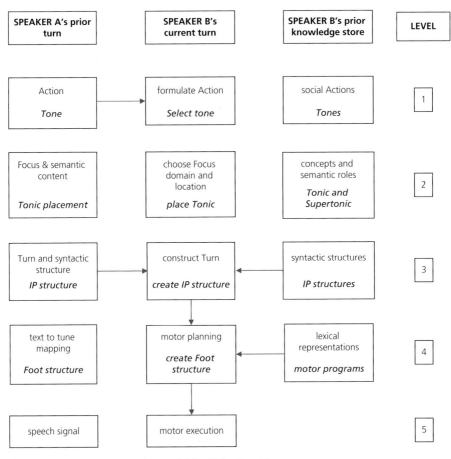

SPEAKER A's prior turn	SPEAKER B's current turn	SPEAKER B's prior knowledge store	LEVEL
Action *Tone*	formulate Action *Select tone*	social Actions *Tones*	1
Focus & semantic content *Tonic placement*	choose Focus domain and location *place Tonic*	concepts and semantic roles *Tonic and Supertonic*	2
Turn and syntactic structure *IP structure*	construct Turn *create IP structure*	syntactic structures *IP structures*	3
text to tune mapping *Foot structure*	motor planning *create Foot structure*	lexical representations *motor programs*	4
speech signal	motor execution		5

Figure 12.1 Intonation processing model for Ricky: line 62.

other hand, there is no evidence that he has selected a Tone to match or not to match, his mother – in fact, because he has overlapped her, he has not yet heard her produce a Tone. Even though interactional alignment is evident in other modalities at line 62 – Ricky nods his head and he repeats his mother's words - there is no evidence that he is drawing on a stored system of Tone choice to back up this up, so we have not drawn an arrow at Level 1 from the right-hand box. Since he does not produce a Tonic here, there is no evidence to suggest that he can use Tonic placement for the purposes of Focus, so there are no arrows at Level 2. In terms of Turn construction, line 62 does not provide evidence that he is able to generate an appropriate IP structure with a Head and final Tonic, to show that he has produced a complete turn. However, it does provide evidence that he can start at turn in overlap when it is warranted: here, his mother has produced the relevant semantic information for her turn before she has actually completed the IP and Ricky has legitimately anticipated what she intends to say, helping her out with her sentence formulation. Elsewhere, for example in line 60, there is clear evidence that Ricky can use Tonic-like pitch movement and that his mother, as in line 61, responds to it as marking the end of his turn. For these reasons, we have included arrows at Level 3. At Level 4, Ricky displays a rudimentary mapping of text (the monosyllabic words TRAIN and FAST, onto a 'tune', since each word has its own pitch contour.

The psycholinguistic modelling of this single turn of Ricky's supports conclusions that we can draw from his IIP (Appendix 8), namely, that there is rather little evidence of his using the intonation systems of English in a consistent way. He may draw on prosodic features from his mother's prior turn, but apparently with limited understanding how they should be used to construct an IP and thus a turn. Elsewhere in the passage, as captured on the IIP, he shows some ability to construct turns with Tonic-like pitch movements, which are responded to as complete by his mother. There was also evidence that he responds to his mother's use of the Tonic to delimit her turn. This suggests that he has stored some pitch patterns and has some knowledge of how to use them for turn-taking. However, there is little evidence that he has any knowledge or command of the system of Tonic placement for Focus or the system of Tone matching for Action alignment.

Extract (12.10.4) suggests that Ricky is able to establish a direction for the conversation (the fast train) that is different from the one his mother has embarked on (Japan) , and eventually to bring his mother round to his own agenda and topic. He manages to do this with very limited resources in terms of intelligible vocabulary and grammatical structure. We might expect a child with more linguistic resources to make use of the Tonic/Focus system to sort out an interactional issue like the one that Ricky and his mother are engaged with here, which is about identifying and establishing a topic. In Chapter 8, we saw that typically developing school-aged children routinely manipulate Tonic placement to identify the topic. Moreover, earlier in this chapter Extract (12.4), we noted that W, despite his hearing impairment, was able to use Tonic placement to correct or contradict his father in conversation. Some of the school-aged children with cochlear implants in O'Halpin's study demonstrated this ability under experimental conditions. However, Ricky only produces TCUs of at most two or three words, often unintelligible even to his mother, and there is no evidence in the recordings that he is able to manipulate the placement of the Tonic at all; instead his Tonic occurs in final position in the IP, thereby usefully marking a TRP, i.e. potentially the end of his turn. This is a pattern we noted in some of the deaf children described by Parker and Rose (1992), as well as in early typical development (Chapter 7) and cases of delayed intonation development such as David (Chapter 5).

In the final part of Extract (12.10.4), reproduced here as (12.10.6), following their convergence on the shared topic of the fast train, Ricky's mother now reverts to her original topic from lines 56 and 58, requesting him to provide the name of the country depicted on the page.

```
(12.10.6)
63  M:  =   ||['where] is 'this dyou 'know where this `is|| (0.5)
64  R:  ≠   [?m    ]
65  M:  ≠   ||its 'Ja`pan ||
66  R:  =   `ıeeee
67  M:  =   ||`yes||nononono`no ≠ ||this ˇcoun:try =||⇒ˇnot where
            erm Eu'gene is ||
69      =   ||'this ˇcountry||(.)is Ja^pan||(.) where they have
            the 'fast `trains||(.)
```

The start of her turn in line 63 is in overlap with a short turn from Ricky, who drops out immediately. She reformulates her original question, "where is this?" as "do you know where this is". Recycling of this kind is common in everyday talk when a speaker emerges from overlap (Schegloff, 2000; Kurtić et al., 2013). After a brief pause, in line 65 she provides the answer to her own question, using slow tempo and marking each syllable as distinct. However, in this instance, Ricky, in line 66, does not echo her as he had done in line 62. Instead, he produces a turn with a single long vowel that has more in common phonetically with his earlier versions of TRAIN. He produces it with a falling pitch, which, while matching the pitch of his earlier productions of "train" also matches the Tone of his mother's turns in lines 63 and 65. This may be one reason why in line 67 his mother initially appears not to recognize line 66 as TRAIN, responding with "yes", which suggests she accepts Ricky's turn in line 66 as an appropriate acknowledgement of her "Japan". She seems to treat his matching Tone as displaying alignment with her agenda, as predicted by the Tone matching system of English. However, in line 67, she immediately revises her understanding with "ˋyes‖nononono`no" , on realizing that Ricky is still focussed on where Eugene is (i.e. on the train) rather than on the name of the country (Japan). She makes this quite explicit both verbally and with gesture in lines 67–69, at the end of the turn making an overt verbal connection between the two topics that have been at issue during the sequence: Japan and the fast train. Her misinterpretation of Ricky's Tone matching is further evidence that he is not yet in command of this aspect of English intonation.

Finally, it is noteworthy that in line 65, his mother answers her own question from line 63: "Do you know where this is? It's Japan." This time she has not provided Ricky with access to her turn by inviting him to complete it, as she had in the case of SMALL in (12.10.2), where she had designed her IP as unfinished, producing the Head only and leaving him to supply the Tonic. As a result, following line 65, a misunderstanding arises as to what they are talking about, which necessitates an explicit repair from his mother in lines 67–69 and which does not elicit any further talk from Ricky about this page of the book. The breakdown suggests that Ricky is highly dependent on his mother's intonational support: without it, the progress of their conversation is at risk.

It is important to consider the issue of overlapping talk, since this is a striking feature of the interaction in Extract (12.10) and it involves intonation. While some overlaps may be accidental by-products of the turn-taking system, as mentioned in Chapter 2, both competitive and non-competitive overlaps happen frequently in everyday conversation. Although this might at first glance be thought to indicate a problem with the Turn-taking system, this is not entirely true. The use of both competitive and non-competitive overlaps to enable shared participation plays a large part in the interaction of Ricky and his mother. The strategies they use ensure that they can maintain collaboration in the activity. We saw that the placement of turns in overlap was instrumental in ensuring that the two participants knew where they were at a given point in the interaction. First, Ricky's speaking in overlap with his mother's reading aloud marked his introduction of a new topic, which his mother picked upon once she had completed her turn. Second, his mother's competitive overlaps indicated that she was initiating a pedagogical sequence where the agenda was work on Ricky's linguistic production, rather than progressing with the book reading. Thus, by being locally competitive, Ricky's mother is able to keep the unfolding interaction on track. Mutual understanding is thus maintained. Third, the overlaps that come about as a result of his mother's offer of conditional access to the floor indicated that both participants were aligned and agreed on the form and meaning of a particular word. Thus, it can be seen that overlap contributes to mutual understanding and can thereby serve to progress the talk where there is a range of possible actions that might be pursued, even within a restricted type of activity such as shared book reading.

In terms of temporal placement, Ricky produced competitive overlaps midway through a turn in progress from his mother. Their prosodic design was relatively high in pitch and volume, reflecting the typical system (French & Local, 1983; Kurtić, Brown, & Wells, 2013). Ricky's competitive incomings are mostly very short, just a single word. He does not therefore fight for the floor until the current speaker drops out, as often happens in talk (Schegloff, 2000). Instead, he allows his mother to complete her turn. However, on completing her turn, his mother often returns to the topic that was raised earlier by Ricky in his overlapping incoming. This suggests that they have established a routine way of managing his incomings. By contrast, where his mother comes in competitively in overlap, Ricky typically drops out, leaving the floor to her. There thus appears to be an asymmetry in handling of turn-competitive incomings by Ricky and his mother, though both of them use practices that have been reported in the literature on overlap.

In the case of non-competitive overlaps, Ricky responds to phonetically designed invitations from his mother to complete her turn; this often happens in overlap and is sometimes done by Ricky with a pitch pattern that matches his mother's. It may be further accompanied by a nod or other gesture of assent. Taken together, Ricky's behaviours indicate that he is orienting to the overlapping turns as an embodiment of interactional alignment between himself and his mother: he displays that at this point in the interaction they share the same agenda. These prosodic and nonverbal practices are ones found widely in talk-in-interaction to indicate alignment (Stivers, 2008; Gorisch et al., 2012). This evidence that Ricky can manage the occurrence of overlaps in ways that are common in typical talk-in-interaction suggests that in some respects at least, he is able to attend to pitch and loudness features of his mother's talk and also to deploy these features in his own talk in ways that are conventional for British English. This is noteworthy, given the difficulties that people with AN, even after cochlear implantation, are known to have with the perception of pitch patterns, as discussed earlier in this chapter. What the case of Ricky strikingly demonstrates is that control and understanding of the precise timing of turns can be just as important as the command and understanding of the intonation systems themselves.

Although we have seen that with his mother, Ricky can communicate without other resources, it nevertheless remains the case that Ricky's spoken repertoire is very limited. In the terms of the developmental phase model of intonation, he has not yet progressed beyond the Paradigmatic phase, since he does not yet have command over Tone matching, although there is some evidence from his use of intonation for turn-taking that he may be able to progress to the Syntagmatic phase. An alternative to speech, such as signing or a communication aid, may therefore be beneficial. However, this would lead to Ricky losing what he does have going for him in terms of the timing and prosodic construction of his turns. His use of these resources allows him to participate in interaction, if this is facilitated by his mother's management of the context, the timing of her turns and her own use of specific prosodic features. The case of Ricky illustrates that a hearing impairment does not necessarily exist in isolation but may be accompanied by other difficulties in speech and language development that also have a major impact on the child's communication. The book-reading episode between Ricky and his mother also underlines the crucial role of the co-participant(s) in maximizing the CI user's full participation in the cut and thrust of conversation. This motivates the inclusion of family members of CI users in interventions targeted at communication skills.

Summary

The cases presented in this chapter have highlighted the following key points about intonation in children with hearing impairments:

- There is diversity among deaf children using conventional aids in their understanding and use of intonation systems.
- By signalling Turns, Focus and Action alignment, a child's use of intonation can help to compensate for reduced speech intelligibility.
- Cochlear implants currently convey to the user only a limited amount of the speech signal that would be relevant to intonation.
- Users of Cis vary in their ability to perceive and access the intonationally relevant parameters of pitch, loudness and duration.
- Some CI users may nevertheless be able to communicate intonation systems, such as Tonic for Focus, although individuals differ in the prosodic parameters they draw on to do so.
- For CI users, the relation between perception and production of intonation features is often not a direct one.
- Intervention should focus on intonational functions in interaction, so that the CI user can understand how intonation may be used to help manage conversational exchanges.
- Control over the precise timing of turns is interactionally important and may compensate for lack of knowledge of intonation systems per se.
- For those children who already understand intonation systems but whose production of them in their own speech is idiosyncratic, intervention using visual feedback may improve control over phonetic parameters of pitch, loudness and duration.

Key to Activity 12.1

1 Decide if you can identify changes in terms of:
    a *Pitch*. It is possible to hear that different syllables are pronounced on different pitch levels: some are higher than others. The pitch can be heard to fall or to rise on certain syllables.
    b *Loudness*. Some syllables are perceptibly louder than neighbouring syllables.
    c *Timing and duration*. There are variations in tempo, with short silences; some filled pauses, i.e. sustained "er" type syllables are also audible at some points. Some syllables are perceptibly longer than neighbouring syllables.

2 Consider what intonational information the listener might be able to access that is relevant to:
  a *Turns*. The recording is a monologue, so Turn-taking is not at issue. Nevertheless, it is possible to detect IP structure which in another context would be relevant to a listener to identify the end of a turn. It is possible to hear 'Tonic' syllables, as these are louder and longer than surrounding syllables and have moving pitch. Any following syllables can be heard as the Tail, and preceding syllables as the Head. The filled pauses noted under (1) seem to occur in the Head. Silences seem to occur at IP boundaries.
  b *Focus*. As noted for Turns, some Tonic syllables are identifiable, which would be a guide to the speaker's Focus.
  c *Actions*. The recording is a monologue, so Tone matching for interactional alignment is not at issue. Nevertheless, it is possible to detect Tones (rising or falling) which in another context would be relevant to a listener to tell whether the speaker is aligning or initiating a new action.

Key to Activity 12.2

1 Decide if you can identify changes in terms of:
  a *Pitch*. It is not possible to hear whether different syllables are pronounced on different pitch levels or whether the pitch falls or rises on certain syllables.
  b *Loudness*. Some syllables are perceptibly louder than neighbouring syllables.
  c *Timing and duration*. There are variations in tempo, with short silences. Some syllables are perceptibly longer than their neighbouring syllables.
2 Consider what intonational information the listener might be able to access that is relevant to:
  a *Turns*. The recording is a monologue, so turn-taking is not at issue. However, it would be relevant to detect IP structure which in another context would be relevant to a listener to identify the end of a turn. It is possible to hear some syllables as stressed, and therefore as starting a Foot, on the basis of their rhythmic prominence where the syllable is louder and longer than surrounding syllables. However, the lack of pitch information makes it hard to identify a stressed syllable as a Tonic. Silences can be heard. The listener could hypothesize that these are associated with IP boundaries.
  b *Focus*. As noted for Turns, Tonic syllables are not readily identifiable, so there is little guidance about the speaker's Focus.
  c *Actions*. It is not possible to detect Tones as rising or falling, which in another context would be relevant to a listener to tell whether the speaker is aligning or initiating a new action.

References

Abberton, E., & Fourcin, A. (1997). Electrolaryngography. In M. J. Ball, & C. Code (Eds.), *Instrumental clinical phonetics*. London: Whurr.

Anstey, J., & Wells, B. (2013). The uses of overlap: carer-child interaction involving a nine-year-old boy with auditory neuropathy. *Clinical Linguistics & Phonetics, 27*(10–11), 746–769. doi:10.3109/02699206.2013.803602

Arrowsmith, D. R. (2005). An analysis of conversations between children and teachers in nursery counting activities. PhD thesis, University of Leeds. Retrieved from http://etheses.whiterose.ac.uk/id/eprint/805

Astruc, L., Payne, E., Post, B., Vanrell, M. D. M., & Prieto, P. (2013). Tonal targets in early child English, Spanish, and Catalan. *Language and Speech, 56*(2), 229–253. doi:10.1177/0023830912460494

Atkinson-King, K. (1973). Children's acquisition of phonological stress contrasts. *UCLA Working Papers in Phonetics, 25*.

Baker, E., Croot, K., McLeod, S., & Paul, R. (2001). Psycholinguistic models of speech development and their application to clinical practice. *Journal of Speech, Language and Hearing Research, 44*(3), 685–702.

Balog, H. L. (2010). A comparison of maternal and child intonation: does adult input support child production? *Infant Behavior & Development, 33*(3), 337–45. doi:10.1016/j.infbeh.2010.04.001

Balog, H. L., & Snow, D. (2007). The adaptation and application of relational and independent analyses for intonation production in young children. *Journal of Phonetics, 35*(1), 118–133. doi:10.1016/j.wocn.2005.10.002

Baltaxe, C. (1984). Use of contrastive stress in normal, aphasic and autistic children. *Journal of Speech and Hearing Research, 21*, 97–105.

Baltaxe, C., Simmons, J., & Zee, E. (1984). Intonation patterns in normal, aphasic and autistic children. In A. Cohen & B. M. D. R. V. D. (Eds.), *Proceedings of the Tenth International Conference of Phonetic Sciences*. Dordrecht: Foris Publications.

Barry, J., Blamey, P., Martin, L., Lee, K., Tang, T., Ming, Y., & van Hasselt, C. (2002). Tone discrimination in Cantonese-speaking children using a cochlear implant. *Clinical Linguistics & Phonetics, 16*(2), 79–99.

Beach, C., Katz, W., & Skowronski, A. (1996). Children's processing of prosodic cues for phrasal interpretation. *The Journal of the Acoustical Society of America, 99*(2), 1148. doi:10.1121/1.414599

Behrens, H., & Gut, U. (2005). The relationship between prosodic and syntactic organization in early multiword speech. *Journal of Child Language, 32*(1), 1–34. doi:10.1017/S0305000904006592

Benjamin, R. G., & Schwanenflugel, P. J. (2010). Text complexity and oral reading. *Reading Research Quarterly, 45*(4), 388–404.

Benjamin, R. G., Schwanenflugel, P. J., Meisinger, E. B., Groff, C., Kuhn, M. R., & Steiner, L. (2013). A spectrographically grounded scale for evaluating reading expressiveness. *Reading Research Quarterly, 48*(2), 105–133. doi:10.1002/rrq.43

Bergeson, T. R., Miller, R. J., & McCune, K. (2006). Mothers' speech to hearing-impaired infants and children with cochlear implants. *Infancy, 10*(3), 221–240. doi:10.1207/s15327078in1003_2

Children's Intonation: A Framework for Practice and Research, First Edition. Bill Wells and Joy Stackhouse.
© 2016 John Wiley & Sons, Ltd. Published 2016 by John Wiley & Sons, Ltd.
Companion website: www.wiley.com/go/childintonation

Bishop, D. (1989). *Test for Reception of Grammar (TROG)* (2nd ed.). Manchester: University of Manchester.

Bishop, D. (1997). *Uncommon understanding: Development and disorders of language comprehension in children*. Hove: Psychology Press.

Boersma, P., & Weenink, D. (2014). Praat: doing phonetics by computer. *Praat: Doing Phonetics by Computer [Computer Program]. Version 5.4.01.* Amsterdam: University of Amsterdam. Retrieved from http://www.praat.org/

Bone, D., Lee, C.-C., Black, M. P., & Williams, M. E. (2014). The psychologist as an interlocutor in autism spectrum disorder assessment: Insights from a study of spontaneous prosody. *Journal of Speech, Language and Hearing Research, 57.*, 1162–1178.

Branigan, G. (1979). Some reasons why successive single word utterances are not. *Journal of Child Language, 6*(03), 411–421. doi:10.1017/S0305000900002452

Broerse, J., & Elias, G. (1994). Changes in the content and timing of mothers' talk to infants. *British Journal of Developmental Psychology, 12*, 131–145.

Bryant, G., & Barrett, H. C. (2007). Recognizing intentions in infant-directed speech: evidence for universals. *Psychological Science, 18*(8), 746–51. doi:10.1111/j.1467-9280.2007.01970.x

Bryant, G., & Fox Tree, J. (2005). Is there an ironic tone of voice ? *Language and Speech, 48*(3), 257–277.

Bull, D., Eilers, R. E., & Oller, D. K. (1984). Infants' discrimination of intensity variation in multisyllabic stimuli. *Journal of the Acoustical Society of America, 76*, 13–17.

Camarata, S., & Gandour, J. (1985). Rule invention in the acquisition of morphology by a language impaired child. *Journal of Speech and Hearing Research, 50*, 40–45.

Capelli, C., Nakagawa, N., & Madden, C. (1990). How children understand sarcasm: The role of context and intonation. *Child Development, 61*(6), 1824–1841.

Catterall, C., Howard, S., Stojanovik, V., Szczerbinski, M., & Wells, B. (2006). Investigating prosodic ability in Williams syndrome. *Clinical Linguistics & Phonetics, 20*(7-8), 531–8. doi:10.1080/02699200500266380

Clarke, M., & Wilkinson, R. (2007). Interaction between children with cerebral palsy and their peers 1: Organizing and understanding VOCA use. *Augmentative and Alternative Communication (Baltimore, Md. : 1985), 23*(4), 336–48. doi:10.1080/07434610701390350

Consortium for Research into Deaf Education. (2014). *CRIDE report on 2013 survey on educational provision for deaf children in England*. Retrieved from http://www.ndcs.org.uk/professional_support/national_data/uk_education_.html

Corrin, J. (2002). *The emergence of early grammar: a conversation analytic perspective*. PhD thesis, University of London. Retrieved from ethos.bl.uk

Corrin, J. (2010a). Hm? what? Maternal repair and early child talk. In H. Gardner & M. Forrester (Eds.), *Analysing interactions in childhood: Insights from conversation analysis* (pp. 23–41). Chichester: Wiley-Blackwell.

Corrin, J. (2010b). Maternal repair initiation at MLU Stage I: The developmental power of "hm?". *First Language, 30*(3–4), 312–328. doi:10.1177/0142723710370526

Corrin, J., Tarplee, C., & Wells, B. (2001). Interactional linguistics and language development: a conversation analytic perspective on emergent syntax. In M. Selting, & E. Couper-Kuhlen (Eds.), *Studies in Interactional Linguistics* (pp. 199–255). Amsterdam and Philadelphia: Benjamins.

Couper-Kuhlen, E. (1996). The prosody of repetition: on quoting and mimicry. In E. Couper-Kuhlen, & M. Selting (Eds.), *Prosody in conversation: Interactional studies* (pp. 366–405). Cambridge: Cambridge University Press.

Couper-Kuhlen, E. (2009). A sequential approach to affect: The case of "disappointment." In J. Haakana, M. Laakso, & M. Lindström (Eds.), *Talk in interaction: Comparative dimensions* (pp. 94–123). Helsinki: Finnish Literature Society.

Couper-Kuhlen, E. (2012). Some truths and untruths about final intonation in conversational questions. In J. de Ruiter (Ed.), *Questions: Formal, functional and interactional perspectives* (pp. 123–145). Cambridge: Cambridge University Press.

Cowie, R., Douglas-Cowie, E., & Wichmann, A. (2002). Prosodic characteristics of skilled reading: fluency and expressiveness in 8-10-year-old readers. *Language and Speech, 45*(1), 47–82. doi:10.1177/00238309020450010301

Cruttenden, A. (1985). Intonation comprehension in ten-year-olds. *Journal of Child Language, 12*(03), 643–661. doi:10.1017/S030500090000670X

Cruttenden, A. (1994). Phonetic and prosodic aspects of baby talk. In C. Gallaway, & B. J. Richards (Eds.), *Input and interaction in language acquisition* (pp. 135–152). Cambridge: Cambridge University Press.

Cruttenden, A. (1997). *Intonation* (2nd ed.). Cambridge: Cambridge University Press.

Crystal, D. (1969). *Prosodic systems and intonation in English.* Cambridge: Cambridge University Press.

Crystal, D. (1982). *Profiling linguistic disability.* London: Edward Arnold.

Crystal, D. (1987). *Clinical linguistics.* London: Edward Arnold.

Cutler, A., & Swinney, D. a. (1987). Prosody and the development of comprehension. *Journal of Child Language, 14*(01), 145–167. doi:10.1017/S0305000900012782

Dankovičová, J. (1997). The domain of articulation rate variation in Czech. *Journal of Phonetics, 25*(3), 287–312. doi:10.1006/jpho.1997.0045

Dankovičová, J., Pigott, K., Wells, B., & Peppé, S. (2004). Temporal markers of prosodic boundaries in children's speech production. *Journal of the International Phonetic Association, 34*(1), 17–36. doi:10.1017/S0025100304001525

Demuth, K. (1995). Problems in the acquisition of tonal systems. In J. Archibald (Ed.), *The acquisition of non-linear phonology* (pp. 111–134). Hillsdale, NJ: Lawrence Erlbaum Associates.

Dickie, C., Ota, M., & Clark, A. (2012). Revisiting the phonological deficit in dyslexia: Are implicit nonorthographic representations impaired? *Applied Psycholinguistics, 34*(04), 649–672. doi:10.1017/S0142716411000907

Diehl, J. J., & Paul, R. (2013). Acoustic and perceptual measurements of prosody production on the profiling elements of prosodic systems in children by children with autism spectrum disorders. *Applied Psycholinguistics, 34*(01), 135–161. doi:10.1017/S0142716411000646

Drew, P. (2005). Conversation analysis. In K. Fitch, & R. Sanders (Eds.), *Handbook of language and social interaction* (pp. 71–102). Mahwah, NJ: Lawrence Erlbaum Associates.

Dunn, L. M., Dunn, L., Whetton, C., & Pintillie, O. (1982). *The British Picture Vocabulary Scales.* Windsor: NFER-Nelson.

Dunn, L., Whetton, C., & Burley, J. (1997). *The British Picture Vocabulary Scales* (2nd ed.). Windsor: NFER Nelson.

Ebbels, S. (2000). Psycholinguistic profiling of a hearing-impaired child. *Child Language Teaching and Therapy, 16*(3), 3–22. doi:10.1177/026565900001600102

Edwards, S. (1990). Conversational interaction between adults and young severely mentally handicapped children. PhD thesis, University of Reading. Retrieved from http://ethos.bl.uk

Eilers, R. E., Bull, D. H., Oller, D. K., & Lewis, D. C. (1984). The discrimination of vowel duration by infants. *Journal of the Acoustical Society of America, 75*, 1213–1218.

Elias, G., & Broerse, J. (1996). Developmental changes in the incidence and likelihood of simultaneous talk during the first two years: a question of function. *Journal of Child Language, 23*(01), 201–217. doi:10.1017/S0305000900010151

Esteve-Gibert, N., & Prieto, P. (2012). Prosody signals the emergence of intentional communication in the first year of life: Evidence from Catalan-babbling infants. *Journal of Child Language, 40*(5), 1–26. doi:10.1017/S0305000912000359

Fernald, A. (1989). Intonation and communicative intent in mothers' speech to infants: Is the melody the message? *Child Development, 60*, 1497–1510. doi:10.1111/1467-8624.ep9772504

Fernald, A., & Mazzie, C. (1991). Prosody and focus in speech to infants and adults. *Developmental Psychology, 27*(2), 209–221. doi:10.1037//0012-1649.27.2.209

Ferrand, C., & Bloom, R. (1996). Gender differences in children's intonational patterns. *Journal of Voice, 10*, 284–291.

Filipi, A. (2009). *Toddler and parent interaction: The organisation of gaze, pointing and vocalisation.* Amsterdam: John Benjamins.

Firth, G. (2006). Intensive interaction: A research review. *Mental Health and Learning Disabilities Research and Practice, 3*(1), 53–62.

Flax, J., Lahey, M., Harris, K., & Boothroyd, A. (1991). Relations between prosodic variables and communicative functions. *Journal of Child Language, 18*(1), 3–19. doi:10.1017/S030500090001326X

Fletcher, P. (1985). *A child's learning of English.* London: Blackwell.

Ford, C., & Thompson, S. (1996). Interactional units in conversation: syntactic, intonational, and pragmatic resources for the management of turns. In E. Ochs, E. Schegloff, & S. Thompson (Eds.), *Interaction and grammar* (pp. 134–184). Cambridge: Cambridge University Press.

French, P., & Local, J. (1983). Turn-competitive incomings. *Journal of Pragmatics, 7,* 17–38.

Frota, S., Butler, J., & Vigário, M. (2014). Infants' perception of intonation: Is it a statement or a question? *Infancy, 19*(2), 194–213. doi:10.1111/infa.12037

Gerhardt, K. J., & Abrams, R. M. (2000). Fetal exposures to sound and vibroacoustic stimulation. *Journal of Perinatology, 20,* S20–S29.

Ginsburg, G. P., & Kilbourne, B. K. (1988). Emergence of vocal alternation in mother-infant interchanges. *Journal of Child Language, 15*(02), 221–235. doi:10.1017/S0305000900012344

Glenwright, M., Parackel, J. M., Cheung, K. R. J., & Nilsen, E. S. (2014). Intonation influences how children and adults interpret sarcasm. *Journal of Child Language, 41*(2), 472–484. doi:10.1017/S0305000912000773

Gorisch, J., Wells, B., & Brown, G. J. (2012). Pitch contour matching and interactional alignment across turns: An acoustic investigation. *Language and Speech, 55*(1), 57–76. doi:10.1177/0023830911428874

Grabe, E., Post, B., Nolan, F., & Farrar, K. (2000). Pitch accent realization in four varieties of British English. *Journal of Phonetics, 28,* 161–185. doi:10.006/jpho.2000.0111

Gratier, M., & Devouche, E. (2011). Imitation and repetition of prosodic contour in vocal interaction at 3 months. *Developmental Psychology, 47*(1), 67–76. doi:10.1037/a0020722

Graven, S. N., & Browne, J. V. (2008). Auditory development in the fetus and infant. *Newborn and Infant Nursing Reviews, 8*(4), 187–193. doi:10.1053/j.nainr.2008.10.010

Gussenhoven, C. (2004). *The phonology of tone and intonation.* Cambridge: Cambridge University Press.

Gut, U. (2000). *The acquisition of intonation by German/English bilingual children.* Tübingen: Niemayer.

Gut, U. (2004). Nigerian English prosody. *English World Wide, 26*(2), 153–176.

Halliday, M. A. K. (1975). *Learning how to mean: Explorations in the development of language.* London: Edward Arnold.

Halliday, M. A. K. (2003). *The language of early childhood.* New York: Continuum.

Hargrove, P., & Sheran, C. (1989). The use of stress by language-impaired children. *Journal of Communication Disorders, 22,* 361–373.

Hellermann, J. (2003). The interactive work of prosody in the IRF exchange: Teacher repetition in feedback moves. *Language in Society, 32*(01), 79–104. doi:10.1017/S0047404503321049

Heselwood, B. C., Bray, M., & Crookston, I. (1995). Juncture, rhythm and planning in the speech of an adult with Down's syndrome. *Clinical Linguistics & Phonetics, 9*(2), 121–137. doi:10.3109/02699209508985328

Hirst, D., & Di Cristo, A. (1998). *Intonation systems.* Cambridge: Cambridge University Press.

Hornby, P. (1971). Surface structure and the topic-comment distinction: a developmental study. *Child Development, 42,* 1975–1988.

Hornby, P., & Hass, W. (1970). Use of contrastive stress by preschool children. *Journal of Speech and Hearing Research, 13,* 395–399.

Howard, S., & Heselwood, B. (2011). Instrumental and perceptual phonetic analyses: The case for two-tier transcriptions. *Clinical Linguistics & Phonetics, 25*(11–12), 940–948. doi:10.3109/026992 06.2011.616641

Hua, Z. (2002). *Phonological Development in Specific Contexts: Studies of Chinese-Speaking Children.* Clevedon: Multilingual Matters.

Ingold, T. (2000). Speech, writing and the modern origins of "language origins." In T. Ingold *The perception of the environment: essays on livelihood, dwelling and skill* (pp. 392–405). London: Routledge.

Ito, K., Bibyk, S. A., Wagner, L., & Speer, S. R. (2014). Interpretation of contrastive pitch accent in six- to eleven-year-old English-speaking children (and adults). *Journal of Child Language, 41*(1), 84–110. doi:10.1017/S0305000912000554

Jefferson, G. (1984). Notes on some orderlinesses of overlap onset. In V. D'Urso, & P. Leonardi (Eds.), *Discourse analysis and natural rhetoric* (pp. 11–38). Padua: Cleup Editore.

Jefferson, G. (1987). Notes on "latency" in overlap onset. *Human Studies, 9,* 153–183.

Jun, S.-A. (2005). *Prosodic typology: The phonology of intonation and phrasing.* Oxford: Oxford University Press.

Juszczyk, P. (1997). *The discovery of spoken language.* Cambridge, MA: MIT Press.

Karzon, R. G., & Nicholas, J. G. (1989). Syllabic pitch perception in 2- to 3-month-old infants. *Perception and Psychophysics, 45,* 10–14.

Katz, W., Beach, C., Jenouri, K., & Verma, S. (1996). Duration and fundamental frequency correlates of phrase boundaries in productions by children and adults. *Journal of the Acoustical Society of America, 99,* 3179–3191.

Keenan, E. O. (1983). Making it last: Repetition in children's discourse. In *Acquiring conversational competence* (pp. 26–39). London: Routledge & Kegan Paul.

Kellett, M. (2000). Sam's story: Evaluating Intensive Interaction in terms of its effect on the social and communicative ability of a young child with severe learning difficulties. *Support for Learning, 15*(4), 165–171. doi:10.1111/1467-9604.00170

Kelly, D., & Beeke, S. (2011). The management of turn taking by a child with high-functioning autism: Re-examining atypical prosody. In V. Stojanovik, & J. Setter (Eds.), *Speech prosody in atypical populations: Assessment and remediation* (pp. 71–98). Guildford: J & R Press.

Kent, R., & Vorperian, H. (1995). Development of the craniofacial–oral–laryngeal anatomy: A review. *Journal of Medical Speech-Language Pathology, 3,* 145–190.

Kitamura, C., Thanavishuth, C., Burnham, D., & Luksaneeyanawin, S. (2002). Universality and specificity in infant-directed speech: Pitch modifications as a function of infant age and sex in a tonal and non-tonal language. *Infant Behavior & Development, 24,* 372–392.

Kurtić, E., Brown, G. J., & Wells, B. (2013). Resources for turn competition in overlapping talk. *Speech Communication, 55*(5), 721–743.

Ladd, D. R. (2008). *Intonational phonology* (2nd ed.). Cambridge: Cambridge University Press.

Laver, J. (1994). *Principles of phonetics.* Cambridge: Cambridge University Press.

Levelt, W. J. M. (1989). *Speaking: From intention to articulation.* Cambridge, MA: MIT Press.

Li, C., & Thompson, S. (1977). The acquisition of tone in Mandarin-speaking children. *Journal of Child Language, 4*(02), 185–199. doi:10.1017/S0305000900001598

Local, J. (1982). Modelling intonational variability in children's speech. In S. Romaine (Ed.), *Sociolinguistic variation in speech communities* (pp. 85–103). London: Edward Arnold.

Local, J., Kelly, J., & Wells, W. (1986). Towards a phonology of conversation: turn-taking in Tyneside English. *Journal of Linguistics, 22*(02), 411–437. doi:10.1017/S0022226700010859

Local, J., & Walker, G. (2004). Abrupt-joins as a resource for the production of multi-unit, multi-action turns. *Journal of Pragmatics, 36*(8), 1375–1403. doi:10.1016/j.pragma.2004.04.006

Local, J., & Walker, G. (2008). Stance and affect in conversation: On the interplay of sequential and phonetic resources. *Text & Talk: An Interdisciplinary Journal of Language, Discourse Communication Studies, 28*(6), 723–747. doi:10.1515/TEXT.2008.037

Local, J., & Walker, G. (2012). How phonetic features project more talk. *Journal of the International Phonetic Association, 42*(03), 255–280. doi:10.1017/S0025100312000187

Local, J., Wells, B., & Sebba, M. (1985). Phonetic aspects of turn delimitation in London Jamaican. *Journal of Pragmatics, 9,* 309–330.

Local, J., & Wootton, T. (1995). Interactional and phonetic aspects of immediate echolalia in autism: A case study. *Clinical Linguistics & Phonetics, 9*(2), 155–184. doi:10.3109/02699209508985330

Lodge, K. (2001). *Eugene the plane spotter.* London: Bloomsbury.

MacWhinney, B., & Bates, E. (1978). Sentential devices for conveying givenness and newness: A cross-cultural developmental study. *Journal of Verbal Learning and Verbal Behaviour, 17,* 539–558.

Mahon, M. (1997). *Conversational interactions between young deaf children and their families in homes where English is not the first language.* PhD Thesis, University of London.

Mahon, M. (2003). Conversations with young deaf children in families where English is an additional language. In S. Gallaway, & C.Young (Eds.), *Deafness and education in the UK: Research perspectives* (pp. 35–53). London: Whurr.

Mampe, B., Friederici, A. D., Christophe, A., & Wermke, K. (2009). Newborns' cry melody is shaped by their native language. *Current Biology: CB, 19*(23), 1994–1997. doi:10.1016/j.cub.2009.09.064

Marschark, M., Rhoten, C., & Fabich, M. (2007). Effects of cochlear implants on children's reading and academic achievement. *Journal of Deaf Studies and Deaf Education, 12*(3), 269–282. doi:10.1093/deafed/enm013

Marshall, C. R., Harcourt-Brown, S., Ramus, F., & van der Lely, H. K. J. (2009). The link between prosody and language skills in children with specific language impairment (SLI) and/or dyslexia. *International Journal of Language & Communication Disorders, 44*(4), 466–488. doi:10.1080/13682820802591643

Mattock, K., & Burnham, D. (2006). Chinese and English infants' tone perception: Evidence for perceptual reorganization. *Infancy, 10*(3), 241–265. doi:10.1207/s15327078in1003_3

McEwan, I. (2001). *Atonement.* London: Jonathan Cape.

Morgan, J., & Demuth, K. (1996). *Signal to syntax: Bootstrapping from speech to grammar.* Mahwah, NJ: Lawrence Erlbaum.

Morgan, J., Edwards, S., & Wheeldon, L. (2014). The relationship between language production and verbal short-term memory: The role of stress grouping. *Quarterly Journal of Experimental Psychology, 67*(2), 220–246. doi:10.1080/17470218.2013.799216

Most, T., & Peled, M. (2007). Perception of suprasegmental features of speech by children with cochlear implants and children with hearing aids. *Journal of Deaf Studies and Deaf Education, 12*(3), 350–361. doi:10.1093/deafed/enm012

Muskett, T., & Body, R. (2013). The case for multimodal analysis of atypical interaction: Questions, answers and gaze in play involving a child with autism. *Clinical Linguistics & Phonetics, 27*(10–11), 837–850. doi:10.3109/02699206.2013.816780

Muskett, T., Perkins, M., Clegg, J., & Body, R. (2010). Inflexibility as an interactional phenomenon: Using conversation analysis to re-examine a symptom of autism. *Clinical Linguistics & Phonetics, 24*(1), 1–16. doi:10.3109/02699200903281739

Nazzi, T., Floccia, C., & Bertoncini, J. (1998). Discrimination of pitch contours by neonates. *Infant Behavior and Development, 21*(4), 779–784.

Northern, J., & Downs, M. (2002). *Hearing in children* (5th ed.). Baltimore, MD: Lippencott. Williams & Wilkins.

O'Connor, J., & Arnold, G. (1973). *Intonation of colloquial English.* London: Longman.

O'Halpin, R. (2010). *The perception and production of stress and intonation by children with cochlear implants.* PhD thesis, University of London. Retrieved from http://ethos.bl.uk

Ogden, R. (2006). Phonetics and social action in agreements and disagreements. *Journal of Pragmatics, 38*(10), 1752–1775. doi:10.1016/j.pragma.2005.04.011

Papaeliou, C. F., & Trevarthen, C. (2006). Prelinguistic pitch patterns expressing "communication" and "apprehension". *Journal of Child Language, 33*(1), 163–178. doi:10.1017/S0305000905007300

Papoušek, M., & Papoušek, H. (1989). Forms and functions of vocal matching in interactions between mothers and their precanonical infants. *First Language, 9*(6), 137–158.

Parker, A. (1999). *Phonological Evaluation & Transcription of Audio-Visual language - PETAL.* Bicester: Winslow Press.

Parker, A., & Rose, H. (1992). Deaf children's phonological development. In P. Grunwell (Ed.), *Developmental speech disorders: Clinical issues and practical implications* (pp. 83–107). London: Whurr.

Pascoe, M., Randall-Pieterse, C., & Geiger, M. (2013). Speech and literacy development in a child with a cochlear implant: Application of a psycholinguistic framework. *Child Language Teaching and Therapy, 29*(2), 185–200. doi:10.1177/0265659012467197

Patel, R., & Brayton, J. (2009). Identifying prosodic contrasts in utterances produced by 4- ,7- , and 11-year old children. *Journal of Speech, Language and Hearing Research, 52*(June), 790–802.

Patel, R., & Grigos, M. I. (2006). Acoustic characterization of the question–statement contrast in 4, 7 and 11 year-old children. *Speech Communication, 48*(10), 1308–1318. doi:10.1016/j.specom.2006.06.007

Peppé, S. (2009). Why is prosody in speech-language pathology so difficult? *International Journal of Speech-Language Pathology, 11*(4), 258–271. doi:10.1080/17549500902906339

Peppé, S., Cleland, J., Gibbon, F., O'Hare, A., & Castilla, P. M. (2011). Expressive prosody in children with autism spectrum conditions. *Journal of Neurolinguistics, 24*(1), 41–53. doi:10.1016/j.jneuroling.2010.07.005

Peppé, S., Maxim, J., & Wells, B. (2000). Prosodic variation in Southern British English. *Language and Speech, 43*, 309–334.

Peppé, S., & McCann, J. (2003). Assessing intonation and prosody in children with atypical language development: The PEPS-C test and the revised version. *Clinical Linguistics & Phonetics, 17*(4–5), 345–354. doi:10.1080/0269920031000079994

Peppé, S., McCann, J., Gibbon, F., O'Hare, A., & Rutherford, M. (2007). Receptive and expressive prosodic ability in children with high-functioning autism. *Journal of Speech, Language, and Hearing Research, 50*(4), 1015–1028. doi:10.1044/1092-4388(2007/071)

Perera, K. (1984). *Children's writing and reading: Analysing classroom language.* Oxford: Blackwell.

Perera, K. (1989). *The development of prosodic features in children's oral reading.* PhD thesis, University of Manchester. Retrieved from http://ethos.bl.uk

Perkins, M. (1985). Problems in discourse error analysis. In *Papers from the First English Language Teaching Symposium. University of Leeds Working Papers in Linguistics and Phonetics* (pp. 4–8). Dordrecht: Foris Publications.

Pickering, M. J., & Garrod, S. (2004). Toward a mechanistic psychology of dialogue. *Behavioral and Brain Sciences, 27*(02), 169–225. doi:10.1017/S0140525X04000056

Quam, C., & Swingley, D. (2010). Phonological knowledge guides two-year-olds' and adults' interpretation of salient pitch contours in word learning. *Journal of Memory and Language, 62*(2), 135–150. doi:10.1016/j.jml.2009.09.003

Quam, C., Yuan, J., & Swingley, D. (2008). Relating intonational pragmatics to the pitch realizations of highly frequent words in English speech to infants. In V. Love, C. McRae, & K. Sloutsky (Eds.), *Proceedings of the 30th Annual Conference of the Cognitive Science Society* (pp. 217–222). Austin, TS: Cognitive Science Society.

Roach, P. (2009). *English phonetics and phonology* (3rd ed.). Cambridge: Cambridge University Press.

Roush, P., Frymark, T., Venediktov, R., & Wang, B. (2011). Audiologic management of auditory neuropathy spectrum disorder in children: A systematic review of the literature. *American Journal of Audiology, 20*(December), 159–170. doi:10.1044/1059-0889(2011/10-0032)

Rutter, B., & Cunningham, S. (2013). The recording of audio and video data. In N. Müller, & M. Ball (Eds.), *Guide to research methods in clinical linguistics and phonetics.* (pp. 160–176). New York: Wiley.

Rvachew, S., & Brosseau-Lapré, F. (2012). *Developmental phonological disorders: Foundations of clinical practice.* San Diego: Plural Publishers.

Sacks, H., Schegloff, E., & Jefferson, G. (1974). A simplest systematics for the organisation of turn-taking in conversation. *Language, 50*(4), 696–735.

Sarant, J. Z., Holt, C. M., Dowell, R. C., Rickards, F. W., & Blamey, P. J. (2009). Spoken language development in oral preschool children with permanent childhood deafness. *Journal of Deaf Studies and Deaf Education*, 14(2), 205–217. doi:10.1093/deafed/enn034

Schegloff, E. (1996). Turn organisation: One intersection of grammar and interaction. In E. Ochs, E. A. Schegloff, & S. Thompson (Eds.), *Interaction and grammar* (pp. 52–133). Cambridge: Cambridge University Press.

Schegloff, E. (2000). Overlapping talk and the organization of turn-taking for conversation. *Language in Society*, 29(1), 1–63.

Schegloff, E. (2007). *Sequence organisation in interaction: A primer in conversation analysis*. Cambridge: Cambridge University Press.

Semel, E., Wiig, E., & Secord, W. (1987). *Clinical evaluation of language fundamentals: Revised*. London: The Psychological Corporation.

Shriberg, L., Aram, D., & Kwiatkowski, J. (1997). Developmental apraxia of speech : II . Toward a diagnostic marker. *Journal of Speech, Language and Hearing Research*, 40(2), 286–312.

Shriberg, L., Kwiatkowski, J., & Rasmussen, C. (1990). *Prosody-voice screening profile*. Tucson, AZ: Communication Skill Builders.

Snow, D. (1994). Phrase-final syllable lengthening and intonation in early child speech. *Journal of Speech and Hearing Research*, 37, 831–840.

Snow, D. (1995). Formal regularity of the falling tone in children's early meaningful speech. *Journal of Phonetics*, 23(4), 387–405. doi:10.1006/jpho.1995.0030

Snow, D. (1998). Prosodic markers of syntactic boundaries in the speech of 4-year-old children with normal and disordered language development. *Journal of Speech, Language and Hearing Research*, 41(5), 1158–1170.

Snow, D. (2001). Imitation of intonation contours by children with normal and disordered language development. *Clinical Linguistics & Phonetics*, 15(7), 567–584. doi:10.1080/02699200110078168

Snow, D. (2002). Intonation in the monosyllabic utterances of 1-year-olds. *Infant Behavior and Development*, 24, 393–407.

Snow, D. (2004). Falling intonation in the one- and two-syllable utterances of infants and preschoolers. *Journal of Phonetics*, 32(3), 373–393. doi:10.1016/S0095-4470(03)00038-X

Snow, D. (2006). Regression and reorganization of intonation between 6 and 23 months. *Child Development*, 77(2), 281–296. doi:10.1111/j.1467-8624.2006.00870.x

Snow, D., & Balog, H. (2002). Do children produce the melody before the words? A review of developmental intonation research. *Lingua*, 112(12), 1025–1058. doi:10.1016/S0024-3841(02)00060-8

Snow, D., & Ertmer, D. (2009). The development of intonation in young children with cochlear implants: A preliminary study of the influence of age at implantation and length of implant experience. *Clinical Linguistics & Phonetics*, 23(9), 665–679. doi:10.1080/02699200903026555

Snow, D., & Ertmer, D. (2012). Children's development of intonation during the first year of cochlear implant experience. *Clinical Linguistics & Phonetics*, 26(1), 51–70. doi:10.3109/0269920 6.2011.588371

Stacey, P., Fortnum, H., Barton, G., & Summerfield, Q. (2006). Hearing-impaired children in the United Kingdom, I: Auditory performance, communication skills, educational achievements, quality of life, and cochlear implantation. *Ear and Hearing*, 27(2), 161–186.

Stackhouse, J., & Wells, B. (1993). Psycholinguistic assessment of developmental speech disorders. *International Journal of Language & Communication Disorders*, 28(4), 331–348. doi:10.3109/13682829309041469

Stackhouse, J., & Wells, B. (1997). *Children's speech and literacy difficulties Book 1: A psycholinguistic framework*. London: Wiley.

Sterponi, L., & Shankey, J. (2014). Rethinking echolalia: Repetition as interactional resource in the communication of a child with autism. *Journal of Child Language*, 41(2), 275–304. doi:10.1017/S0305000912000682

Stivers, T. (2008). Stance, alignment, and affiliation during storytelling: When nodding is a token of affiliation. *Research on Language & Social Interaction*, *41*(1), 31–57. doi:10.1080/08351810701691123

Stojanovik, V. (2010). Understanding and production of prosody in children with Williams syndrome: A developmental trajectory approach. *Journal of Neurolinguistics*, *23*(2), 112–126. doi:10.1016/j.jneuroling.2009.11.001

Stojanovik, V. (2011). Prosodic deficits in children with Down syndrome. *Journal of Neurolinguistics*, *24*(2), 145–155. doi:10.1016/j.jneuroling.2010.01.004

Stojanovik, V., Perkins, M., & Howard, S. (2004). Williams syndrome and specific language impairment do not support claims for developmental double dissociations and innate modularity. *Journal of Neurolinguistics*, *17*(6), 403–424. doi:10.1016/j.jneuroling.2004.01.002

Stojanovik, V., & Setter, J. (2011). Prosody in two genetic disorders: Williams and Down's syndrome. In V. Stojanovik, & J. Setter (Eds.), *Speech prosody in atypical populations: assessment and remediation* (pp. 25–43). Guildford: J & R Press.

Stojanovik, V., Setter, J., & van Ewijk, L. (2007). Intonation abilities of children with Williams syndrome: A preliminary investigation. *Journal of Speech, Language, and Hearing Research : JSLHR*, *50*(6), 1606–1617. doi:10.1044/1092-4388(2007/108)

Szczepek Reed, B. (2004). Turn-final intonation in English. In E. Couper-Kuhlen, & C. E. Ford (Eds.), *Sound patterns in interaction* (pp. 97–118). Amsterdam: John Benjamins.

Szczepek Reed, B. (2006). *Prosodic orientation in English conversation*. Basingstoke: Palgrave Macmillan.

Tarplee, C. (1993). *Working on talk: The collaborative shaping of linguistic skills within child-adult interaction*. DPhil thesis, Department of Language and Linguistic Science, University of York, York, UK. Retrieved from http://ethos.bl.uk

Tarplee, C. (1996). Working on young children's utterances: Prosodic aspects of repetition during picture labelling. In E. Coupler-Kuhlen, & M. Selting (Eds.), *Prosody in conversation: Interactional studies* (pp. 406–435). Cambridge: Cambridge University Press.

Tarplee, C., & Barrow, E. (1999). Delayed echoing as an interactional resource: A case study of a 3-year-old child on the autistic spectrum. *Clinical Linguistics & Phonetics*, *13*(6), 449–482.

Tempest, A., & Wells, B. (2012). Alliances and arguments: A case study of a child with persisting speech difficulties in peer play. *Child Language Teaching and Therapy*, *28*(1), 57–72. doi:10.1177/0265659011419233

Thomson, J. M., Fryer, B., Maltby, J., & Goswami, U. (2006). Auditory and motor rhythm awareness in adults with dyslexia. *Journal of Research in Reading*, *29*(3), 334–348. doi:10.1111/j.1467-9817.2006.00312.x

Trevarthen, C. (2008). The musical art of infant conversation: Narrating in the time of sympathetic experience, without rational interpretation, before words. *Musicae Scientiae*, *12*(1 Suppl), 15–46. doi:10.1177/1029864908012001021

Tuaycharoen, P. (1977). The phonetic and phonological development of a Thai baby: From early communicative interaction to speech. PhD thesis, University of London.

Tye-Murray, N., & Witt, S. (1996). Conversational moves and conversational styles of adult cochlear-implant users. *Journal of the Academy of Rehabilitative Audiology*, *29*, 11–26.

Vonwiller, J. (1988). *The development of intonation in infants: Working papers*. Macquarie University, Speech, Hearing and Language Research Centre.

Walker, G. (2004). *The phonetic design of turn endings, beginnings, and continuations in conversation*. DPhil thesis, University of York, UK. Retrieved from http://gareth-walker.staff.shef.ac.uk/pubs/2004-Walker-phd.pdf

Walker, G. (2010). The phonetic constitution of a turn-holding practice: Rush-throughs in English talk-in-interaction. In D. Barth-Weingarten, E. Reber, & M. Selting (Eds.), *Prosody in interaction* (pp. 51–72). Amsterdam: John Benjamins.

Walker, G. (2013). Young children's use of laughter after transgressions. *Research on Language & Social Interaction*, *46*(4), 363–382. doi:10.1080/08351813.2013.810415

Waring, R., & Knight, R. (2013). How should children with speech sound disorders be classified? A review and critical evaluation of current classification systems. *International Journal of Language & Communication Disorders, 48*(1), 25–40. doi:10.1111/j.1460-6984.2012.00195.x

Weiner, F. (1979). *Phonological process analysis.* Baltimore, MD: University Park Press.

Wells, B. (1994). Junction in developmental speech disorder: A case study. *Clinical Linguistics & Phonetics, 8*(1), 1–25. doi:10.1080/02699209408985572

Wells, B. (2010). Tonal repetition and tonal contrast in English carer-child interaction. In D. Barth-Weingarten, E. Reber, & M. Selting (Eds.), *Prosody in interaction* (pp. 243–262). Amsterdam: John Benjamins.

Wells, B., & Corrin, J. (2004). Prosodic resources, turn-taking and overlap in children's talk-in-interaction. In E. Couper-Kuhlen, & C. E. Ford (Eds.), *Sound patterns in interaction* (pp. 119 –143). Amsterdam: John Benjamins.

Wells, B., & Local, J. (1993). The sense of an ending: A case of prosodic delay. *Clinical Linguistics & Phonetics, 7*(1), 59–73. doi:10.3109/02699209308985544

Wells, B., & Macfarlane, S. (1998). Prosody as an interactional resource: Turn-projection and overlap. *Language and Speech, 41*(3–4), 269–294.

Wells, B., & Peppé, S. (1996). Ending up in Ulster: Prosody and turn-taking in English dialects. In E. Couper-Kuhlen, & M. Selting (Eds.), *Prosody in conversation: Interactional studies* (pp. 101–130). Cambridge: Cambridge University Press.

Wells, B., & Peppé, S. (2001). Intonation within a psycholinguistic framework. In J. Stackhouse, & B. Wells (Eds.), *Children's speech and literacy difficulties 2: Identification and intervention* (pp. 366–395). London: Wiley.

Wells, B., & Peppé, S. (2003). Intonation abilities of children with speech and language impairments. *Journal of Speech, Language and Hearing Research, 46*(1), 5–20.

Wells, B., Peppé, S., & Goulandris, N. (2004). Intonation development from five to thirteen. *Journal of Child Language, 31*(4), 749–778.

Wells, W. (1986). An experimental approach to the interpretation of focus in spoken English. In C. Johns-Lewis (Ed.), *Intonation in discourse* (pp. 53–75). London: Croom Helm.

Wells, W. (1988). Focus in spoken English. DPhil thesis, Univesity of York, York, UK Retrieved from http://ethos.bl.uk

Whalen, D. H., Levitt, A. G., & Wang, Q. (1991). Intonational differences between the reduplicative babbling of French- and English-learning infants. *Journal of Child Language, 18*(03), 501–506. doi:10.1017/S0305000900011223

Whalley, K., & Hansen, J. (2006). The role of prosodic sensitivity in children's reading development. *Journal of Research in Reading, 29*(3), 288–303. doi:10.1111/j.1467-9817.2006.00309.x

Whiteside, S., & Hodgson, C. (2000). Some acoustic characteristics in the voices of 6- to 10-year-old children and adults: A comparative sex and developmental perspective. *Logopedics Phoniatrics Vocology, 25*, 122–132.

Wieman, L. (1976). Stress patterns of early child language. *Journal of Child Language, 3*(02), 283–286. doi:10.1017/S0305000900001501

Winner, E., & Leekam, S. (1991). Distinguishing irony from deception: Understanding the speaker's second-order intention. *British Journal of Developmental Psychology, 9*, 257–270.

Wootton, A. J. (1999). An investigation of delayed echoing in a child with autism. *First Language, 19*(57), 359–381. doi:10.1177/014272379901905704

Wootton, A. J. (2002). Interactional contrasts between typically developing children and those with autism, Asperger's syndrome , and pragmatic impairment. *Issues in Applied Linguistics, 13*(2), 133–159.

Yip, M. (2002). *Tone.* Cambridge: Cambridge University Press.

Zeng, F., & Liu, S. (2006). Speech perception in individuals with auditory neuropathy. *Journal of Speech, Language and Hearing Research, 49*(April), 367–381.

APPENDIX 1

Transcription conventions and symbols

General conventions

CA: Chronological age, expressed as years; months. e.g. Robin (CA 1;9) = Robin aged 1 year 9 months.

Symbols and diacritics of the International Phonetic Alphabet (IPA) and its extensions (ExtIPA), used throughout, have their conventional interpretations.

In addition, the following conventions adopted in this book series are used:

SMALL CAPITALS:	target form of a word or phrase; gloss of presumed target of child's production
Courier font:	data from speech recordings
Meridien LT Std	data from written texts
< >	encloses written language example

Intonation notation for reading transcriptions (English)

‖	Intonation Phrase (IP) boundary
ˈ	first syllable of Foot (also marks lexical stress placement for isolate word forms)
ˈ_	silent beat
ˋ	falling pitch on Tonic
ˊ	rising pitch on Tonic
ˇ	fall-rise pitch on Tonic
ˆ	rise-fall pitch on Tonic
↑	high onset
‖⇒	rush through at IP boundary

Children's Intonation: A Framework for Practice and Research, First Edition. Bill Wells and Joy Stackhouse.
© 2016 John Wiley & Sons, Ltd. Published 2016 by John Wiley & Sons, Ltd.
Companion website: www.wiley.com/go/childintonation

Phonological notation

Turn-taking: traffic light system

Dark shading	red light, current speaker's turn is in progress
Light shading	yellow light, current speaker signals potential end of turn
No shading	green light, next speaker may start turn, even if this overlaps current speaker.

Focus: Tonic placement system

Location of ordinary Tonic is indicated by Tone diacritic preceding Tonic syllable; or by light shading on Tonic word.

⇑	Supertonic; indicates narrow Focus on following word
{F}	domain of focus
{TF}	domain of Tonic Focus, i.e. Focus implied by location of the Tonic
{SF}	domain of Semantic Focus, i.e. Focus implied by the newness of the content relative to the immediately preceding context.

Actions: Tone matching system

=	matching Tone, aligns with ongoing action/agenda
≠	non-matching Tone, disaligns with ongoing action/agenda
H	High Tone; reaches top of pitch range
L	Low Tone; reaches base of pitch range
Ø	no Tone in the line

Impressionistic transcription

Relative pitch height and pitch movement are marked iconically between staves that represent the speaker's normal pitch range. Example:

2   R: ə n ʌ:: bʊkʰ

[ ]	Overlaps, i.e. instances of simultaneous speech. The brackets extend over the transcript of both speakers, indicating the start and end points of the overlap.
(.)	Silence of less than 100 ms. Silence (time in seconds)
((nods))	Nonverbal action
: : : : : :	Long; very long; extremely long.
{f} {ff} {fff}	Loud; very loud; extremely loud.

{p} {pp} {ppp}	Quiet; very quiet; extremely quiet.
{dim}	(diminuendo) getting quieter
{all}	(allegro) fast
{lento}	Slow
{fls}	Falsetto
{nsal}	Nasal resonance

Background to the recordings of Robin and his mother

Robin (not his real name) was the first-born child of socio-economically advantaged parents from the South-East of England, living in a community where Standard English dialect was typical. Robin's mother was a university-educated professional who cared for him full-time. At interview she described age-appropriate milestones of motor, cognitive, language and social development.

Starting at CA 1;7, when Robin's single-word vocabulary had reached the 50-item level, Juliette Corrin, the researcher, began weekly half-hour video recordings of Robin and his mother over a period of two months, concluding when Robin was CA 1;9. These were backed-up with simultaneous audio-recordings using an external corded microphone. The video films sampled the mother and Robin playing with his customary range of toys in their home environment. Typically, Robin chose to play with puzzles, a set of construction bricks and farm characters, a train set, soldiers, and to look at picture books. Their dog, Elsa, was quite often present. The Sony Handycam Video 8mm was mounted on a tripod at a distance of approximately 4 feet from the participants. The researcher was present during recordings. Robin was noticeably camera-aware during the first recording session, but appeared relaxed thereafter, talking and playing animatedly.

Video recordings of the interactions involving Robin are available for general access from the CAVA (human Communication: an Audio-Visual Archive) repository at University College London: www.ucl.ac.uk/ls/cava/. The relevant project is entitled "Single-word Multiword Transition".

Several publications contain analyses based on these recordings: Corrin et al., (2001); Corrin, (2002; 2010a; 2010b); Wells & Corrin, (2004); Wells, (2010); Walker, (2013).

APPENDIX 3

The Intonation In Interaction Profile (IIP): Proforma

Name:_____   **Length of sample:** _____

Age at sample: ___   **d.o.b:**_____   **Co-participants:** _____

Date & venue of sample: _____   **Activities:** _____

Name of profiler & date of profile: _____   **Comments:** _____

TURNS

Gaining the floor

1 Does C refrain from taking a turn until the current speaker has projected the end of her/his own turn? (C observes red light)

Yes: line	No: line	No evidence:
Comment:		

2 Does C routinely start a turn with minimal pause, following the prior speaker's turn? C observes yellow and green lights)

Yes: line	No: line	No evidence:
Comment:		

3 Does C produce an appropriately designed non-competitive turn in overlap, while the current speaker is still talking?

Yes: line	No: line	No evidence:
Comment:		

4 Does C produce an appropriately designed competitive turn in overlap, in a bid to capture the floor while the current speaker is still talking?

Yes: line	No: line	No evidence:
Comment:		

Children's Intonation: A Framework for Practice and Research, First Edition. Bill Wells and Joy Stackhouse.
© 2016 John Wiley & Sons, Ltd. Published 2016 by John Wiley & Sons, Ltd.
Companion website: www.wiley.com/go/childintonation

Holding the floor

1 Does C produce a turn of more than one word by creating an IP with a Head? (C uses red light)

Yes: line	No: line	No evidence:
Comment:		

2 Does C produce a turn of more than a single IP by creating a non-final IP before the final IP? (C keeps red light on)

Yes: line	No: line	No evidence:
Comment:		

3 Does C produce a turn of more than a single IP by rushing through a projected TRP at end of the first IP? (C keeps red light on)

Yes: line	No: line	No evidence:
Comment:		

4 Does C resist a turn-competitive incoming by using intonation features? (C keeps red light on)

Yes: line	No: line	No evidence:
Comment:		

Giving up the floor

1 Does C project the end of the turn by using the Tonic? (C uses yellow light)

Yes: line	No: line	No evidence:
Comment:		

2 Does C break off to give way to a turn-competitive incoming? (C uses green light)

Yes: line	No: line	No evidence:
Comment:		

3 Does C invite collaborative turn completion by producing an incomplete IP as a prompt?
(C uses red and green lights)

Yes: line	No: line	No evidence:
Comment:		

FOCUS

1 Does C indicate broad Focus over the whole IP by using final Tonic placement?

Yes: line	No: line	No evidence:

Comment:

2 Does C indicate narrow Focus on the final word of the IP by using final Supertonic placement?

Yes: line	No: line	No evidence:

Comment:

3 Does C indicate narrow Focus on a non-final word of the IP by using non-final Supertonic placement?

Yes: line	No: line	No evidence:

Comment:

4 Does C background non-Focus material, by placing it in the Tail after a non-final Tonic?

Yes: line	No: line	No evidence:

Comment:

5 Does C recognize the current speaker's broad and narrow Focus by attending to Tonic and Supertonic placement? Does C design the next turn accordingly?

Yes: line	No: line	No evidence:

Comment:

ACTIONS

Aligning

1 Does C align with the action of the co-participant's prior turn by using Tone matching?

Yes: line	No: line	No evidence:

Comment:

2 If so, what actions does C align with? For example, Assessments; Repairs; Requests; Offers

Comment:

3 Does C extend action to a second TCU in own turn, by using Tone matching within the turn?

Yes: line	No: line	No evidence:

Comment:

Initiating

1 Does C initiate a new action, different from the action underway in the previous speaker's prior turn, by using Tone non-matching?

Yes: line	No: line	No evidence:
Comment:		

2 Does C initiate a new action, different from the action underway in C's preceding IP in his own current turn, by using Tone non-matching?

Yes: line	No: line	No evidence:
Comment:		

3 If so, what actions does C initiate by Tone non-matching? For example, Repair; Request.

Comment:

4 Does C recognize that the prior speaker has initiated a new action by use of Tone non-matching, and respond accordingly?

Yes: line	No: line	No evidence:
Comment:		

APPENDIX 4
The Developmental Phase Model

Children's Intonation: A Framework for Practice and Research, First Edition. Bill Wells and Joy Stackhouse.
© 2016 John Wiley & Sons, Ltd. Published 2016 by John Wiley & Sons, Ltd.
Companion website: www.wiley.com/go/childintonation

	TURNS	FOCUS	ACTIONS
Preverbal	**Birth–0;6**		
Internal Maturation	Vocal tract; respiratory system	Neonate can hear changes in loudness and pitch prominence Unable to control loudness locally - only globally	Hearing for pitch discrimination already in place. Limited ability to control own pitch
Input	IDS (parent, family)	Neonate can hear differences in length of turns he is exposed to. Respiratory capacity limits length of vocalization Carer may respond to vocalization as conveying meaning (e.g. a need, 'request')	Prosodic perception starts to become attuned to ambient language Carer Tone may match infant pitch contour
Output	Nonverbal; cry; cooing	Vocalizations of varying length and phonetic quality	Infant may match carer Tone
Paradigmatic	**0;6–1;6**		
Internal Maturation		Non-verbal pointing; gaze Onset of joint attention Increasing local control over production of pitch, loudness and duration	Prosodic perception becomes attuned to ambient language Increasing control over laryngeal actions allows for more precise pitch movements)
	(Reciprocal turn-taking) Increasing respiratory capacity permits longer vocalizations		

Input	IDS: (family, childcare)	Carer delimits own turns with Tonic Carer responds to infant vocal strings as turns	Carer uses 'Tonic' placement for focus. Carers tend to use Supertonic Carers may respond to any child vocalization as topically relevant (Tonic not important)	Carer matches child Tone In non-Tone languages, Carer versions of adult Tones are exaggerated compared to ADS. This is not so in Tone languages
Output	Babble; Single word stage	Solo babble play: exploratory extension of IP In interaction: child only produces the Tonic 'word' Child uses 'fall' and 'rise' but not always as distinctly as in the adult language Use of intonation gestalts reflecting adult intonation	Variable 'Tonic' placement in solo babble In interaction: Tonic 'word' only (sometimes combined with babble in IP)	Child works out whether ambient language is Tone or non-Tone language If non-Tone language like English, child works out functional value of Tone matching vs. non-matching Child matches or does not match carer's Tone. Child starts to establish Tone inventory for English

Syntagmatic   **1;6–4;6**

Internal Maturation		Increase in working memory span (phonological loop) as articulatory skills mature –allows for longer IPs	Greater control over production of pitch, intensity and duration allow for more precise location of Tonic; differentiation of Tonic vs. Supertonic	Greater control over laryngeal actions allows for more precise pitch movements
Input	CDS (family, childcare) -> Peer	Adult provides online feedback re: 'illegal' incomings, illegal overlap by child Collaborative completions to induct into IP structure	Adult provides online feedback re 'illegal' Tonic placement, by child	Adult models of Tones become less exaggerated and more like ambient ADS

(Continued)

	TURNS	FOCUS	ACTIONS
Language	Multiword -> grammar		
	Dysfluency arises from demands of combining multiple elements within an IP	Turn-final only Tonic 'errors' Double-tonic 'errors'	Tone-matching for interactional alignment is established
	Child extends IP and Turn in interaction: adds non-final IP: use of mid pitch Head: use of level pitch Tail: absence of IP final prominence	Sorts out that (super)Tonic is used for (narrow) Focus Sorts out that only one Tonic allowed per IP	Tonal inventory established Child acquires language-specific phonetic exponents of Tones Later: Tone matching as means of creating alliances, etc. in peer interaction
	Child starts to use overlap functionally		
	Mastery of traffic-light system		
	Later: integration of IP structure with grammatical structure, e.g. Lists; subordinate clauses		
	Turn-taking in multiparty interaction (e.g. peer play)		
Metalinguistic	**4;6–14**		
Internal Maturation	General development of meta awareness Enables child to progressively become more aware of intonation Chunking, e.g. compound nouns	General development of meta awareness Enables child to progressively become more aware of Tonic/Focus (as in PEPS-C Bingo & other Focus experiments)	Laryngeal changes, including puberty General development of meta awareness enables child to progressively become more aware of Interactional role of Tone (as in PEPSC)

Input	Adult – Teacher - Peer	Instruction (explicit/implicit) on Turn-taking in formal situations e.g. classroom Teaching about punctuation and its relation to sentence structure (full stop, comma, etc.) as equivalent to Intonational chunking of spoken turns Teaching of word-by-word decoding and reading aloud	Adult uses Tonic to signal new/important information in complex spoken input e.g. stories read aloud, and lessons on range of subjects .Child has to follow Topic development	Instruction (explicit/implicit) in classroom re matching aligning and non-matching/initiating, around repair & correction sequences Teaching about written language punctuation and its assumed relation to speech acts e.g. Question, Exclamation
Language	Learning to read (aloud); oral narrative; drama	Needs to work out relationship between spoken Turns/TCUs and written sentences Dysfluency induced by demands of orthographic decoding recapitulates dysfluency of early 'Syntagmatic' phase Can lead to 'error' where child recruits List intonation (non-final IPs) to deal with reading aloud a (non-list) sentence word by word	When reading aloud, child needs to work out how the Focus in a sentence can be identified from the sentence itself in relation to the prior written context (given/new); and then apply Tonic or Supertonic accordingly in the right place When reading aloud, can lead to recapitulation of final Tonic 'error' pattern found in early Syntagmatic phase	Child acquires dialect-specific phonetic exponents of Tones Increasing awareness of indexical sociophonetic dimension of intonation Learns 'adult' conventions about mapping between speech act, as indicated by punctuation, and Tone choice .Establishes a Tone 'lexicon' for reading/drama/meta tasks Can lead to 'errors' where child uses spoken language/interactional conventions (e.g. Tone matching for alignment) instead of written language conventions (i.e. a Tonal lexicon)

The Intonation Processing Model

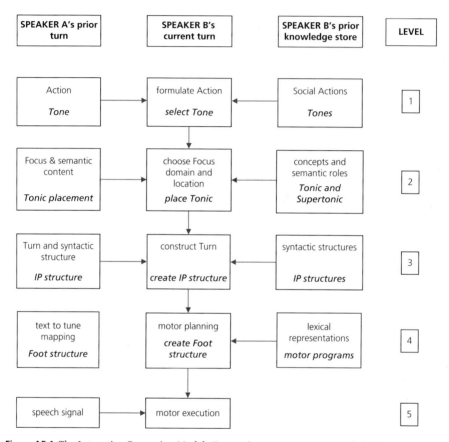

Figure A5.1 The Intonation Processing Model. (Intonation components are in *italics*.)

Children's Intonation: A Framework for Practice and Research, First Edition. Bill Wells and Joy Stackhouse.
© 2016 John Wiley & Sons, Ltd. Published 2016 by John Wiley & Sons, Ltd.
Companion website: www.wiley.com/go/childintonation

The Intonation In Interaction Profile: Mick

Name: Mick

Age at sample: 5 years   d.o.b:____

Date & venue of sample: School room

Name of profiler & date of profile: BW

Length of sample: 8/26 lines

Co-participants: Johnny, Fred

Activities: Peer play (construction)

Comments: _____

TURNS

Gaining the floor

1 Does C refrain from taking a turn until the current speaker has projected the end of her/his own turn? (C observes red light)

Yes: *lines 2; 8; 10; 13; 25*	No: *lines 6; 17*	No evidence:
Comment:		

2 Does C routinely start a turn with minimal pause, following the prior speaker's turn? (C observes yellow and green lights)

Yes: *lines 2; 8; 10; 13; 17; 25*	No: line	No evidence:
Comment:		

3 Does C produce an appropriately designed non-competitive turn in overlap, while the current speaker is still talking?

Yes: *line 6*	No: line	No evidence:
Comment:		

4 Does C produce an appropriately designed competitive turn in overlap, in a bid to capture the floor while the current speaker is still talking?

Yes: line	No: line	No evidence: *X*
Comment:		

Children's Intonation: A Framework for Practice and Research, First Edition. Bill Wells and Joy Stackhouse.
© 2016 John Wiley & Sons, Ltd. Published 2016 by John Wiley & Sons, Ltd.
Companion website: www.wiley.com/go/childintonation

Holding the floor

1 Does C produce a turn of more than one word by creating an IP with a Head? (C uses red light)

Yes: *lines 2; 6; 8; 10; 11; 13; 17; 25*	No: line	No evidence:
Comment:		

2 Does C produce a turn of more than a single IP by creating a non-final IP before the final IP? (C keeps red light on)

Yes: line	No: line	No evidence: *X*
Comment:		

3 Does C produce a turn of more than a single IP by rushing through a projected TRP at end of the first IP? (C keeps red light on)

Yes: line	No: line	No evidence: *X*
Comment:		

4 Does C resist a turn-competitive incoming by using intonation features? (C keeps red light on)

Yes: line	No: line	No evidence: *X*
Comment:		

Giving up the floor

1 Does C project the end of the turn by using the Tonic? (C uses yellow light)

Yes: *lines 2; 8; 11; 13; 17; 25*	No: *line 6*	No evidence:
Comment:		

2 Does C break off to give way to a turn-competitive incoming? (C uses green light)

Yes: line	No: line	No evidence: *X*
Comment:		

3 Does C invite collaborative turn completion by producing an incomplete IP as a prompt? (C uses red and green lights)

Yes: *line 6*	No: line	No evidence:
Comment:		

FOCUS

1 Does C indicate broad Focus over the whole IP by using final Tonic placement?

Yes: *line 2*	No: line	No evidence:

Comment: *Not clear he does this in this extract; most final Tonics sound like Supertonics*
for narrow Focus

2 Does C indicate narrow Focus on the final word of the IP by using final Supertonic placement?

Yes: *lines 8, 10, 25*	No: line	No evidence:

Comment:

3 Does C indicate narrow Focus on a non-final word of the IP by using non-final Supertonic placement?

Yes: *lines 13, 17*	No: line	No evidence:

Comment:

4 Does C background non-Focus material, by placing it in the Tail after a non-final Tonic?

Yes: *lines 13, 17*	No: line	No evidence:

Comment: *Only one word, "one".*

5 Does C recognize the current speaker's broad and narrow Focus by attending to Tonic and Supertonic placement? Does C design the next turn accordingly?

Yes: *lines 9–10; 12–13*	No: line	No evidence:

Comment:

ACTIONS

Aligning

1 Does C align with the action of the co-participant's prior turn by using Tone Matching?

Yes: *lines 5–6; 9–10; 12–13*	No: line	No evidence:

Comment: *Lines 10 = Fall; 13 = Rise; 6 = level Head*

2 If so, what actions does C align with? For example, Assessments; Repairs; Requests; Offers

Comment: *Proposal (lines 5; 9); listing (line 12)*

3 Does C extend action to a second TCU in own turn, by using Tone matching within the turn?

Yes: line	No: line	No evidence:	*X*

Comment:

Initiating

1 Does C initiate a new action, different from the action underway in the previous speaker's prior turn, by using Tone non-matching?

Yes: *lines 2; 25*	No: line	No evidence:

Comment: *Line 2: Following J's proposal in line1, M starts the list*

Comment: *Line 25: M reverts to list following J & F argument in lines 19–24*

2 Does C initiate a new action, different from the action underway in C's preceding IP in his own current turn, by using Tone non-matching?

Yes: *lines 10–11*	No: line	No evidence:

Comment:

3 If so, what actions does C initiate by Tone non-matching? For example, Repair; Request.

Comment: *Line 10 addresses F's proposal; line 11 reverts to listing*

4 Does C recognize that the prior speaker has initiated a new action by use of Tone non-matching, and respond accordingly?

Yes: *lines 9–10?*	No: line	No evidence:

Comment: *Not clear that F initiates a new action in line 9, though he uses non-matching*
Tone; M matches that in line 10

APPENDIX 7

The Intonation In Interaction Profile: Jacob

Name: Jacob

Age at sample: 8 years   d.o.b._____

Date & venue of sample: University clinic

Name of profiler & date of profile: BW

Length of sample: 10/15 lines

Co-participants:
Sally – student

Activities: play (*Thomas the Tank* toys)

Comments:_____

TURNS

Gaining the floor

1 Does C refrain from taking a turn until the current speaker has projected the end of her/his own turn? (C observes red light)

Yes: *lines 2–3; 8–9*	No: line	No evidence:
Comment:		

2 Does C routinely start a turn with minimal pause, following the prior speaker's turn? (C observes yellow and green lights)

Yes: *line 3*	No: *line 9*	No evidence:
Comment: *Inconsistent*		

3 Does C produce an appropriately designed non-competitive turn in overlap, while the current speaker is still talking?

Yes: line	No: line	No evidence:	X
Comment:			

4 Does C produce an appropriately designed competitive turn in overlap, in a bid to capture the floor while the current speaker is still talking?

Yes: line	No: line	No evidence:	X
Comment:			

Children's Intonation: A Framework for Practice and Research, First Edition. Bill Wells and Joy Stackhouse.
© 2016 John Wiley & Sons, Ltd. Published 2016 by John Wiley & Sons, Ltd.
Companion website: www.wiley.com/go/childintonation

Holding the floor

1 Does C produce a turn of more than one word by creating an IP with a Head? (C uses red light)

Yes: *lines 5; 7; 13; 19*	No: line	No evidence:
Comment:		

2 Does C produce a turn of more than a single IP by creating a non-final IP before the final IP? (C keeps red light on)

Yes: *lines 16 (start); 13?*	No: line	No evidence:
Comment:		

3 Does C produce a turn of more than a single IP by rushing through a projected TRP at end of the first IP? (C keeps red light on)

Yes: *line 16 (end)*	No: line	No evidence:
Comment:		

4 Does C resist a turn-competitive incoming by using intonation features? (C keeps red light on)

Yes: *line 5*	No: line	No evidence: *X*
Comment:		

Giving up the floor

1 Does C project the end of the turn by using the Tonic? (C uses yellow light)

Yes: *lines 7; 19*	No: *lines 5; 9; 16; 18*	No evidence:
Comment: *Line 5: mismatch of traffic light and grammar; lines 9; 16; 18: early Tonics make signalling of yellow light unclear*		

2 Does C break off to give way to a turn-competitive incoming? (C uses green light)

Yes: line	No: line	No evidence: *X*
Comment:		

3 Does C invite collaborative turn completion by producing an incomplete IP as a prompt? (C uses red and green lights)

Yes: line	No: line	No evidence: *X*

FOCUS

1 Does C indicate broad Focus over the whole IP by using final Tonic placement?

Yes: *lines 5; 7; 13*	No: line	No evidence:
Comment:		

2 Does C indicate narrow Focus on the final word of the IP by using final Supertonic placement?

Yes: *line 19*	No: line	No evidence:
Comment: *Done with unusually long preceding pause*		

3 Does C indicate narrow Focus on a non-final word of the IP by using non-final Supertonic placement?

Yes: *lines 9; 18*	No: line	No evidence:
Comment: *Tonic on first word of IP results in long Tail*		

4 Does C background non-Focus material, by placing it in the Tail after a non-final Tonic?

Yes:	No: *lines 9; 18*	No evidence:
Comment: *Material in the Tail should also be in Focus in line 9 and line 18*		

5 Does C recognize the current speaker's broad and narrow Focus by attending to Tonic and Supertonic placement? Does C design the next turn accordingly?

Yes: *lines 1–5*	No: *line 8*	No evidence:
Comment:		

ACTIONS

Aligning

1 Does C align with the action of the co-participant's prior turn by using Tone matching?

Yes: *line 3*	No: *lines 7; 9*	No evidence:
Comment: *Inconsistent*		

2 If so, what actions does C align with? For example, Assessments; Repairs; Requests; Offers

Comment: *Request*

3 Does C extend action to a second TCU in own turn, by using Tone matching within the turn?

Yes: *lines 16–19*	No: line	No evidence:
Comment: *Lines 16–19 – matching implies a single agenda, though hard for outsider to follow because of gaps*		

Initiating

1 Does C initiate a new action, different from the action underway in the previous speaker's prior turn, by using Tone non-matching?

Yes: *line 9*	No: line	No evidence:

Comment: *Non-match shows lack of attention to S's question, reverting to his own prior agenda*

2 Does C initiate a new action, different from the action underway in C's preceding IP in his own current turn, by using Tone non-matching?

Yes: *line 9–13*	No: line	No evidence:

Comment: *Possibly, though there are also long gaps*

3 If so, what actions does C initiate by Tone non-matching? For example, Repair; Request.

Comment: *More a change of topical focus*

4 Does C recognize that the prior speaker has initiated a new action by use of Tone non-matching, and respond accordingly?

Yes: line	No: line	No evidence:

Comment: *S's nonmatch invites him to expand on l.5, but he goes to own agenda*

APPENDIX 8

Phonetic transcript: Ricky

(12.10)

```
                  (R turns page)
 1  M:   ‖he 'looked out of the `window‖ (.) (reading)
 2  M:   ‖'everything seemed 'so: ‖
         _____


            ⌐ [     ]


         ___ [ ⟍    ]

 3  R:   ‖`mo: [jɛ   ]‖
 4  M:       ‖'[whats] that ´word‖ [(points] to word)
         _____


            ⌐⟍


         _____

 5  R:   ‖`mo:‖
         (thumb and finger together)
 6  M:   ‖ `sma:ll ‖thats `right ‖ (.)
         (R pushes M's index finger along page with his finger)
 7  M:   ‖['after the 'plane had ˇlanded(.)‖
         the 'first thing 'Eugeneˇspotted‖ (.) (looks at R)


            ⟍
         _____

 8  R:   jɛ
         {ppp} (nods)
 9  M:   ‖was his `luggage ‖ (.) (M takes finger off page)
10  M:   ‖it goes 'rou:nd and 'round youveˇdone this be'fore
         (M circles on page with finger)
    M:   ‖'havent `you‖   (M looks towards R) (R starts to turn turn page)


            ⌣ ‿
         _____

11  R:   ‖mhm ‖
         {pp} (nods)
```

12 M: ‖ˊyes ‖⇒ you ˈget the ˇluggage‖(0.5)
                        (R turns page)
13 M: hhh(.)‖ˈeveryˈwhere he ˈwent Euˈgene[ˈspotted] ˋplanes‖
          (RH opens)
                                              [_____]
                                              [—   ]
                                              [   ]
                                              [_____]
14 R: ‖[ˊnɪʔ] ‖
          (R points to picture)   { f   }
15 M: ‖ˈwhats ˊthis ‖
          ‾‾‾‾‾

          ∧⌐\

          ‾‾‾‾‾
16 R: ‖nəʊŋ‖
17 M: ‖ˈEiffel ˇTower‖ (.)
18 M: ‖ˈwhere ˋis it‖(0.3)
          ‾‾‾‾‾

          ＼

          ‾‾‾‾‾
19 R: ‖ˋk̜ɛ::əm‖
          (points)
20 M: ‖ˋfra:nce‖   (1.0)
          ‾‾‾‾‾
            [   ]
          ⩗   ]
          __[____]
21 R: ‖ˇɑ:[:   ]‖
22 M: [ˈRicky](.)ˋfra:nce ‖
          ‾‾‾‾‾

          ‿

          ‾‾‾‾‾
23 R: ‖frɑ: ‖
24 M: ‖ˈthats r oh[well [ˋdone]Ricky ‖⇒[ˈgood(.)with your ˋef]‖
                      [_____]   [_____]
                      [   ]   [   ]
                      [‿   ]   [‾‾‾‾‾⌐‿‾]
                      [_____]   [_____]
25 R: [ʔe::   ]   [e: ɪ:]
                      {f   f}

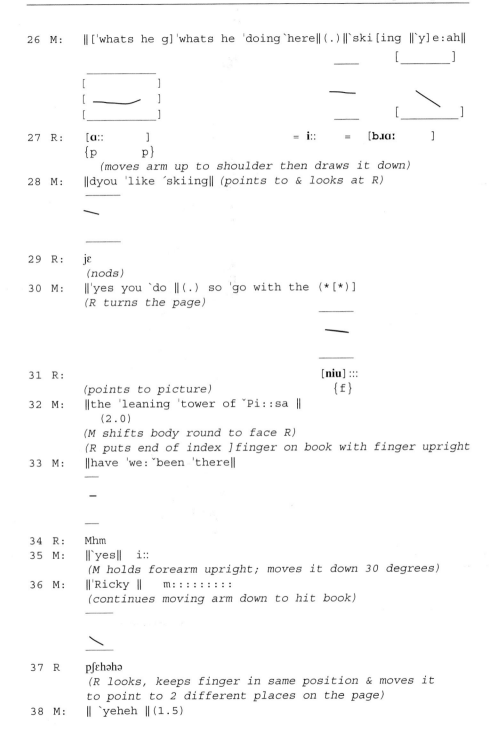

26 M: ‖['whats he g]'whats he 'doing`here‖ (.) ‖`ski[ing ‖`y]e:ah‖

27 R: [ɑ::   ]   = i::   = [bɹɑ:]
       {p   p}
         (moves arm up to shoulder then draws it down)
28 M: ‖dyou 'like ´skiing‖ (points to & looks at R)

29 R: jɛ
       (nods)
30 M: ‖'yes you `do ‖ (.) so 'go with the (*[*)]
       (R turns the page)

31 R: [niu] :::
       (points to picture)   {f}
32 M: ‖the 'leaning 'tower of ˇPi::sa ‖
          (2.0)
       (M shifts body round to face R)
       (R puts end of index]finger on book with finger upright
33 M: ‖have 'we:ˇbeen 'there‖

34 R: Mhm
35 M: ‖`yes‖   i::
       (M holds forearm upright; moves it down 30 degrees)
36 M: ‖'Ricky ‖   m:::::::::
       (continues moving arm down to hit book)

37 R   pʃɛhəhə
       (R looks, keeps finger in same position & moves it
       to point to 2 different places on the page)
38 M: ‖ `yeheh ‖ (1.5)

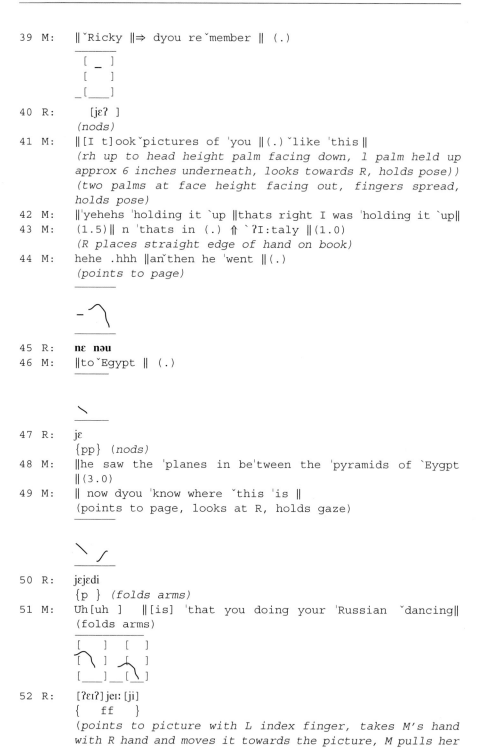

```
39  M:   ‖ ˇRicky ‖⇒ dyou re ˇmember ‖ (.)
            _____
            [ _ ]
            [   ]
           _[___]
40  R:      [jɛʔ ]
            (nods)
41  M:   ‖[I t]ook ˇpictures of 'you ‖(.) ˇlike 'this ‖
            (rh up to head height palm facing down, 1 palm held up
            approx 6 inches underneath, looks towards R, holds pose))
            (two palms at face height facing out, fingers spread,
            holds pose)
42  M:   ‖'yehehs 'holding it ˋup ‖thats right I was 'holding it ˋup‖
43  M:   (1.5)‖ n 'thats in (.) ⇑ ˋʔI:taly ‖(1.0)
            (R places straight edge of hand on book)
44  M:   hehe .hhh ‖anˇthen he 'went ‖(.)
            _____
            (points to page)
```

```
45  R:   nɛ nəʊ
46  M:   ‖to ˇEgypt ‖ (.)
            _____
```

```
47  R:   jɛ
         {pp} (nods)
48  M:   ‖he saw the 'planes in be'tween the 'pyramids of ˋEygpt
         ‖(3.0)
49  M:   ‖ now dyou 'know where ˇthis 'is ‖
         (points to page, looks at R, holds gaze)
            _____
```

```
50  R:   jɛjɛdi
         {p } (folds arms)
51  M:   Uh[uh ]  ‖[is] 'that you doing your 'Russian ˇdancing‖
         (folds arms)
            _____
            [   ] [  ]
            [ \ ] [  ]
            [___]_[ \ ]
52  R:   [ʔɛɪʔ] jeɪː [ji]
         {   ff   }
         (points to picture with L index finger, takes M's hand
         with R hand and moves it towards the picture, M pulls her
         hand back, R points to picture with both index fingers)
```

```
53  M:    ‖Eugene spotted ꞌplanes over the ꞌonion ꞌdomes of ꞌMoscow‖
54  M:    ‖there he ´is yes ‖
          ─────
```

```
              ╱

55  R:    nǝu
56  M:    ‖an  dyou ꞌknow ꞌwhere ´this is ‖(0.5)
          (points to picture, turns body towards R)
          ──  ┌─────────────────────┐
          ┌   [                     ]
           ╲  [   ⌒⌒        ⌒        ]
          ──  [_____⌐]
57  R:    bæʔ (.) [ tse ɪ :          j e ɪ: ]
                  [    { f }               ]
58  M:            ‖ [dyou know wherèthis is]‖
                    (2.0)
59  M:    ‖´there[he is]‖
          [(points to pi]cture)
              ───────────
            [ ⌒    ]
            [  ⌒  ]⌒
            [_____]  ╲
60  R:         [jɛ:   ] jei:
               {ff          f}
61  M:    ‖the ꞌtrain the ꞌfa:st[ˆtrain‖ꞌyes]‖
                        ──────────
                        [          ]
                        [ ⌒  ⌒    ]
                        [_____]
62  R:                  [fɑ:   deɪ   ]  (nods)
63  M:    ‖[ꞌwhere] is ꞌthis dyou ꞌknow where this ꞌis‖ (0.5)
          ──────
            [ _ ]
            [ ⁻ ]
            [___]
64  R:    [ʔm   ]
65  M:    ‖its ꞌJaꞌpan ‖
          ─────

            ╲

66  R:    ɟeeee
67  M:    ‖ ꞌyes‖nononono`no‖this˅coun:try ‖⇒˅not where em Euꞌgene is‖
68        (makes circles on page with index finger:::)
69  M:    ‖ ꞌthis˅country‖(.)is Jaˆpan‖(.) where they have the
          ꞌfast ꞌtrains ‖(.)
          (R turns over page)
```

(12.10.1) Phonological transcript

```
 1  M:  L   ‖he 'looked out of the `window‖ (.)
 2  M:  Ø   ‖'everything seemed 'so:‖
 3  R:  =   ‖`mo:[ jɛ  ]  ‖
 4  M:  ≠      ‖ '[whats] that ´word ‖
 5  R:  ≠   ‖`mo:‖
 6  M:  =   ‖`sma:ll ‖thats `right ‖(.)
 7          ‖after the 'plane had ˇlanded‖(.)
            ‖the 'first thing 'Eugene ˇspotted‖(.)
 8  R:      jɛ
 9  M:      ‖was his `luggage ‖(.)
10          ‖it goes 'rou:nd and 'round youve ˇdone this be'fore‖
            ‖'havent `you‖
11  R:  =   ‖`mhm ‖
12  M:      ‖´yes ‖⇒ you 'get the ˇluggage‖(0.5)
13      L   hhh (.)‖everywhere he went Eugene['spotted] `planes‖
14  R:  ≠                                ‖[ ´nɪʔ  ]‖
15  M:  =   ‖'whats ´this‖
16  R:  Ø   ‖nəuŋ‖
17  M:      ‖'Eiffel ˇTower‖ (.)
18      ≠   ‖'where `is it ‖(0.3)
19  R:  =   ‖`k̩ɛ::əm ‖
20  M:  =   ‖`fra:nce‖  (1.0)
21  R:  ≠   ‖ˇɑ:[:     ] ‖
22  M:  ≠        ['Ricky](.)`fra:nce‖=
23  R:  =   ‖frɑ:‖
24  M:  =   ‖thats r oh[well `done]Ricky ‖⇒[good(.)with your `ef]‖
25  R:  ≠          [?e::    ]      [e:   ɪ:     ]
26  M:      ‖['whats he g]'whats he 'doing `here‖(.)=‖`ski[ing =‖`y]eh‖
27  R:      [ɑ::     ]            = i::  = [bɹɑ:    ]
28  M:  ≠   ‖dyou 'like ´skiing‖
29  R:      jɛ
30  M:      ‖'yes you `do ‖(.) so 'go with the (*[*])‖
31  R:                                [niu]:::
32  M:      ‖the 'leaning 'tower of ˇPi::sa ‖
            (2.0)
33          ‖have 'we ˇbeen 'there‖
34  R:      Mhm
35  M:      ‖`yes ‖  i::
36          ‖'Ricky ‖    m::::::::::
37  R       pʃɛhəhə
38  M:  =   ‖`yeheh ‖(1.5)
39      ≠   ‖ˇRicky ‖⇒dyou reˇmember ‖ (.)
40  R:  =   [jɛʔ ]
41  M:  =   ‖[I t]ook ˇpictures of 'you ‖(.) ˇlike 'this ‖
42      ≠   ‖'yehehs 'holding it `up ‖ thats right I was 'holding it
            `up‖ (1.5)
```

```
43    =    ‖n 'thats in (.) ⇑`?I:taly ‖(1.0)
44    ≠    hehe .hhh ‖anˇthen he 'went ‖(.)
45 R: ≠    nε nəu
46 M: ≠    ‖toˇEgypt ‖(.)
47 R:      jε
48 M:      ‖he saw the 'planes in be'tween the 'pyramids of `Eygpt
           ‖(3.0)
49    ≠    ‖now dyou 'know whereˇthis 'is‖
50 R:      jεjεdi
51 M:      Uh[uh ]  ‖[is] 'that you doing your 'Russianˇdancing‖
52 R: ≠      [?εɪ?] jeɪ:[ji]
53 M: ≠    ‖Eu'gene spotted 'planes over the 'onion 'domes of ` Moscow‖
54    ≠    ‖there he ´is yes ‖
55 R: =    nəu
56 M: =    ‖an  dyou 'know 'where ´this is ‖(0.5)
57 R: ≠    bæ?  (.) [ts e ɪ:     j e ɪ:      ]
58 M: =           ‖[dyou know where `this is]‖
                  (2.0)
59    ≠    ‖´there[he is]‖
60 R: ≠          [jε:   ]jeɪ:
61 M: =    ‖the 'train the 'fa:st[`train ‖`yes]‖
62 R: =                  [ fɑ:      deɪ ]
63 M: =    ‖['where] is 'this dyou 'know where this `is‖ (0.5)
64 R: ≠    [ ?m  ]
65 M: ≠    ‖its 'Ja`pan ‖
66 R: =    ɟeeee
67 M: =    ‖`yes‖nononono`no ≠ ‖this ˇcoun:try =‖⇒ˇnot where erm
           Eu'gene is ‖
69    =    ‖ 'this ˇcountry ‖(.)is Ja^pan‖(.) where they have the
           'fast `trains ‖(.)
```

Intonation In Interaction Profile

Name: Ricky   **Length of sample: 24 spoken turns**

Age at sample: 9;11   **Co-participants: Mother**

Date & venue of sample: R's school   **Activities: shared book reading**

Name of profiler & date of profile: BW   **Comments:** _____

TURNS

Gaining the floor

1 Does C refrain from taking a turn until the current speaker has projected the end of her/his own turn? (C observes red light)

Yes: *lines 5; 15–16; 29; 40; 50; 55; 66*	*No: line 14*	No evidence:
Comment:		

2 Does C routinely start a turn with minimal pause, following the prior speaker's turn? (C observes yellow and green lights)

Yes: *lines 2-3; 5; 11; 16; 23; 29; 34; 40; 47; 50; 55; 66*	No: *lines 18–19; 20–21; 64*	No evidence:
Comment: *Lines 12–13; 44–45: R completes M's IP; lines 18-19 (0.3); 20-21 (1.0)*		

3 Does C produce an appropriately designed non-competitive turn in overlap, while the current speaker is still talking?

Yes: *lines 31; 52; 62*	No: line	No evidence:
Comment: *Line 31: M is fading out, so overlap OK; line 52: at potential TRP*		

4 Does C produce an appropriately designed competitive turn in overlap, in a bid to capture the floor while the current speaker is still talking?

Yes: *lines 14; 25; 27; 60*	No: line	No evidence:
Comment:		

Holding the floor

1 Does C produce a turn of more than one word by creating an IP with a Head? (C uses red light)

Yes: *lines 27; 52; 57; 60*	No: line	No evidence:
Comment: *Lines 27; 57; 60 in overlap*		

2 Does C produce a turn of more than a single IP by creating a non-final IP before the final IP? (C keeps red light on)

Yes: *line 25*	No: line	No evidence:
Comment: *Line 25: in overlap*		

3 Does C produce a turn of more than a single IP by rushing through a projected TRP at end of the first IP? (C keeps red light on)

Yes: line	No: line	No evidence:	*X*
Comment:			

4 Does C resist a turn-competitive incoming by using intonation features? (C keeps red light on)

Yes: line	No: line	No evidence:	*X*
Comment:			

Giving up the floor

1 Does C project the end of the turn by using the Tonic? (C uses yellow light)

Yes: *lines 5–6; 19–20*	No: *line 4?*	No evidence:
Comment:		

2 Does C break off to give way to a turn-competitive incoming? (C uses green light)

Yes: line	No: *line 58*	No evidence:
Comment: *Line 58: R continues after completing*		

3 Does C invite turn completion by producing an incomplete IP as a prompt? (Red and green lights)

Yes: line	No: line	No evidence:
Comment:		

FOCUS

1 Does C indicate broad Focus over the whole IP by using final Tonic placement?

Yes: *lines 27; 52?; 57; 60*	No: *lines 25; 63*	No evidence:
Comment: *Line 27; in overlap*		

2 Does C indicate narrow Focus on the final word of the IP by using final Supertonic placement?

Yes: line	No: line	No evidence:	*X*
Comment:			

3 Does C indicate narrow Focus on a non-final word of the IP by using non-final Supertonic placement?

Yes: line	No: line	No evidence:	*X*
Comment:			

4 Does C background non-Focus material, by placing it in the Tail after a non-final Tonic?

Yes: line	No: line	No evidence:	*X*
Comment:			

5 Does C recognize the current speaker's broad and narrow Focus by attending to Tonic and Supertonic placement? Does C design the next turn accordingly?

Yes: *lines 61–62; 18–19*	No: *lines 56–57*	No evidence:

Comment:

ACTIONS

Aligning

1 Does C align with the action of the co-participant's prior turn by using Tone matching?

Yes: *lines 3; 19; 23; 25; 50; 55; 60*	No: *lines 16; 21*	No evidence:

Comment: *Line 28 in overlap*

2 If so, what actions does C align with? For example, Assessments; Repairs; Requests; Offers

Comment: *Lines 19; 27; 50 - request; line 23 - repair; lines 55; 60 – offer*

3 Does C extend action to a second TCU in own turn, by using Tone matching within the turn?

Yes: line	No: line	No evidence: *X*

Comment:

Initiating

1 Does C initiate a new action, different from the action underway in the previous speaker's prior turn, by using Tone non-matching?

Yes: *lines 5; 14; 30; 60*	No: line	No evidence:

Comment:

2 Does C initiate a new action, different from the action underway in C's preceding IP in his own current turn, by using Tone non-matching?

Yes: line	No: line	No evidence: *X*

Comment:

3 If so, what actions does C initiate by Tone non-matching? For example, Repair; Request.

Comment: *Line 5; lines 14; 31 – repair; line 60 – topic shift*

4 Does C recognize that the prior speaker has initiated a new action by use of Tone non-matching, and respond accordingly?

Yes: line	No: *line 45?*	No evidence:

Comment:

Index

Children's Intonation: A Framework for Practice and Research, First Edition. Bill Wells and Joy Stackhouse.
© 2016 John Wiley & Sons, Ltd. Published 2016 by John Wiley & Sons, Ltd.
Companion website: www.wiley.com/go/childintonation